Hypersomnia

Guest Editor

ALON Y. AVIDAN, MD, MPH

SLEEP MEDICINE CLINICS

www.sleep.theclinics.com

June 2012 • Volume 7 • Number 2

SAUNDERS an imprint of ELSEVIER, Inc.

W.B. SAUNDERS COMPANY
A Division of Elsevier Inc.

1600 John F. Kennedy Boulevard • Suite 1800 • Philadelphia, PA 19103-2899

http://www.sleep.theclinics.com

SLEEP MEDICINE CLINICS Volume 7, Number 2
June 2012, ISSN 1556-407X, ISBN-13: 978-1-4557-3934-9

Editor: Katie Hartner
Developmental Editor: Donald E. Mumford

Sleep Medicine Clinics (ISSN 1556-407X) is published quarterly by Elsevier Inc., 360 Park Avenue South, New York, NY 10010-1710. Months of issue are March, June, September and December. Business and Editorial Offices: 1600 John F. Kennedy Blvd., Ste. 1800, Philadelphia, PA 19103-2899. Customer Service Office: 3251 Riverport Lane, Maryland Heights, MO 63043. Periodicals postage paid at New York, NY and additional mailing offices. Subscription prices are $174.00 per year (US individuals), $86.00 (US residents), $368.00 (US institutions), $214.00 (foreign individuals), $120.00 (foreign residents), and $406.00 (foreign institutions). Foreign air speed delivery is included in all *Clinics* subscription prices. All prices are subject to change without notice. **POSTMASTER:** Send change of address to *Sleep Medicine Clinics*, Elsevier Health Sciences Division, Subscription Customer Service, 3251 Riverport Lane, Maryland Heights, MO 63043. Customer Service: **Tel: 1-800-654-2452 (U.S. and Canada); 314-447-8871 (outside U.S. and Canada). Fax: 314-447-8029. E-mail: journalscustomerservice-usa@elsevier.com (for print support); journalsonlinesupport-usa@elsevier.com (for online support).**

Reprints. For copies of 100 or more of articles in this publication, please contact the Commercial Reprints Department, Elsevier Inc., 360 Park Avenue South, New York, NY 10010-1710. Tel.: 212-633-3812; Fax: 212-462-1935; E-mail: reprints@elsevier.com.

Printed and bound by CPI Group (UK) Ltd, Croydon, CR0 4YY

Transferred to Digital Print 2012

GOAL STATEMENT

The goal of *Sleep Clinics of North America* is to keep practicing physicians up to date with current clinical practice by providing timely articles reviewing the state of the art in patient care.

ACCREDITATION

The *Sleep Clinics of North America* is planned and implemented in accordance with the Essential Areas and Policies of the Accreditation Council for Continuing Medical Education (ACCME) through the joint sponsorship of the University of Virginia School of Medicine and Elsevier. The University of Virginia School of Medicine is accredited by the ACCME to provide continuing medical education for physicians.

The University of Virginia School of Medicine designates this enduring material activity for a maximum of 15 *AMA PRA Category 1 Credit(s)*™ for each issue, 60 credits per year. Physicians should only claim credit commensurate with the extent of their participation in the activity.

The American Medical Association has determined that physicians not licensed in the US who participate in this CME enduring material activity are eligible for a maximum of 15 *AMA PRA Category 1 Credit(s)*™ for each issue, 60 credits per year.

Credit can be earned by reading the text material, taking the CME examination online at http://www.theclinics.com/home/cme, and completing the evaluation. After taking the test, you will be required to review any and all incorrect answers. Following completion of the test and evaluation, your credit will be awarded and you may print your certificate.

FACULTY DISCLOSURE/CONFLICT OF INTEREST

The University of Virginia School of Medicine, as an ACCME accredited provider, endorses and strives to comply with the Accreditation Council for Continuing Medical Education (ACCME) Standards of Commercial Support, Commonwealth of Virginia statutes, University of Virginia policies and procedures, and associated federal and private regulations and guidelines on the need for disclosure and monitoring of proprietary and financial interests that may affect the scientific integrity and balance of content delivered in continuing medical education activities under our auspices.

The University of Virginia School of Medicine requires that all CME activities accredited through this institution be developed independently and be scientifically rigorous, balanced and objective in the presentation/discussion of its content, theories and practices.

All authors/editors participating in an accredited CME activity are expected to disclose to the readers relevant financial relationships with commercial entities occurring within the past 12 months (such as grants or research support, employee, consultant, stock holder, member of speakers bureau, etc.). The University of Virginia School of Medicine will employ appropriate mechanisms to resolve potential conflicts of interest to maintain the standards of fair and balanced education to the reader. Questions about specific strategies can be directed to the Office of Continuing Medical Education, University of Virginia School of Medicine, Charlottesville, Virginia.

The faculty and staff of the University of Virginia Office of Continuing Medical Education have no financial affiliations to disclose.

The authors/editors listed below have identified no professional or financial affiliations for themselves or their spouse/partner:

Imran Ahmed, MD; Claudio L. Bassetti, MD; Michel Billiard, MD; Marcia E. Braun, PhD; Cynthia Brown, MD (Test Author); Peter R. Buchanan, MD, FRACP; Shintaro Chiba, MD, PhD; Pamela Cines, MD; Dierdre A. Conroy, PhD, CBSM; Maryann C. Deak, MD; Carl Deguzman; Neil Freedman, MD; Carmella G. Gonzales, MD; Ronald R. Grunstein, MD, PhD, FRACP; Irma Gvilia, PhD; Shelby Harris, PsyD; Katie Hartner, (Acquisitions Editor); Christer Hublin, MD, PhD; Takashi Kanbayashi, MD, PhD; Douglas B. Kirsch, MD; Suresh Kotagal, MD; Arlie Loughnan, BA, LLB, LLM, PhD; Tony J. Masri, MD; Seiji Nishino, MD, PhD; Danielle M. Novick, PhD; Paul Reading, FRCP, PhD; Mikael Sallinen, PhD; Leslie M. Swanson, PhD; and Wataru Yamadera, MD, PhD.

The authors/editors listed below identified the following professional or financial affiliations for themselves or their spouse/partner:

Alon Y. Avidan, MD, MPH (Guest Editor) is a consultant and is on the Advisory Board for Purdue Pharmaceuticals, and is on the Speakers' Bureau for Teva and GSK.

Nalaka S. Gooneratne, MD, MSc has an unrestricted educational grant from Respironics.

Meeta Goswami, BDS, MPH, PhD receives grants to publish newsletters from Jazz Pharmaceuticals and Cephahon.

Clete A. Kushida, MD, PhD is an Industry funded research/investigator for ResMed, Pacific Medico, and Merck.

Teofilo Lee- Chiong, Jr, MD (Consulting Editor) is employed by Respironics, and is an industry funded research/investigator for Respironics and Embla.

Sebastiaan Overeem, MD, PhD is on the Speakers' Bureau for UCB Pharma, Boehringer Ingelheim, and Novartis Pharma.

Thomas Roth, PhD receives grant support from Apnex and Merck, is a consultant for Abbott, AstraZenca, Intec, Jazz, Merck, Neurocrine, Proctor and Gamble, Pfizer, Purdue, Sepracor, Shire, Somaxon, Somnus, Steady Sleep Rx, and Transcept, and is on the Speakers' Bureau for Sepracor and Somaxon.

Ronald Szymusiak, PhD's spouse is employed by Parexcel.

Michael Thorpy, MB is on the Advisory Board for Jazz and TEVA Pharaceuticals.

Disclosure of Discussion of Non-FDA Approved Uses for Pharmaceutical Products and/or Medical Devices.

The University of Virginia School of Medicine, as an ACCME provider, requires that all faculty presenters identify and disclose any off-label uses for pharmaceutical and medical device products. The University of Virginia School of Medicine recommends that each physician fully review all the available data on new products or procedures prior to clinical use.

TO ENROLL

To enroll in the Sleep Clinics of North America Continuing Medical Education program, call customer service at 1-800-654-2452 or visit us online at www.theclinics.com/home/cme. The CME program is available to subscribers for an additional fee of $114.00.

SLEEP MEDICINE CLINICS

Contributors

CONSULTING EDITOR

TEOFILO LEE-CHIONG Jr, MD
Professor of Medicine and Chief, Division
of Sleep Medicine, National Jewish Health;
Associate Professor of Medicine, University
of Colorado Denver School of Medicine,
Denver, Colorado

GUEST EDITOR

ALON Y. AVIDAN, MD, MPH
Professor of Neurology, Department of
Neurology; Director, Sleep Disorders Center,
University of California, Los Angeles,
Los Angeles, California

AUTHORS

IMRAN AHMED, MD
Assistant Professor, Neurology, Montefiore
Medical Center, Albert Einstein College
of Medicine; Neurology Department,
Sleep-Wake Disorders Center, Bronx,
New York

ALON Y. AVIDAN, MD, MPH
Professor of Neurology, Department of
Neurology; Director, Sleep Disorders Center,
University of California, Los Angeles,
Los Angeles, California

CLAUDIO L. BASSETTI, MD
Chairman and Director, Department of
Neurology, University Hospital (Inselspital),
Bern; Director of Neuroscience,
Neurocenter of Southern Switzerland,
Lugano, Switzerland

MICHEL BILLIARD, MD
Honorary Professor of Neurology, Department
of Neurology, Gui de Chauliac Hospital,
Montpellier, France

MARCIA E. BRAUN, PhD
Postdoctoral Fellow, Division of Sleep and
Chronobiology, Unit for Experimental
Psychiatry, Perelman School of Medicine at the
University of Pennsylvania, Philadelphia,
Pennsylvania

PETER R. BUCHANAN, MD, FRACP
Senior Clinical Research Fellow, Senior Staff
Specialist and Consultant Sleep Medicine
Physician, Sleep and Circadian Research
Group, NHMRC Centre for Integrated
Research and Understanding of Sleep,
Woolcock Institute of Medical Research,
University of Sydney; Department of
Respiratory Medicine, Liverpool Hospital,
Liverpool; Sleep Disorders Service, St
Vincent's Clinic, Sydney, New South Wales,
Australia

SHINTARO CHIBA, MD, PhD
Stanford University Sleep and Circadian
Neurobiology Laboratory, Visiting Assistant
Professor, Department of Psychiatry and
Behavioral Sciences, Stanford University
School of Medicine, Palo Alto, California

PAMELA CINES, MD
Division of Geriatric Medicine, Department
of Medicine, University of Pennsylvania School
of Medicine, Philadelphia, Pennsylvania

DEIRDRE A. CONROY, PhD, CBSM
Clinical Assistant Professor, Department
of Psychiatry, University of Michigan; Clinical
Director, Behavioral Sleep Medicine Program,
University of Michigan Hospital and Health
Systems, Ann Arbor, Michigan

MARYANN C. DEAK, MD
Clinical Instructor, Division of Sleep Medicine,
Harvard Medical School; Medical Director,
Sleep HealthCenters, Brighton,
Massachusetts

CARL DEGUZMAN
Stanford University Sleep and Circadian
Neurobiology Laboratory, Department of
Psychiatry and Behavioral Sciences, Stanford
University School of Medicine, Palo Alto,
California

NEIL FREEDMAN, MD
Division of Pulmonary and Critical Care
Medicine, Department of Medicine,
NorthShore University Healthcare System,
Evanston, Illinois

CARMELLA G. GONZALES, MD
Neurology Resident, Neurology Department,
Case Western Reserve University, Cleveland,
Ohio

NALAKA S. GOONERATNE, MD, MSc
Division of Geriatric Medicine, Department of
Medicine; Center for Sleep and Circadian
Neurobiology, University of Pennsylvania
School of Medicine, Philadelphia,
Pennsylvania

MEETA GOSWAMI, BDS, MPH, PhD
Director, Narcolepsy Institute, Sleep-Wake
Disorders Center, Montefiore Medical Center;
Assistant Professor, Department of Neurology,
Albert Einstein College of Medicine, Bronx,
New York

RONALD R. GRUNSTEIN, MD, PhD, FRACP
Professor of Sleep Medicine, Sleep and
Circadian Research Group, NHMRC Centre for
Integrated Research and Understanding of
Sleep, Woolcock Institute of Medical
Research, University of Sydney and Royal
Prince Alfred Hospital; Sleep Disorders
Service, St Vincent's Clinic, Sydney,
New South Wales, Australia

IRMA GVILIA, PhD
Research Service, Veterans Affairs Greater
Los Angeles Healthcare System, Los Angeles;
Research Service, Veterans Affairs Greater
Los Angeles Healthcare System, North Hills,
California; Department of Neurophysiology,
Ilia State University, Tbilisi, Georgia

SHELBY HARRIS, PsyD
Assistant Professor, Neurology and Psychiatry,
Montefiore Medical Center, Albert Einstein
College of Medicine; Neurology Department,
Sleep-Wake Disorders Center, Bronx,
New York

CHRISTER HUBLIN, MD, PhD
Centre of Expertise for Human Factors at Work,
Finnish Institute of Occupational Health;
Adjunct Professor in Neurology, Department
of Clinical Neurosciences, Helsinki University,
Helsinki, Finland

TAKASHI KANBAYASHI, MD, PhD
Associate Professor, Department of
Neuropsychiatry, Akita University Graduate
School of Medicine, Akita, Japan

DOUGLAS B. KIRSCH, MD
Clinical Instructor, Division of Sleep Medicine,
Harvard Medical School; Regional Medical
Director, Sleep HealthCenters, Brighton,
Massachusetts

SURESH KOTAGAL, MD
Professor, Departments of Neurology;
Department of Pediatrics and Center for Sleep
Medicine, Mayo Clinic, Rochester, Minnesota

CLETE A. KUSHIDA, MD, PhD
Professor of Psychiatry and Behavioral
Science, Director of the Stanford Sleep Center,
Stanford University, Stanford Sleep Medicine
Center, Redwood City, California

ARLIE LOUGHNAN, BA, LLB, LLM, PhD
Senior Lecturer, Faculty of Law, The University of Sydney, Sydney, New South Wales, Australia

TONY J. MASRI, MD
Sleep Medicine Fellow, Stanford University, Stanford Sleep Medicine Clinic, Redwood City, California

SEIJI NISHINO, MD, PhD
Director, Stanford University Sleep and Circadian Neurobiology Laboratory; Professor, Department of Psychiatry and Behavioral Sciences, Stanford University School of Medicine, Palo Alto, California

DANIELLE M. NOVICK, PhD
Post-doctoral Fellow, Department of Psychiatry, University of Michigan, Ann Arbor, Michigan

SEBASTIAAN OVEREEM, MD, PhD
Department of Neurology, Donders Institute for Brain, Cognition and Behaviour, Radboud University Nijmegen Medical Centre, Nijmegen; Sleep Medicine Centre 'Kempenhaeghe', Heeze, The Netherlands

PAUL READING, FRCP, PhD
Department of Neurology, The James Cook University Hospital, Middlesbrough, United Kingdom

THOMAS ROTH, PhD
Henry Ford Hospital Sleep Center, Detroit, Michigan

MIKAEL SALLINEN, PhD
Centre of Expertise for Human Factors at Work, Finnish Institute of Occupational Health, Helsinki; Research Professor, Agora Center, University of Jyväskylä, Jyväskylä, Finland

LESLIE M. SWANSON, PhD
Clinical Lecturer, Department of Psychiatry, University of Michigan, Ann Arbor, Michigan

RONALD SZYMUSIAK, PhD
Research Service, Veterans Affairs Greater Los Angeles Healthcare System, Los Angeles; Research Service, Veterans Affairs Greater Los Angeles Healthcare System, North Hills; Department of Medicine, David Geffen School of Medicine, University of California, Los Angeles, Los Angeles, California

MICHAEL THORPY, MD
Professor, Neurology, Montefiore Medical Center, Albert Einstein College of Medicine; Neurology Department, Sleep-Wake Disorders Center, Bronx, New York

WATARU YAMADERA, MD, PhD
Stanford University Sleep and Circadian Neurobiology Laboratory, Visiting Assistant Professor, Department of Psychiatry and Behavioral Sciences, Stanford University School of Medicine, Palo Alto, California

Contents

Hypersomnia can result from deficits in 1 or more of the arousal systems or through excessive activation of sleep-promoting systems. What is known about brain abnormalities in clinical disorders with hypersomnia suggests that arousal deficiency is a common culprit. This article reviews the neurophysiology, functional anatomy, and neurochemistry of brain arousal systems that have been implicated in excessive sleepiness in human disorders. Chronically increased production of the endogenous somnogens interleukin 1 and tumor necrosis factor has been implicated in hypersomnia associated with infection and chronic inflammatory disease, and the mechanisms of action of these 2 neuromodulators are also discussed.

The term hypersomnia is used to identify disorders that are associated with excessive sleepiness, such as idiopathic hypersomnia or narcolepsy. Sleepiness is considered excessive when there is an increased amount of sleep or an increased drive toward sleep during the wake period, making a person unable to sustain wakefulness or alertness. Patients who have excessive sleepiness tend to have involuntary sleep episodes during activities. The hypersomnias either shorten or fragment the major sleep period or are a manifestation of central nervous system dysfunction. This article discusses disorders, including the hypersomnias, that should be considered when evaluating individuals with excessive sleepiness.

Hypersomnia is a common symptom of many medical disorders, including several sleep disorders. Although patients with hypersomnia may not always have examination abnormalities, certain sleep disorders have specific physical findings that an experienced clinician should be comfortable evaluating. In combination with an appropriate clinical history taking, a sleep-specific physical examination leads to more appropriate diagnostic testing and patient management. This article reviews the physical examination findings linked with sleep disorders causing hypersomnia, aiding physicians in their ability to effectively manage their patients.

Although there are several objective and subjective tests available for the assessment of daytime sleepiness in both clinical practice and research settings, none of the available tests accurately differentiate sleepiness in normal individuals from sleepiness in patients with various sleep disorders or accurately predict safety in real world situations. Typically, a combination of subjective and objective testing in combination with the clinical history is necessary to best determine the degree and clinical significance of a given patient's daytime sleepiness.

condition is rare. The rarity of idiopathic hypersomnia has precluded any systematic studies or randomized-controlled trials on the subject, and as a result, ability to fully understand and treat this condition is greatly limited. This review covers the major points regarding the clinical features and diagnosis of idiopathic hypersomnia and discusses current evidence supporting the available treatment options for this condition.

treatment approach for patients with hypersomnia may involve both medication and behavioral components. This article focuses on the behavioral and psychological therapies for hypersomnolence that can be considered independent or adjunctive interventions.

Pharmacotherapy of Excessive Sleepiness
333

Thomas Roth

Excessive sleepiness (ES) has significant morbidity. The role of stimulants in alleviating this morbidity needs to be more specifically defined. Several stimulants are effective for managing ES. They act, at least in part, through inhibition of dopamine reuptake. Stimulants have efficacy but hypothesized differential safety and abuse liability. Large-scale clinical trials are needed to measure their relative efficacy and safety profile. US Food and Drug Administration-approved indications for stimulants covers only a small part of the ES population. There are no indications for ES associated with neurologic, psychiatric, or other medical disorders. Large-scale clinical trials are needed in these populations.

Quality of Life in Narcolepsy
341

Meeta Goswami

Theoretical constructs defining quality of life (QOL) and the significance of measuring quality of life in chronic illnesses are discussed. Narcolepsy can be a very disabling condition with negative consequences on the physical, mental, and social well-being of some affected individuals. Pharmacologic treatment may not be optimal. To alleviate the compound effects of this disorder, a comprehensive, person-centered and family-centered approach incorporating pharmacologic and psychosocial management with multidisciplinary clinicians working as a team will improve the quality of care and QOL of people with narcolepsy.

Inappropriate Situational Sleepiness and the Law
353

Peter R. Buchanan, Arlie Loughnan, and Ronald R. Grunstein

Sleepiness causes adverse personal consequences and inconvenience to individuals but may also impact on performance with sequelae that have potential to cause harm to others. Such harm has individual and societal consequences and the community has reasonable grounds from which to use legal and other frameworks to mitigate such adverse events and sanction against their occurrence. Where sleepiness, mediated by impaired performance, is the promoter of potential and actual harmful outcomes, communities have reacted by amending the law and using existing legal measures to protect society in general. This article presents an overview of some aspects of the interaction between sleepiness and various facets of the law.

Hypersomnia in Older Patients
365

Marcia E. Braun, Pamela Cines, and Nalaka S. Gooneratne

Hypersomnia is a common clinical complaint in older patients that has many characteristics unique to this population. Such features are related in part to the effects of comorbid medical conditions and their associated medications, changes in work patterns from retirement or part-time employment, increased prevalence rates of sleep disorders, and biological changes in the sleep-wake drive associated with aging. Assessment of hypersomnia in older patients is also affected by many of these factors. Despite these challenges, hypersomnia warrants evaluation and management because the adverse impact of hypersomnia can be considerable in older adults.

Suresh Kotagal

Daytime sleepiness is a common symptom during childhood and adolescence. It may be related to a variety of disorders, such as inadequate sleep hygiene, narcolepsy, sleep-disordered breathing, and circadian rhythm disorders. Consequent daytime sleepiness can lead to impaired mood and cognition and slowing of motor reaction time, with increased propensity to accidents. This article discusses some general aspects of childhood hypersomnia and provides an update on specific sleep disorders.

Foreword
Hypersomnia

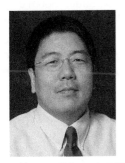

Teofilo Lee-Chiong Jr, MD
Consulting Editor

Hypersomnia is conventionally defined as an inability to consistently attain and sustain wakefulness and alertness necessary to meet the demands and accomplish the tasks of daily living. This definition, however, poses major challenges to a clinician who attempts to establish its presence and grade its severity. Needless to say, it is essential to distinguish among hypersomnia in which alertness mechanisms fail, leading to potentially dangerous sleep attacks; weak alerting systems in which a sleepy person has to put extra effort to stay awake; and overactive sleep-promoting processes.

Foremost among these dilemmas are applying parameters of what is considered "pathologic sleepiness" for a person across time as well as between persons. Similar to sleep deprivation, hypersomnia is associated with significant intra- and interindividual variability in performance deficits and subjective impairment. Vulnerability to occupational, academic, and social consequences also differs based, in large measure, to daily tasks that have to be accomplished and the subjective demands on living that have to be met. Thus, what could be considered clinically inconsequential hypersomnia for a specific individual at a specific period of time may be critical either for the same person at a different time period or for other individuals.

Second, hypersomnia can manifest in various ways, such as frequent napping, sleep attacks, microsleep episodes, automatic behavior, or hyperactivity (the latter particularly among children). Depending on cultural perceptions, employer expectations, career ambitions, domestic apprehensions, personal agenda, and demand characteristics, a pattern of hypersomnia can be regarded as "normal" or "problematic." Equally pertinent are the perception of hypersomnia's permanence or temporariness, its underlying physiologic origin(s), and the availability, effectiveness, and ease of therapy.

Last, our current tools to identify excessive sleepiness and to distinguish it from fatigue, weakness, or lassitude are neither sensitive nor specific enough to be applicable across all situations, individuals, occupations, or life stages at all times.

I would like to propose a new screening questionnaire for hypersomnia—the North America Predictor of Sleepiness (NAPS) scale. This is a six-item tool that addresses diverse facets of excessive sleepiness, namely, introspective-general (i), introspective-temporal (ii), introspective-goal oriented (iii), manifest-objective (iv), manifest-descriptive (v), and physiologic-self-report (vi).

i. *Have you felt that your daytime functioning is affected by sleepiness?*
ii. *Do you feel sleepier now than in the past?*
iii. *Have you taken steps to improve your alertness?*
iv. *Do you fall asleep frequently without wanting to do so?*

Sleep Med Clin 7 (2012) xv–xvi
doi:10.1016/j.jsmc.2012.04.003
1556-407X/12/$ – see front matter

sleep.theclinics.com

v. *Have you been told that you appear excessively sleepy?*

vi. *Would you fall asleep within 8 minutes if allowed to do so during the daytime?*

A positive response to any of these questions should prompt a more thorough evaluation into the presence, severity, and cause of excessive sleepiness. I hope you find this questionnaire helpful.

Teofilo Lee-Chiong Jr, MD
Division of Sleep Medicine
National Jewish Health
University of Colorado Denver School of Medicine
1400 Jackson Street, Room J221
Denver, CO 60206, USA

E-mail address:
Lee-ChiongT@NJC.ORG

Preface
Hypersomnia

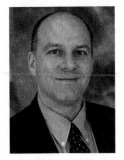

Alon Y. Avidan, MD, MPH
Guest Editor

*"Sleep Medicine is at the stage of where we
stand on the rock of knowledge and continue
to look into the abyss of the unknown."*
Modified from "A naturalist in Borneo"
—By Robert Walter

I am honored and delighted to serve as guest editor
for the *Sleep Medicine Clinics* issue focusing on
hypersomnia. The term hypersomnia is applied
clinically to describe a state of pathological or inappropriate somnolence (sleepiness) and is inter-
changeable with excessive daytime sleepiness.
Discussion of all causes of hypersomnia in sleep
medicine would have been very challenging in
a single issue and for this reason I have narrowed
the focus to hypersomnia related to central nervous system (CNS) causes. The issue is organized
according to a parallel scheme provided by the
second edition of the International Classifications
of Sleep Disorders (ICSD-2).[1] The ICSD-2 defines
hypersomnia of central origin as a category of hypersomnia not due to a sleep-related breathing
disorder, a circadian rhythm sleep disorder, or
other causes of disturbed nocturnal sleep. While
other sleep disorders may be present, they must
first be properly treated prior to establishing diagnoses in this category.

Patients with hypersomnia continue to challenge sleep experts for a number of reasons.
Some of these may be related to nomenclature
used to describe hypersomnia, while others are
related to diagnostic tests for sleepiness, health
care infrastructure used to care for these patients,
and access to pharmacotherapy that is sometimes
hindered.

CHALLENGES IN THE CARE OF PATIENTS WHO COMPLAIN OF HYPERSOMNIA

1. Nomenclature: Not all patients with clinically
   significant "hypersomnia" present to the sleep
   disorders clinic complaining of this precise
   symptom. In 2000, Ron Chervin published
   an interesting study demonstrating that, when
   clinically significant hypersomnia is present,
   patients may choose a variety of words to describe their problem—in particular, sleepiness,
   fatigue, tiredness, or lack of energy.[2]
2. Education: Given the high prevalence of sleep
   disorders in the primary clinic setting and
   ever-expanding knowledge about sleep disorders, one would have expected a parallel evolution in teaching about sleep disorders during
   medical school and residency. Unfortunately
   this has not been the case as most graduating
   physicians receive about 2 hours of sleep
   during the medical school curriculum, which is
   unlikely to meet the needs of the practicing
   physician. Physicians are not taught about fatigue management in their own lives while
   they practice in a culture that traditionally has
   not fostered adequate sleep. This is on the
   trajectory of change as the Accreditation Council for Graduate Medical Education contem-
   plates the benefits of altering physician work
   hours.[3]
3. Clinical infrastructure: Patients with hypersomnia are routinely asked to adapt to a clinic infrastructure that does not always cater to their
   needs. Patients who complain about excessive
   sleepiness are asked to arrive for consultation

Sleep Med Clin 7 (2012) xvii–xx
doi:10.1016/j.jsmc.2012.04.002
1556-407X/12/$ – see front matter

sleep.theclinics.com

during operating hours that may not be appropriate for them. For example, scheduling patients with narcolepsy to arrive to an 8 AM appointment may lead to missed appointments due to severe sleepiness. We have also encountered sleepy patients who fall asleep in the waiting room, never remembering to sign in when they arrive, leading staff to assume the patient has canceled the visit.

4. Testing: Subjective and objective assessments of hypersomnia are not perfect. The most universally used test for the subjective assessment of excessive sleepiness, the Epworth Sleepiness Scale, does not correlate well with the gold standard test—the multiple sleep latency test (MSLT).[4] As discussed in this issue, finding sleep onset REM periods, or very short sleep latencies, on MSLTs is not always indicative of narcolepsy.[5] On occasions, we may have to "undiagnose" patients who were previously told they have narcolepsy as testing was conducted during a week of sleep deprivation, or in some who were abruptly taken off their antidepressants a few days prior to testing. Similarly, the absence of pathologically short sleep latencies or SOREMPs does not always "rule out" narcolepsy.

5. The practice of and care for the patient with hypersomnia differs among clinics:
   a. The use of polysomnogram and MSLT in the diagnosis of CNS hypersomnia: Sleep clinicians sometime encounter patients who were previously diagnosed with narcolepsy based on clinical grounds alone. While the ICSD-2 allows for the diagnosis of narcolepsy with cataplexy based on the presence of hypersomnia with bone fide cataplexy, all patients with suspected narcolepsy should have a polysomnogram with a follow-up MSLT. The MSLT should not follow positive airway pressure titration or be conducted while on CNS-acting medications (unless other compelling reasons arise). Similarly, the MSLT may not be conducted following sleep studies using "split night protocols."
   b. Hypocretin assay: The measurement of cerebrospinal fluid hypocretin, while it can be used as an alternative to the MSLT, is not universally available in most sleep disorders clinics.
   c. Analeptics: Patients who are prescribed CNS stimulant medication need to be screened and followed up carefully. Certain medications (like modafinil and armodafinil) have the potential to induce the hepatic cytochrome (P450) system and render steroidal contraceptive treatment ineffective. Women of childbearing age who are prescribed these agents must be counseled about this potential interaction.

6. Patient advocacy: We are not only our patient's physicians, but also their advocates. The care of patients with hypersomnia should not be limited to diagnosis and treatment. After all, we have all needed to write letters of medical necessity for patients with narcolepsy who were told that our prescribed treatment was not approved. It is our duty to use these as opportunities to educate our colleagues, whether they are trainees, pharmacists, or insurance administrators who may need additional information and education about the condition. I have seen these efforts bear fruit after providing the prior authorization officers information and review papers about the condition. We may be asked to complete short-term disability forms for a patient with narcolepsy who lost his job after falling asleep at the wheel and was instructed to avoid driving. These issues are just as important as determining how many SOREMPs are on the patient's MSLT.

Hypersomnia is a unique point of intersection of many specialties in sleep medicine: it draws on the neurophysiologists to explain its neurophysiology; the psychiatrists to differentiate it from depression; the pediatrician to recognize it early in life; the psychologist, social worker, and all other sleep specialists to confirm diagnosis, entertain multidisciplinary management strategies, and provide ongoing costumer service for sufferers.

When beginning work on this issue, I have enlisted the help of outstanding and distinguished authorities in sleep medicine. The author list illustrates the rich geographic and multidisciplinary diversity that reflects the field itself. While many are neurologists, some are psychiatrists, neurophysiologists, psychologists, pediatricians, geriatricians, and pulmonologists. This is an international group of authors further pointing to the fact that hypersomnia is a global disorder in a society that is facing more frequent sleep deprivation and more frequent sleep disturbances.

The issue begins with a discussion of the neuroanatomy and neurophysiology of sleepiness and wakefulness by Ronald Szymusiak and Irma Gvilia from UCLA. Their review provides evidence that hypersomnia is due to a dysfunction in one or more of the ascending arousal systems located in the rostral brainstem, posterior hypothalamus, and basal forebrain. Imran Ahmed, Shelby Harris, and Michael Thorpy from the Albert Einstein College of Medicine discuss the differential diagnosis of hypersomnia in patients who present to the clinic with the chief complaint of excessive daytime sleepiness. Neil Freedman from the NorthShore University Healthcare System presents the measurement of sleep and describes their utility, limitations, and potential indications in clinical and research settings. Seiji Nishino, Carl Deguzmana, Wataru Yamadera, and Shintaro Chiba from Stanford University, and Takashi Kanbayashi from Akita University, deliver a window into the neurochemistry of excessive sleepiness and an updated review of surrogate biomarkers for hypersomnia.

The next several articles in this issue provide the reader with the spectrum of clinical disorders, comorbidities, consequences, and managements of hypersomnia. Sebastiaan Overeem from Radboud University Nijmegen, Paul Reading from The James Cook University Hospital, and Claudio Bassetti from University Hospital, Inselspital, Bern provide an appraisal of the narcolepsies focusing on clinical aspects and diagnostic approaches. Idiopathic hypersomnia is discussed next by Tony Masri and Clete Kushida from Stanford University and Carmella Gonzales from Case Western Reserve University, who report on the etiology, clinical features, and management. Claudio Bassetti returns with an assessment of primary and secondary neurogenic hypersomnias focusing on clinical spectrum, pathophysiology, differential diagnosis, and management guided with images drawn from clinical practice. I then consider several important comorbidities encountered in patients with hypersomnia, specifically focusing on those in narcolepsy where data are more plentiful. Hypersomnia in children is described by Suresh Kotagal from the Mayo Clinic, listing the causes and consequences of excessive sleepiness. Kotagal also touches on the challenges of assessment of sleepiness in children due to limited data. Hypersomnia in older patients is evaluated by Marcia Braun, Pamela Cines, and Nalaka Gooneratne from the University of Pennsylvania, focusing on the assessment of sleepiness in this population and consideration of a multimodal therapeutic approach. One of the rarest but distinguishable forms of hypersomnias is Kleine–Levin syndrome, a fascinating form of recurrent hypersomnia, presented by Michel Billiard from Gui de Chauliac Hospital. Christer Hublin and Mikael Sallinen from Helsinki University discuss a pervasive cause of excessive sleepiness, the phenomenon of behaviorally induced insufficient sleep. Deirdre Conroy, Danielle Novick, and Leslie Swanson from the University of Michigan examine behavioral management of hypersomnia reviewing psychological and behavioral interventions that might be effective as primary treatment or in combination with pharmacological treatment. Thomas Roth from Henry Ford Hospital offers a review of the armamentarium used in the pharmacotherapy of excessive sleepiness discussing the historical perspective of the stimulants and indication for the various medications used to manage hypersomnia. Meeta Goswami from Albert Einstein College of Medicine touches on an important, yet sometimes neglected area of consideration—that of quality-of-life issues facing patients suffering from hypersomnia. Peter Buchanan, Arlie Loughnan, and Ronald Grunstein from the University of Sydney appropriately conclude this issue with a discussion on one of the most challenging issues to address when caring for patients complaining of hypersomnia—inappropriate situational sleepiness and the law. Metaphorically perhaps, as we conclude the visit of the patient with hypersomnia, it is incumbent on us to discuss the risk of hypersomnia given the risk to patient and public alike.

I would like to conclude by thanking Katie Hartner Editor of *Sleep Medicine Clinics*, as well as all of the authors for their outstanding contributions. I have had the pleasure of working with many of them as colleagues and friends in this ever-evolving and exciting field. While this issue is not meant to be used as a textbook on narcolepsy or hypersomnia, it is intended to serve as a practical review of the data regarding etiology, diagnosis, and treatment approach to patients who complain of this chronic debilitating, but fortunately manageable, condition.

Alon Y. Avidan, MD, MPH
Sleep Disorders Center and
Department of Neurology
University of California, Los Angeles
710 Westwood Boulevard
Room 1-169 RNRC
Los Angeles, CA 90095-6975, USA

E-mail address:
avidan@mednet.ucla.edu

REFERENCES

1. American Academy of Sleep Medicine A. The International Classification of Sleep Disorders, 2nd edition. Diagnostic and coding manual. Westchester (IL): American Academy of Sleep Medicine;2005.

2. Chervin RD. Sleepiness, fatigue, tiredness, and lack of energy in obstructive sleep apnea. Chest 2000; 118(2):372–9.

3. Iglehart JK. Revisiting duty-hour limits–IOM recommendations for patient safety and resident education. New Engl J Med 2008;359(25):2633–5.

4. Chervin RD, Aldrich MS. The Epworth Sleepiness Scale may not reflect objective measures of sleepiness or sleep apnea. Neurology 1999;52(1):125–31.

5. Chervin RD, Aldrich MS. Sleep onset REM periods during multiple sleep latency tests in patients evaluated for sleep apnea. Am J Respir Crit Care Med 2000;161(2 Pt 1):426–31.

Neurophysiology and Neurochemistry of Hypersomnia

Ronald Szymusiak, PhD[a,b,c,*], Irma Gvilia, PhD[a,b,d]

KEYWORDS

- Excessive sleepiness • Monoamines • Hypocretin • Orexin • Cytokines

KEY POINTS

- Hypersomnia can be a consequence of dysfunction in 1 or more of the arousal systems in the rostral brainstem, posterior hypothalamus, and basal forebrain.
- Reduced HA neurotransmission has been identified as a potential cause of excessive sleepiness, both in combination with hypocretin (HCT) deficiency in narcolepsy/cataplexy syndrome, and in disorders such as idiopathic hypersomnia, in which HCT function is preserved.
- The pharmacology brain dopamine (DA) systems show a potent role for this neurotransmitter in regulating generalized brain activation. It seems likely that DA deficiency contributes to excessive sleepiness in Parkinson disease (PD), but direct causal links are difficult to establish because of comorbid sleep disorders and the sleep-promoting effects of some DA receptor agonists used to treat PD.

Generalized electroencephalographic (EEG) and behavioral activation during waking emerges from the collective activity of multiple, neurochemically specified ascending arousal systems located in the rostral brainstem, posterior hypothalamus, and basal forebrain. Hypersomnia can be a consequence of dysfunction in one or more of these arousal systems. Experimental and clinical lesions of the rostral brainstem frequently destroy ascending projections of brainstem cholinergic, monoaminergic, and/or glutamatergic neurons, causing disturbance of consciousness ranging from hypersomnia to coma, depending on lesion size and location. Hypocretin-containing neurons in the lateral hypothalamus exert powerful activating effects on the EEG and behavior through excitatory connections with monoaminergic and cholinergic nuclei in the hypothalamus and brainstem. Loss of hypocretin neurons is central to the pathophysiology of narcolepsy. Hypocretin deficiency may also contribute to hypersomnia in advanced Parkinson disease and in traumatic brain injury that involves the posterior hypothalamus. Reduced histamine in cerebrospinal fluid has been identified as a correlate of excessive sleepiness, both in combination with hypocretin deficiency in narcolepsy/cataplexy syndrome, and in disorders such as idiopathic hypersomnia when hypocretin function is preserved. The pharmacology of brain dopamine systems demonstrate a potent role for this neurotransmitter in regulating generalized brain activation, and dopamine deficiency may contribute to sleepiness in Parkinson disease. Although deficits in arousal seem to be

This work was supported by the Department of Veterans Affairs and Grant #MH63323 from the National Institutes of Health. The authors have nothing to disclose.

[a] Research Service, V.A. Greater Los Angeles Healthcare System, Los Angeles, CA, USA; [b] Research Service, V.A. Greater Los Angeles Healthcare System, 16111 Plummer Street, North Hills, CA 91343, USA; [c] Department of Medicine, David Geffen School of Medicine, University of California, Los Angeles, Los Angeles, CA, USA; [d] Department of Neurophysiology, Ilia State University, Tiblisi, Georgia
* Corresponding author. Research Service, V.A. Greater Los Angeles Healthcare System, 16111 Plummer Street, North Hills, CA 91343.
E-mail address: rszym@ucla.edu

a central component of many clinical disorders associated with hypersomnia, increased expression of sleep-promoting cytokines, both in the periphery and in the brain, are likely mediators of excessive sleepiness accompanying acute infection and chronic inflammation.

OVERVIEW OF THE REGULATORY MECHANISMS OF AROUSAL AND SLEEP

Since the pioneering studies of Morruzzi and Magoun,[1] global brain activation during waking has been believed to be achieved by an ascending arousal system located in the rostral brainstem reticular formation that broadly targets the forebrain. It is now understood that a network of chemically defined neuronal systems, located in the brainstem and hypothalamus, function to promote both behavioral and electrographic aspects of arousal (**Fig. 1**). This network includes monoaminergic neurons in the rostral pons, midbrain, and posterior hypothalamus, cholinergic neurons in the brainstem and basal forebrain, dopaminergic neurons in the ventral tegmentum

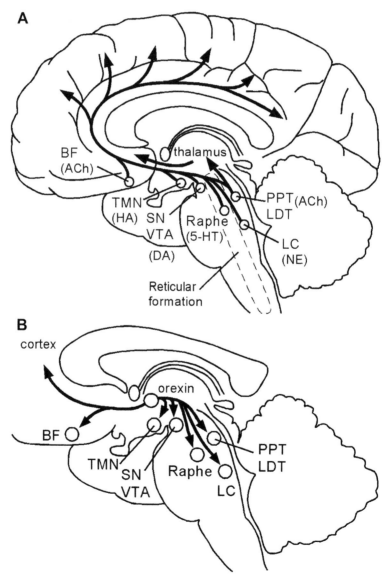

Fig. 1. (*A, B*) Sagittal view of the human brain indicating the location of arousal-regulatory neuronal groups as described in text. ACh, acetylcholine; BF, basal forebrain; DA, dopamine; LC, locus coeruleus; LDT, laterodorsal tegmentum; NE, norepinephrine; PPT, pedunculopontine tegmentum; SN, substantia nigra; VTA, ventral tegmental area; 5HT, serotonin; Raphe, dorsal and median raphe nuclei. Orexin is referred to as HCT in text. (*Adapted from* Espana RA, Scammell TE. Sleep neurobiology for the clinician. Sleep 2004;27:811–20; with permission.)

and periaqueductal gray (PAG) and hypocretin (HCT)-containing (orexin-containing) neurons in the lateral hypothalamus (reviewed in Refs.[2–5]). Collective activity in arousal systems during waking imparts a tonic background level of activation that is reflected in low voltage, fast frequency cortical electroencephalographic (EEG) patterns. Neuronal activity in these systems is characterized by high levels of tonic or phasic discharge during waking and quiescence during sleep.[3,5,6] Neurons in some arousal systems (eg, cholinergic) show increased discharge during waking and rapid eye movement (REM) sleep and minimum activity during non-REM sleep. Others (eg, monoaminergic) show discharge rates during REM sleep that are as low as or lower than rates observed during non-REM sleep (REM-off discharge pattern). What is common to all of the arousal systems is a rapid decline in neuronal activity just before, or at the time of, sleep onset.

Brain mechanisms that generate sleep must achieve a coordinated inhibition of arousal-regulatory neuronal groups. Transitions from wakefulness to sleep are accomplished through interactions among 3 cellular and neurochemical mechanisms: (1) a system of sleep-promoting neurons located in the preoptic hypothalamus, (2) endogenous sleep-regulatory substances, and (3) the circadian timing system.

The anatomic distribution of sleep-regulatory neurons has been determined by visualization of the protein product of the *c-fos* gene, a marker of neuronal activity, in the brains of animals that are asleep during the 1 to 2 hours before they are killed. This approach identified 2 subregions of the preoptic area that contain high densities of sleep-active neurons: the ventrolateral preoptic area (VLPO) and the median preoptic nucleus (MnPN).[7,8] VLPO and MnPN neurons show increased discharge rates during non-REM and REM sleep compared with waking.[9,10] These neurons synthesize the inhibitory neurotransmitter γ-aminobutyric acid (GABA).[11,12] GABAergic (GABA-mediated) neurons in the preoptic area participate in regulating homeostatic increases in sleep amount and sleep depth that occur as a consequence of sustained waking.[3] VLPO and MnPN neurons send direct axonal projections to monoaminergic nuclei, to brainstem cholinergic areas, and to HCT neurons.[2,3] Mechanisms of sleep induction by preoptic area neurons, thus, entail GABAergic inhibition of arousal systems. Lesions of the preoptic area suppress sleep and suppress EEG slow-wave activity (SWA) during sleep (**Fig. 2**).[13,14]

A second feature of sleep-wake control is the contribution of endogenous sleep regulatory substances that exert inhibitory effects on arousal

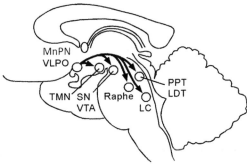

Fig. 2. Sagittal view of human diencephalon and brain stem, indicating descending projection from sleep regulatory neurons in the VLPO and MnPN, MnPN and VLPO neurons are identified as being sleep active, both from electrophysiologic recordings and from sleep-related *c-fos* expression. MnPN neurons co-localize sleep-related c-Fos and markers of GABAergic neurons. VLPO neurons are GABAergic and also express the inhibitory neuropeptide galanin. Activation of MnPN and VLPO GABAergic neurons is a critical short-latency event in switching from wakefulness to sleep, because these neurons can orchestrate rapid and powerful inhibition of cholinergic, monoaminergic, and HCTergic arousal systems via descending monosynaptic projections to the neuronal groups. (*Adapted from* Espana RA, Scammell TE. Sleep neurobiology for the clinician. Sleep 2004;27:811–20; with permission.)

systems or activate sleep-regulatory neurons. Adenosine, a product of brain metabolism, is the most extensively studied sleep regulatory substance. Adenosine levels in the brain are increased as a consequence of waking brain activity.[6,15,16] The sleep generating effects of adenosine entail A_1 adenosine receptor-mediated inhibition of arousal systems, including basal forebrain cholinergic neurons.[6,15] Adenosine may also activate sleep regulatory neurons in the preoptic area, as a result of A_1 receptor-mediated disinhibition and A_{2A} receptor-mediated excitation of preoptic neurons.[17,18]

Several cytokines, including, interleukin 1β (IL1) and tumor necrosis factor α (TNF), are also sleep-promoting and augment EEG SWA during sleep, the latter being a reliable marker of sleep depth.[19] Antagonism of IL1 and TNF can disrupt normal sleep and impair homeostatic responses to sleep deprivation. Expression of IL1 and TNF is increased in multiple brain regions in response to waking neuronal activity.[19,20] Cellular mechanisms of cytokine-mediated sleep generation are not completely understood, but may involve a combination of arousal system inhibition and activation of preoptic neurons.[21–25] Additional, well-characterized endogenous somnogens include prostaglandin D_2 and growth hormone-releasing hormone.[19] Both substances activate sleep-regulatory neurons in the preoptic hypothalamus.[26,27]

The temporal organization of sleep and wakefulness is controlled by the master circadian oscillator in the suprachiasmatic nucleus (SCN) of the hypothalamus (reviewed in Refs.[4,28,29]). Output of the SCN actively promotes waking during certain times of the day (ie, during the night in diurnal species and during the day in nocturnal species). The mechanism of this SCN-dependent alerting seems to be excitation of a subset of the arousal systems through secretion of neurohormones by the SCN and via an excitatory multisynaptic pathway originating in the SCN that targets arousal systems.[28] During sustained waking driven by the SCN, homeostatic pressure for sleep accumulates through increased expression of endogenous sleep factors (eg, adenosine and cytokines) that occur as a result of waking brain activity. At the end of the active period, when SCN output begins to decline, activity in arousal systems declines as a result of diminution of clock-dependent alerting and to increased arousal-suppressing effects of sleep factors. The increase in activity of GABAergic neurons in the MnPN and VLPO is a critical, short-latency event in switching from wakefulness to non-REM sleep, because these neurons can orchestrate rapid and powerful inhibition of several key arousal systems via their direct synaptic projections to these systems (see **Fig. 2**).

Given current knowledge of brain mechanisms that regulate sleep and waking, hypersomnia can result from deficits in 1 or more of the arousal systems or through excessive activation of sleep-promoting systems. What is known about brain abnormalities in clinical disorders with hypersomnia suggests that arousal deficiency is a common culprit. What follows is a review of the neurophysiology, functional anatomy, and neurochemistry of brain arousal systems that have been implicated in excessive sleepiness in human disorders. Chronically increased production of the endogenous somnogens IL1 and TNF has been implicated in hypersomnia associated with infection and chronic inflammatory disease, and the mechanisms of action of these 2 neuromodulators are also discussed.

Hypersomnia as a Consequence of Brainstem Lesions

Morruzi and Magoun[1] were the first to show that electrical stimulation of the rostral brainstem reticular core, and not of the primary sensory pathways, evoked generalized neocortical EEG activation from a background of EEG SWA. Experimental lesions of the rostral pontine and midbrain reticular formation in cats yielded persistent EEG SWA and behavioral immobility, which indicates coma.[30] By tracing degenerating axons from brainstem lesion sites that resulted in coma, it was shown that arousal pathways bifurcated into dorsal and ventral ascending components at the midbrain/diencephalic junction.[31] The dorsal pathway targeted the thalamus and the ventral pathway innervated the hypothalamus and basal forebrain. The rostral-most component of the ascending reticular activating system (RAS) involved projections from the thalamus, lateral hypothalamus, and basal forebrain to the neocortex (reviewed in Ref.[5]). Subsequent clinical observations confirmed that damage of the oral pontine and midbrain reticular formation, or damage to the oral pontine tegmentum alone, results in hypersomnia or coma (reviewed in Ref.[32]).

Subsequent anatomic and neurochemical studies showed that ascending pathways from the rostral pontine and midbrain reticular core contained axons from noradrenalin (NA)-containing neurons in the locus coeruleus (LC), serotonin (5HT)-containing neurons in the dorsal raphe nucleus (DRN) and acetylcholine (ACH)-containing neurons in the laterodorsal tegmental and pedunculopontine tegmental nuclei (LDT/PPT; reviewed in Ref.[5]). The activity of LC and DRN neurons is strongly sleep-wake state-dependent, with maximum discharge rate observed during wakefulness and dramatically reduced discharge rates during non-REM and REM sleep.[33] Discharge of LDT/PPT neurons is correlated with activated EEG patterns, showing high rates of discharge during waking and REM sleep and reduced activity during non-REM sleep.[34] Given the ability of ACH, 5HT, and NA to activate thalamocortical neurons and to activate neurons in the lateral hypothalamus and basal forebrain, ascending arousal influences originating from the rostral brainstem reticular formation were attributed to cholinergic and monoaminergic neurons (reviewed in Refs.[5,28,35]). However, lesions that selectively target each of these neurochemical systems individually have only modest effects on amounts of waking and sleep and on the EEG.

Recently, glutamatergic neurons in the parabrachial nucleus and the adjacent precoeruleus area of the rostral pontine tegmentum have been identified as a component of the ventral RAS, with projections targeting the basal forebrain.[36] Cell specific lesions of the parabrachial-precoeruleus complex in rats cause arousal deficits ranging from hypersomnia to coma depending on lesion size.

The RAS contains important ascending cholinergic, monoaminergic, and glutamatergic components. With the possible exception of the glutamate-containing neurons in the parabrachial nucleus, selective loss of 1 neurochemical component in experimental animals can have only small effects on global sleep-wake amounts, suggesting that brainstem damage encompassing multiple neurochemical cell types is required to produce persistent hypersomnia. Clinical lesions of the rostral brainstem typically affect multiple neurochemical systems, causing deficits ranging from hypersomnia to coma depending on lesion size and location.

Hypersomnia Because of HCT (Orexin) Insufficiency

Reduced HCT signaling is central to the pathophysiology of human narcolepsy and has been implicated in neurologic/neurodegenerative disorders associated with excessive sleepiness. The HCTs are excitatory neuropeptides (HCT-1 and HCT-2; also known as orexin-A and orexin-B) synthesized by neurons located in the posterior lateral hypothalamus and in the adjacent dorsomedial hypothalamus (see **Fig. 1**B).[37,38] HCT neurons have widespread projections to the neocortex, hypothalamus, brainstem, and spinal cord.[39] Among the targets of HCT neurons are several nuclei implicated in generalized brain arousal/activation, including histamine (HA) neurons in the tuberomammillary nucleus (TMN), dopamine (DA) neurons in the ventral tegmental area (VTA), NA neurons in the LC, 5HT neurons in DRN, and ACH neurons in the LDT/PPT (see **Fig. 1**B). HCT evokes excitatory responses among neurons in these nuclei, and the HCT system has the ability to promote global brain activation through these excitatory connections[37,40–43] HCT neurons are most strongly activated during waking, particularly during waking associated with intense motor activity and during reward-seeking behaviors.[44–46] Discharge rates of HCT neurons during quiet waking and non-REM and REM sleep are greatly reduced compared with active waking states.[44,45] Consistent with known activity patterns, levels of HCT in cerebrospinal fluid (CSF) are increased during times of day when waking predominates (ie, during the dark phase in rats).[47,48] Microinjections of HCT peptides into several forebrain and brainstem nuclei promote wakefulness and suppress non-REM and REM sleep.[41,49,50] Selective optogenetic activation of HCT neurons can evoke short-latency awakenings from sleep.[51] Systemic administration of HCT receptor antagonists increases total sleep time.[52]

Experimental HCT deficiency in dogs and mice results in a narcolepsylike syndrome that includes cataplexy and excessive sleepiness. Canine narcolepsy occurs in dogs with a mutation of the HCT-2 receptor.[53] Mice lacking HCT peptides or HCT receptors show cataplexy and increased time spent asleep in the active (dark) phase of the light-dark cycle.[54,55] Human narcolepsy/cataplexy syndrome is associated with severe loss (85%–95%) of HCT immunopositive neurons in the lateral hypothalamus[56,57] and low or undetectable levels of HCT peptides in the CSF.[58] Severity of daytime sleepiness is correlated with CSF levels of HCT-1 in patients with narcolepsy-cataplexy.[59] In cases of symptomatic narcolepsy with excessive sleepiness, most were found to have reduced CSF levels of HCT.[60] Loss of HCT neurons has been observed in other disorders associated with excessive sleepiness, including Parkinson disease (PD), multiple system atrophy, and traumatic brain injury that involves the posterior hypothalamus (reviewed in Ref.[61]).

HA Insufficiency and Hypersomnia

The only group of HA-containing neurons in the brain is located in the TMN, adjacent to the mammillary bodies in the ventral-posterior hypothalamus (see **Fig. 1**A). HA neurons project widely to other hypothalamic nuclei, to the limbic telencephalon and neocortex.[62] HA neurons show tonic levels of discharge during waking, greatly reduced discharge rate during non-REM sleep, and near-cessation of discharge during REM sleep.[63,64] The TMN receives a dense projection from GABA/galanin-containing neurons in the VLPO.[65] VLPO neurons are activated during sleep, and the sleep-related suppression of HA neuronal activity is mediated by inhibitory inputs from the VLPO.[7,9,66] Administration of HA or H1 receptor agonist increases cortical activation and wakefulness and suppresses sleep.[67] H1 receptor antagonists have sleep-promoting effects.[68–70] HA neurons express an H3 inhibitory autoreceptor, and administration of H3 agonists promotes sleep, whereas H3 antagonists are alerting.[71] Mice with deletion of the histidine decarboxylase gene, a gene that codes for an HA-synthesizing enzyme, show relatively normal amounts of spontaneous sleep-wake, but have impaired ability to sustain wakefulness when exposed to a novel environment.[72]

Recent findings support a mechanistic role for HA deficiency in clinical syndromes associated with excessive sleepiness. HA levels in CSF are reduced in HCT-deficient narcolepsy with cataplexy.[59,73] Excitatory inputs from HCT neurons to the TMN are believed to be important in driving HA neuronal activity in the intact brain,[70] and reduced CSF levels of HA in narcolepsy can be viewed as a consequence of reduced HCT signaling. However, CSF levels of HA are also significantly reduced in HCT nondeficient narcolepsy with cataplexy, in HCT nondeficient narcolepsy without cataplexy, and in idiopathic hypersomnia.[73,74] Hence, reduced HA signaling may be contributory to symptoms of excessive sleepiness in several disorders independent of loss of HCT function.

DA Neurotransmission and Arousal

DA has been implicated in several important waking brain functions, including motor activity, motivation, and reward.[75] Acute and chronic pharmacologic manipulation of DA signaling in the brain can have a profound impact on sleep and arousal.[4] DA deficiency in PD is associated with symptoms of disturbed nocturnal sleep and excessive daytime sleepiness.[76]

The largest concentration of DA neurons in the brain is located in the substantia nigra (SN) and VTA in the ventral midbrain, just dorsal to the cerebral peduncles (see **Fig. 1**).[77] These DA neurons innervate the frontal cortex, striatum, thalamus, and limbic system. State-dependent activity of DA neurons differs from the other monoaminergic arousal systems, such as HA. Discharge of DA neurons in the SN is not strongly sleep-wake state-dependent.[78] DA neurons in the VTA do show a wake/REM active discharge pattern, although the activity of these neurons is not as strongly state-dependent as other wake/REM active neuronal populations.[79] However, DA neurons in the VTA discharge high-frequency bursts of action potentials in waking and REM sleep, and burst firing augments DA release from axon terminals.[79] Release of DA in the frontal cortex is higher during waking than during sleep.[80]

Other DA neurons implicated in the regulation of arousal are located in the midline ventral PAG in the midbrain. These DA neurons have been shown to be more active during waking compared with sleep; activity during REM sleep has not been characterized.[81] DA neurons in the PAG project to hypothalamic and basal forebrain regions implicated in sleep-wake regulation. Selective lesions of DA neurons in the PAG cause an arousal deficit.[81]

Sleepiness is a common adverse effect of antipsychotic drugs that function as DA receptor antagonists.[82,83] The actions of DA agonists on sleep and arousal are complex. DA released from presynaptic terminals is removed from the synaptic cleft through reuptake by the membrane-bound DA transporter (DAT).[84] Compounds in clinical use for the treatment of excessive sleepiness bind to and suppress the activity of the DAT,

thereby suppressing DA reuptake and enhancing DA signaling. Alerting drugs that act at the DAT include amphetamine and modafanil.[84–87] In rats, selective D1 DA receptor agonists can promote wakefulness, whereas D2 agonists can cause sleepiness through activation of autoinhibitory D2 receptors that suppress release of DA.[88] The effects of D2 agonists on sleep in rats are biphasic, with low doses causing increased sleep and higher doses promoting arousal.

Daytime sleepiness is a common finding in PD, occurring in approximately 30% of patients.[89] Daytime sleepiness in PD is correlated with age and disease progression. The contribution of DA deficiency to excessive sleepiness in PD is controversial. The well-established associations of increased DA signaling with activated brain states and the alerting effects of drugs that block the DAT suggest that chronic DA deficiency should lead to increased sleepiness. However, there are multiple causes of daytime sleepiness in PD that cannot be directly linked to insufficient DA-mediated arousal.[89,90] These causes include nocturnal sleep disturbance as a result of painful dystonia and nocturia, and comorbid sleep disorders such as restless legs, REM sleep behavior disorder, and sleep apnea. In addition, drug-induced sleepiness may occur in patients treated with DA receptor agonists, either alone or in combination with levodopa.[76,89] As disease progresses, there may be loss of additional neuronal systems implicated in arousal, including HCT neurons in the lateral hypothalamus.[91,92] It seems that central DA deficiency is one of several factors contributing to hypersomnia in PD.

Cytokines and Hypersomnia Associated with Immune System Activation

Cytokines are immune signaling molecules that are synthesized and released by cells in the peripheral immune system during infection. Several cytokines have been shown to alter sleep when administered to experimental animals, but IL1 and TNF have been studied most extensively (reviewed in Ref.[25]). One mechanism by which increased levels of cytokines in the periphery are detected by the brain is through cytokine-mediated activation of the vagus nerve. Systemic administration of IL1 evokes an increase in IL1 mRNA in the hypothalamus, an effect blocked by vagotomy.[93] Peripheral IL1 and TNF can also be detected directly from blood to brain at the circumventricular organs. IL1 and TNF act through specific receptors located in several brain regions including hypothalamus, brainstem, hippocampus, and neocortex.[94] In addition to synthesis by cells of the peripheral immune system, IL1 and TNF are synthesized and released in the brain.[95,96] Cells that are immunoreactive for IL1 and TNF (neurons and glia) are located in the hypothalamus, brainstem, hippocampus, and cortex.

There is considerable evidence in support of the hypothesis that IL1 and TNF function as endogenous sleep regulators. Administration of IL1 and TNF by various routes increases non-REM sleep in several species of laboratory animals (reviewed in Refs.[19,25]) Non-REM sleep induced by IL1 and TNF is frequently associated with increased EEG SWA. In most instances, cytokine administration acutely suppresses REM sleep. Blocking the actions of IL1 or TNF with antibodies, antagonists, or soluble receptors reduces amounts of spontaneous sleep and suppresses recovery sleep after sleep deprivation.[19,25] Sleep deprivation increases IL1 mRNA expression in the hypothalamus and brainstem of rats.[97] Knockout mice lacking IL1 receptors and TNF receptors have reduced non-REM sleep time compared with wild-type mice.[98] Diurnal rhythms of cytokine production are consistent with sleep-promoting functions. IL1 and TNF mRNA levels in rats are maximal around the time of lights-on, the beginning of the major rest period of the day in this species.[99] In humans, plasma levels of IL1 peak at the time of habitual sleep onset.[100]

The mechanisms through which IL1 and TNF increase sleep are not completely understood, but probably involve actions in multiple brain regions. One mechanism involves suppression of arousal, because IL1 has been shown to inhibit activity in subcortical wake-active neuronal populations. Local perfusion of IL1 into cholinergic regions of the rat basal forebrain caused reductions in discharge rate in 79% of wake-active neurons recorded.[101] Local microinjection of IL1 into the rat DRN increases sleep.[23] In brainstem slices containing the DRN, application of IL1 inhibits 5HT neurons by enhancing GABAergic postsynaptic potentials.[24] IL1 inhibits putative cholinergic neurons in the LDT/PPT recorded in rat brainstem slices.[102] Microinjection of IL1 into the LDT/PPT in vivo suppresses REM sleep. Inhibition of brainstem cholinergic neuronal activity is a mechanism by which IL1 can both reduce ascending activation of the thalamus and cortex and suppress the generation of REM sleep by brainstem circuits.[6]

In addition to inhibiting ACH-mediated and 5HT-mediated arousal, IL1 can have excitatory effects on preoptic sleep regulatory neurons. Local perfusion of IL-1 activates a subset of sleep-active neurons recorded in the lateral preoptic area of rats.[101] Sleep induced by intracerebroventricular infusion of IL1 during the dark phase in rats is accompanied by increased c-Fos expression in the MnPN.[22]

Sleep-promoting actions of IL1 and TNF are not confined to subcortical sites. In the neocortex, waking neuronal activity drives the production of cytokines, establishing a link between local changes in the sleep EEG and previous waking activity. Expression of TNF and IL1 is increased in the rat somatosensory cortex in response to intense whisker stimulation.[103,104] Both neurons and astrocytes are potential sources of cytokines in neocortex.[20] Application of IL1[105] and TNF[106] directly to the cortex evokes ipsilateral increases in EEG SWA during non-REM sleep. Antagonism of TNF within the neocortex locally suppresses SWA during sleep.[107] Hence, IL1 and TNF can deactivate cortex and promote sleep oscillations in the EEG via suppression of subcortical activating inputs to the cortex originating in the brainstem and basal forebrain, as well as through local actions in the neocortex.

Cytokines are implicated in pathologic sleep and are a key component of the mechanisms by which sleep is increased in response to infection.[25,108] Most preclinical studies of infection and sleep use bacterial cell wall components such as lipopolysaccharide and muramyl dipeptide to activate the immune system, because these provide better temporal control over the immune response than can be achieved with replicating pathogens.[25] These endotoxins evoke strong innate immune responses and cause upregulation of proinflammatory cytokine mRNAs, including IL1 and TNF mRNAs, in the periphery and in brain.[109] When endotoxins are administered to mice, rats, and rabbits, they cause increases in non-REM sleep and suppression of REM sleep (reviewed in Ref.[110]). Endotoxin-induced changes in sleep in rats and rabbits are attenuated by IL1 receptor antagonists.[111] In humans, high doses of endotoxin that evoke fever and neuroendocrine responses cause fragmentation of sleep, but lower doses that are not fever-producing cause increases in non-REM sleep.[112] Increased TNF production is hypothesized to underlie these endotoxin-induced changes in sleep.

Chronic inflammatory diseases such as rheumatoid arthritis and human immunodeficiency virus infection are associated with sleep fragmentation, sleepiness, and fatigue.[113–115] Increased circulating levels of TNF in these disorders have been hypothesized to underlie sleep abnormalities. Symptoms of disturbed sleep and fatigue in fibromyalgia have been attributed to chronic upregulation of cytokines.[116] Increased production of TNF has been linked to excessive daytime sleepiness in obstructive sleep apnea syndrome (reviewed in Ref.[108]). Levels of TNF are increased in narcoleptic patients compared with controls matched for age, sex, and body mass index (calculated as weight in kilograms divided by the square of height in meters).[117] In human traumatic brain injury, IL1 and TNF levels are acutely increased in brain, peaking within 1 to 3 days of trauma (reviewed in Ref.[118]). Neuroinflammatory responses can be more persistent in certain types of diffuse brain injury,[119,120] and chronically increased cytokine levels in brain may contribute to posttraumatic hypersomnia observed in some patients.[121]

SUMMARY

Generalized activation in the awake brain emerges from the collective activity of multiple, neurochemically specified ascending arousal systems located in the rostral brainstem, posterior hypothalamus, and basal forebrain (see **Fig. 1**). Hypersomnia can be a consequence of dysfunction in 1 or more of these arousal systems. Experimental and clinical lesions of the rostral brainstem often destroy ascending projections of brainstem cholinergic, monoaminergic, or glutamatergic neurons, causing disturbance of consciousness, ranging from excessive sleepiness to coma, depending on lesion location and size. Neurons located in the posterior lateral hypothalamus that contain the HCT peptides exert powerful activating effects on the EEG and behavior through monosynaptic excitatory connections with monoaminergic and cholinergic nuclei (see **Fig. 1**B). Selective loss of HCT peptides or HCT receptors in mice and dogs yields a narcolepsy phenotype, including excessive sleepiness and cataplexy. Loss of HCT neurons is central to the pathophysiology of human narcolepsy. HCT deficiency may also contribute to hypersomnia in advanced PD and in traumatic brain injury that involves the posterior hypothalamus. Reduced HA neurotransmission has been identified as a potential cause of excessive sleepiness, both in combination with HCT deficiency in narcolepsy/cataplexy syndrome, and in disorders such as idiopathic hypersomnia, in which HCT function is preserved. The pharmacology of DA indicates a potent role for this neurotransmitter in regulating generalized brain activation. It seems likely that DA deficiency contributes to excessive sleepiness in PD, but direct causal links are difficult to establish because of comorbid sleep disorders and the sleep-promoting effects of some DA receptor agonists used to treat PD. Although arousal deficiency seems to be a central component of many important clinical disorders associated with hypersomnia, increased expression of sleep-promoting cytokines, both in the periphery and in the brain, are likely mediators of excessive sleepiness accompanying acute infection and chronic inflammation.

REFERENCES

1. Moruzzi G, Magoun H. Brainstem reticular formation and activation of the EEG. Electroencephalogr Clin Neurophysiol 1949;1:455–73.
2. Saper CB, Fuller P, Pedersen N, et al. Sleep state switching. Neuron 2010;68:1023–42.
3. Szymusiak R, Gvilia I, McGinty D. Hypothalamic control of sleep. Sleep Med 2007;8:291–301.
4. Espana RA, Scammell TE. Sleep neurobiology from a clinical perspective. Sleep 2011;34:845–58.
5. Jones BE. Basic mechanisms of sleep-wake states. In: Kryger MH, Roth T, Dement WC, editors. Principles and practice of sleep medicine. Philadelphia: Elsevier Saunders; 2005. p. 136–53.
6. McCarley RW. Neurobiology of REM and NREM sleep. Sleep Med 2007;8:302–30.
7. Sherin JE, Shiromani PJ, McCarley RW, et al. Activation of ventrolateral preoptic neurons during sleep. Science 1996;271:216–9.
8. Gong H, Szymusiak R, King J, et al. Sleep-related c-Fos protein expression in the preoptic hypothalamus: effects of ambient warming. Am J Physiol 2000;279:R2079–88.
9. Szymusiak R, Alam N, Steininger TL, et al. Sleep-waking discharge patterns of ventrolateral preoptic/anterior hypothalamic neurons in rats. Brain Res 1998;803:178–88.
10. Suntsova N, Szymusiak R, Alam MN, et al. Sleep-waking discharge patterns of median preoptic nucleus neurons. J Physiol 2002;543:665–77.
11. Gong H, McGinty D, Guzman-Marin R, et al. Activation of c-Fos in GABAergic neurones in the preoptic area during sleep and in response to sleep deprivation. J Physiol 2004;556:935–46.
12. Gaus SE, Strecker RE, Tate BA, et al. Ventrolateral preoptic nucleus contains sleep-active, galaninergic neurons in multiple mammalian species. Neuroscience 2002;115:285–94.
13. Lu J, Greco MA, Shiromani P, et al. Effect of lesions of the ventrolateral preoptic nucleus on NREM and REM sleep. J Neurosci 2000;20:3830–42.
14. John J, Kumar V. Effect of NMDA lesions of the medial preoptic neurons on sleep and other functions. Sleep 1998;21:587–98.
15. Basheer R, Strecker RE, Thakkar MM, et al. Adenosine and sleep-wake regulation. Prog Neurobiol 2004;73:379–96.
16. Porkka-Heiskanen T, Strecker RE, McCarley RW. Brain site specificity of extracellular adenosine concentration changes during sleep deprivation and spontaneous sleep: an in vivo microdialysis study. Neuroscience 2000;99:507–17.

17. Morairty S, Rainnie D, McCarley RW, et al. Disinhibition of ventrolateral preoptic area sleep-active neurons by adenosine: a new mechanism for sleep promotion. Neuroscience 2004;123:451–7.

18. Scammell T, Gerashchenko D, Mochizuki T, et al. An adenosine A2a agonist increases sleep and induces Fos in ventrolateral preoptic area neurons. Neuroscience 2001;107:663.

19. Obal F Jr, Krueger JM. Biochemical regulation of non-rapid-eye-movement sleep. Front Biosci 2003;8:d520–50.

20. Krueger JM, Rector D, Roy S, et al. Sleep as a fundamental property of neuronal assemblies. Nat Rev Neurosci 2008;9:910–9.

21. Alam MN, McGinty D, Imeri L, et al. Effects of interleukin 1-beta on sleep- and wake-related preoptic/anterior hypothalamic neurons in unrestrained rats. Sleep 2001;24:A59.

22. Baker FC, Shah S, Stewart D, et al. Interleukin 1b enhances non-rapid eye movement sleep and increases c-Fos protein expression in the median preoptic nucleus of the hypothalamus. Am J Physiol Regul Integr Comp Physiol 2005;288:R998–1005.

23. Brambilla D, Bianchi S, Mariotti M, et al. Interleukin-1b enhances non-rapid eye movement sleep when microinjected into the dorsal raphe nucleus and inhibits serotonergic neurons in vitro. Eur J Neurosci 2003;18:1041–9.

24. Brambilla D, Franciosi S, Opp M, et al. Interleukin-1 inhibits firing of serotonergic neurons in the dorsal raphe nucleus and enhances GABAergic inhibitory post synaptic potentials. Eur J Neurosci 2007;26:1862–9.

25. Imeri L, Opp M. How (and why) the immune system makes us sleep. Nat Rev Neurosci 2009;10:199–210.

26. Scammell T, Gerashchenko D, Urade Y, et al. Activation of ventrolateral preoptic neurons by the somnogen prostaglandin D_2. Proc Natl Acad Sci U S A 1998;95:7754–9.

27. Peterfi Z, McGinty D, Sarai E, et al. Growth hormone-releasing hormone activates sleep regulatory neurons of the rat preoptic hypothalamus. Am J Physiol Regul Integr Comp Physiol 2010;298:R147–56.

28. Saper CB, Scammel T, Lu J. Hypothalamic regulation of sleep and circadian rhythms. Nature 2005;437:1257–63.

29. Moore RY. Suprachiasmatic nucleus in sleep-wake generation. Sleep Med 2007;8:S27–33.

30. Lindsley D, Bowden J, Magoun H. Effect upon the EEG of acute injury to the brain stem activating system. Electroencephalogr Clin Neurophysiol 1949;1:475–86.

31. Nauta WJ, Kuypers H. Some ascending pathways in the brain stem reticular formation. In: Jasper H, Proctor L, Knighton R, editors. Reticular formation of the brain. Boston: Little, Brown; 1958. p. 31.

32. Parviai J, Damasio A. Neuroanatomical correlates of brainstem coma. Brain 2003;126:1524–36.

33. McGinty D, Szymusiak R. Neuronal unit activity patterns in behaving animals: brainstem and limbic system. Annu Rev Psychol 1988;39:135–68.

34. Steriade M, Datta S, Pare D, et al. Neuronal activities in brain stem cholinergic nuclei related to tonic activation processes in thalamocortical systems. J Neurosci 2010;10:2541–59.

35. McCormick DA, Bal T. Sleep and arousal: thalamocortical mechanisms. Annu Rev Neurosci 1997;20:185–215.

36. Fuller P, Sherman D, Pedersen N, et al. Reassessment of the structural basis of the ascending arousal system. J Comp Neurol 2010;519:933–56.

37. de Lecea L, Kilduff TS, Peyron C, et al. The hypocretins: hypothalamus-specific peptides with neuroexcitatory activity. Proc Natl Acad Sci U S A 1998;95:322–7.

38. Sakurai T, Amemiya A, Ishii M, et al. Orexins and orexin receptors: a family of hypothalamic neuropeptides and G protein-coupled receptors that regulate feeding behavior. Cell 1998;92:573–85.

39. Peyron C, Tighe DK, van Den Pol AN, et al. Neurons containing hypocretin (orexin) project to multiple neuronal systems. J Neurosci 1998;18:9996–10015.

40. Horvath TL, Peyron C, Diano S, et al. Hypocretin (orexin) activation and synaptic innervation of the locus coeruleus noradrenergic system. J Comp Neurol 1999;415:145–59.

41. Hagan JJ, Leslie RA, Patel S, et al. Orexin A activates locus coeruleus cell firing and increases arousal in the rat. Proc Natl Acad Sci U S A 1999;96:10911–6.

42. Wu M, Zaborszky L, Hajszan T, et al. Hypocretin/orexin innervation and excitation of identified septohippocampal cholinergic neurons. J Neurosci 2004;24:3527–36.

43. Liu R, van Den Pol AN, Aghajanian G. Hypocretins (orexins) regulate serotonin neurons in the dorsal raphe nucleus by excitatory direct and inhibitory indirect actions. J Neurosci 2002;22:9453–64.

44. Lee MG, Hassani OK, Jones BE. Discharge of identified orexin/hypocretin neurons across the sleep-waking cycle. J Neurosci 2005;25:6716–20.

45. Mileykovskiy BY, Kiyashchenko LI, Siegel JM. Behavioral correlates of activity in identified hypocretin/orexin neurons. Neuron 2005;46:787–98.

46. McGregor R, Wu M, Barber G, et al. Highly specific role of hypocretin (orexin) neurons: differential activation as a function of diurnal phase, operant reinforcement versus operant avoidance and light level. J Neurosci 2011;31:15455–67.

47. Fujiki N, Yoshida Y, Ripley B, et al. Changes in CSF hypocretin-1 (orexin-A) levels in rats across 24 hours and in response to food deprivation. Neuroreport 2001;12:993–7.

48. Desarnaud F, Murillo-Rodriguez E, Lin L, et al. Diurnal rhythms of hypocretin in young and old F344 rats. Sleep 2004;27:851–6.

49. Espana R, Baldo B, Kelley A, et al. Wake-promoting and sleep suppressing actions of hypocretin (orexin): basal forebrain sites of action. Neuroscience 2001;106:699–715.

50. Methippara MM, Alam MN, Szymusiak R, et al. Effects of lateral preoptic area application of orexin-A on sleep-wakefulness. Neuroreport 2000; 11:3423–6.

51. Adamantidis A, Zhang F, Aravanis A, et al. Neural substrates of awakening probed with optogenetic control of hypocretin neurons. Nature 2007;450: 420–4.

52. Scammell T, Winrow C. Orexin receptors: pharmacology and therapeutic opportunities. Annu Rev Pharmacol Toxicol 2011;51:243–66.

53. Lin L, Faraco J, Li R, et al. The sleep disorder canine narcolepsy is caused by a mutation in the hypocretin (orexin) receptor 2 gene [see comments]. Cell 1999;98:365–76.

54. Chemelli RM, Willie JT, Sinton CM, et al. Narcolepsy in orexin knockout mice: molecular genetics of sleep regulation. Cell 1999;98:437–51.

55. Mochizuki T, Crocker A, McCormack S, et al. Behavioral state instability in orexin knock-out mice. J Neurosci 2004;24:6291–300.

56. Thannickal TC, Moore RY, Nienhuis R, et al. Reduced number of hypocretin neurons in human narcolepsy. Neuron 2000;27:469–74.

57. Peyron C, Faraco J, Rogers W, et al. A mutation in a case of early onset narcolepsy and a generalized absence of hypocretin peptides in human narcoleptic brains. Nat Med 2000;6:991–7.

58. Nishino S, Ripley B, Overeem S, et al. Low cerebrospinal fluid hypocretin (orexin) and altered energy homeostasis in human narcolepsy. Ann Neurol 2001;50:381–8.

59. Nishino S. Clinical and neurobiological aspects of narcolepsy. Sleep Med 2007;8:373–99.

60. Ritchie C, Okuro M, Kanabayashi T, et al. Hypocretin ligand deficiency in narcolepsy: recent basic and clinical insights. Curr Neurol Neurosci Rep 2010;10:180–9.

61. Fronczek R, Baumann C, Lammers GJ, et al. Hypocretin/orexin disturbances in neurological disorders. Sleep Med Rev 2009;13:9–22.

62. Inagaki N, Yamatodani A, Ando-Yamamoto M, et al. Organization of histaminergic fibers in the rat brain. J Comp Neurol 1988;273:283–300.

63. Vanni-Mercier G, Sakai K, Lin JS, et al. Mapping of cholinoceptive brainstem structures responsible for the generation of paradoxical sleep in the cat. Arch Ital Biol 1989;127:133–64.

64. Steininger TL, Alam MN, Gong H, et al. Sleep-waking discharge of neurons in the posterior lateral hypothalamus of the albino rat. Brain Res 1999; 840:138–47.

65. Sherin JE, Elmquist JK, Torrealba F, et al. Innervation of histaminergic tuberomammillary neurons by GABAergic and galaninergic neurons in the ventrolateral preoptic nucleus of the rat. J Neurosci 1998;18:4705–21.

66. Yang QZ, Hatton GI. Electrophysiology of excitatory and inhibitory afferents to rat histaminergic tuberomammillary nucleus neurons from hypothalamic and forebrain sites. Brain Res 1997;773: 162–72.

67. Monti JM, Jantos H, Leschke C, et al. The selective histamine H1-receptor agonist 2-(3-trifluoromethylphenyl)histamine increases waking in the rat. Eur Neuropsychopharmacol 1994;4:459–62.

68. Tasaka K, Chung Y, Sawada K, et al. Excitatory effects of histamine on the arousal system and its inhibition by H1 blockers. Brain Res Bull 1989;22: 271–5.

69. Krystal A, Lankford A, Durrence H, et al. Efficacy and safety of doxepin 3 and 6 mg in a 35 day sleep laboratory trial in adults with chronic primary insomnia. Sleep 2011;34:1433–42.

70. Yamanaka A, Tsujino N, Funahashi H, et al. Orexins activate histaminergic neurons via orexin 2 receptor. Biochem Biophys Res Commun 2002; 290:1237–45.

71. Lin JS, Segeeva O, Hass H. Histamine H3 receptors and sleep-wake regulation. J Pharmacol Exp Ther 2011;336:17–23.

72. Parmentier M, Ohtsu H, Djebbara-Hannas Z, et al. Anatomical, physiological and pharmacological characteristics of histidine decarboxylase knock-out mice: evidence for the role of brain histamine in behavioral and sleep-wake control. J Neurosci 2002;22:7695–711.

73. Nishino S, Sakurai T, Nevsimalova S, et al. Decreased CSF histamine in narcolepsy with and without low CSF hypocretin-1 in comparison to healthy controls. Sleep 2009;32:175–80.

74. Kanabayashi T, Kodama T, Kondo H, et al. CSF histamine contents in narcolepsy, idiopathic hypersomnia and obstructive sleep apnea syndrome. Sleep 2009;32:181–7.

75. Schultz W. Multiple dopamine functions at different time courses. Annu Rev Neurosci 2007;30:259–88.

76. Knie B, Mitra M, Logishetty K, et al. Excessive daytime sleepiness in patients with Parkinson's disease. CNS Drugs 2011;25:203–12.

77. Lindvall O, Bjorklund A. Neuroanatomy of central dopamine pathways: review of recent progress. In: Keal M, editor. Advances in dopamine research. New York: Pergamon; 1982. p. 297–311.

78. Steinfels G, Heym J, Strecker RE, et al. Behavioral correlates of dopaminergic unit activity in freely moving cats. Brain Res 1983;258:217–28.

79. Dahan L, Astier B, Vautrelle N, et al. Prominent burst firing of dopaminergic neurons in the ventral tegmental area during paradoxical sleep. Neuropsychopharmacology 2007;32:1232–41.

80. Feenstra M, Botterblom M, Mastenbroek S. Dopamine and noradrenalin efflux in prefrontal cortex in the light and dark period: effects of novelty and handling and comparison to the nucleus accumbens. Neuroscience 2000;100:741–8.

81. Lu J, Jhou T, Saper CB. Identification of wake-active dopaminergic neurons in the ventral periaqueductal gray matter. J Neurosci 2006;26:193–202.

82. Ongini E, Bonizzoni E, Ferri N, et al. Differential effects of dopamine D-1 and D-2 receptor antagonist antipsychotics on sleep-wake patterns in the rat. J Pharmacol Exp Ther 1993;266:726–31.

83. Neylan T, vanKammen D, Kelley M, et al. Sleep in schizophrenic patients on and off haloperidol therapy. Clinically stable versus relapsed patients. Arch Gen Psychiatry 1992;49:643–9.

84. Schmitt K, Reith M. Regulation of the dopamine transporter aspects relevant to psychostimulant drugs of abuse. Ann N Y Acad Sci 2010;1187:316–40.

85. Wisor J, Nishino S, Sora I, et al. Dopaminergic role in stimulant-induced wakefulness. J Neurosci 2001;21:1787–94.

86. Zolkowska D, Jain R, Rothman R, et al. Evidence for the involvement of dopamine transporters in behavioral stimulant effects of modafinil. J Pharmacol Exp Ther 2009;329:738–46.

87. Qu WM, Huang ZL, Xu X, et al. Dopaminergic D1 and D2 receptors are essential for the arousal effect of modafinil. J Neurosci 2008;28:8462–9.

88. Monti JM, Monti D. The involvement of dopamine in the modulation of sleep and waking. Sleep Med Rev 2007;11:113–33.

89. DeCock V, Vidailhet M, Arnulf I. Sleep disturbances in patients with parkinsonism. Nat Clin Pract Neurol 2008;4:254–66.

90. Verbaan D, vanRooden S, Visser M, et al. Nighttime sleep problems and daytime sleepiness in Parkinson's disease. Mov Disord 2008;23:35–41.

91. Thannickal TC, Lai Y, Siegel JM. Hypocretin (orexin) cell loss in Parkinson's disease. Brain 2007;130:1586–95.

92. Fronczek R, Overeem S, Lee S, et al. Hypocretin (orexin) loss in Parkinson's disease. Brain 2007;130:1577–85.

93. Hansen M, Taishi P, Chen Z, et al. Vagotomy blocks the induction of interleukin-1 beta mRNA in the brain of rats in response to systemic interleukin-1 beta. J Neurosci 1998;18:2247–53.

94. Ban E. Interleukin-1 receptors in the brain: characterization by quantitative in situ autoradiography. Immunomethods 1994;5:31–40.

95. Breder C, Dinarello C, Saper CB. Interleukin-1 immunoreactive innervation of the human hypothalamus. Science 1988;240:321–4.

96. Breder C, Tsujimoto M, Terano Y, et al. Distribution and characterization of tumor necrosis-like immunoreactivity in the murine central nervous system. J Comp Neurol 1993;337:543–67.

97. Mackiewicz M, Sollars P, Ogilvie M, et al. Modulation of IL-1 beta gene expression in the rat CNS during sleep deprivation. Neuroreport 1996;31:529–33.

98. Baracchi F, Opp M. Sleep-wake behavior and responses to sleep deprivation of mice lacking both interleukin-1beta and tumor necrosis factor alpha receptor. Brain Behav Immun 2008;22:982–93.

99. Cearley C, Churchill L, Krueger JM. Time of day differences in IL1B and TNFa mRNA levels in specific regions of the rat brain. Neurosci Lett 2003;352:61–3.

100. Moldofsky H, Lue F, Eisen J, et al. The relationship of interleukin-1 immune functions to sleep in humans. Psychosom Med 1986;48:309–18.

101. Alam MN, McGinty D, Bashir T, et al. Interleukin-1beta modulates state-dependent discharge activity of preoptic area and basal forebrain neurons: role in sleep regulation. Eur J Neurosci 2004;29:207–16.

102. Brambilla D, Barajon I, Bianchi S, et al. Interleukin-1 inhibits putative cholinergic neurons in vitro and REM sleep when microinjected into the rat laterodorsal tegmental nucleus. Sleep 2010;33:919–29.

103. Churchill L, Rector D, Yasusda K, et al. Tumor necrosis factor a: activity dependent expression and promotion of cortical column sleep in rats. Neuroscience 2008;156:71–80.

104. Hallett H, Churchill L, Taishi P, et al. Whisker stimulation increases expression of nerve growth factor- and interleukin-1-beta immunoreactivity in the rat somatosensory cortex. Brain Res 2010;1333:48–56.

105. Yasusda K, Churchill L, Yasuda T, et al. Unilateral cortical application of interleukin-1b induces asymmetry in fos, IL1b and nerve growth factor immunoreactivity: implications for sleep regulation. Brain Res 2007;1131:44–59.

106. Yoshida H, Peterfi Z, Garcia-Garcia F, et al. State-specific asymmetries in EEG slow wave activity induced by local application of TNFa. Brain Res 2004;1009:129–36.

107. Taishi P, Churchill L, Wang M, et al. TNFa siRNA reduces brain TNF and EEG delta wave activity in rats. Brain Res 2007;1156:125–32.

108. Kapsimalis F, Basta M, Varouchakis G, et al. Cytokines and pathological sleep. Sleep Med 2008;9:603–14.

109. Turrin N, Gayle D, Ilyin S, et al. Pro-inflammatory and anti-inflammatory cytokine mRNA induction in the periphery and brain following intraperitoneal

administration of bacterial lipopolysaccharide. Brain Res Bull 2001;54:443–53.

110. Krueger JM, Majde J. Microbial products and cytokines in sleep and fever regulation. Crit Rev Immunol 1994;14:355–79.

111. Imeri L, Opp M, Krueger JM. An IL-1 receptor and an IL-1 receptor antagonist attenuate muramyl dipeptide and IL-1 induced sleep and fever. Am J Physiol 1993;265:R907–13.

112. Schuld A, Haack M, Hinze-Selch D, et al. Experimental studies on the interaction between sleep and the immune system. Psychother Psychosom Med Psychol 2005;55:29–35.

113. Hirsch M, Carlander B, Verge M, et al. Objective and subjective sleep disturbances in patients with RA: a reappraisal. Arthritis Rheum 1994;37:37–41.

114. Silva L, Ortigosa L, Benard G. Anti-TNF-a agents in the treatment of immune-mediated inflammatory diseases: mechanisms of action and pitfalls. Immunotherapy 2010;2:817–33.

115. Darko D, Miller J, Gallen C, et al. Sleep electroencephalogram delta frequency amplitude, night plasma levels of TNF-alpha and human immuno-deficiency virus infection. Proc Natl Acad Sci U S A 1995;92:12080–4.

116. Moldofsky H. Fibromyalgia, sleep disorder and chronic fatigue syndrome. Ciba Found Symp 1993;173:262–71.

117. Himmerich H, Beitinger P, Fulda S, et al. Plasma levels of tumor necrosis factor alpha and soluble tumor necrosis factor receptors in patients with narcolepsy. Arch Intern Med 2006;166:1739–43.

118. Helmy A, De Simoni M, Guilfoyle M, et al. Cytokines and innate inflammation in the pathogenesis of human traumatic brain injury. Prog Neurobiol 2011;95:352–72.

119. Zink B, Szmydynger-Chodobska J, Chodobski A. Emerging concepts in the pathophysiology of traumatic brain injury. Psyhiatr Clin North Am 2010;33:741–56.

120. Kelley B, Lifshitz J, Povlishock J. Neuroinflammatory responses after experimental diffuse traumatic brain injury. J Neuropathol Exp Neurol 2007;66:989–1001.

121. Castriotta R, Murthy J. Sleep disorders in patients with traumatic brain injury: a review. CNS Drugs 2011;25:175–85.

Differential Diagnosis of Hypersomnias

Imran Ahmed, MD[a,b,*], Shelby Harris, PsyD[a,b],
Michael Thorpy, MD[a,b]

KEYWORDS

- Hypersomnia • Narcolepsy • Idiopathic hypersomnia • Recurrent hypersomnia
- Kleine-Levin syndrome • Menstrual-related hypersomnia
- Behaviorally induced insufficient sleep syndrome

KEY POINTS

- Excessive sleepiness can occur with several disorders: self-inflicted as in insufficient sleep syndrome; secondary to sleep fragmentation as in obstructive sleep apnea; as a result of a central cause as in narcolepsy; as a result of a comorbid medical condition as in Parkinson disease; or as a result of medications.
- Overnight polysomnography with or without a multiple sleep latency test can be a useful adjunct to a thorough history in helping to arrive at the diagnosis.
- Treatment of these disorders usually requires stimulants; treatment of symptoms associated with these disorders, such as cataplexy, may require additional medications.
- OSA, on the other hand, is initially treated nonpharmaceutically (eg, continuous positive airway pressure or other device).

The term hypersomnia is used to identify disorders that are associated with excessive sleepiness, such as idiopathic hypersomnia or narcolepsy. Sleepiness is considered excessive when there is an increased amount of sleep or an increased drive toward sleep during the wake period, making a person unable to sustain wakefulness or alertness in situations in which it is required. Patients who have excessive sleepiness tend to have involuntary sleep episodes that occur during activities such as when relaxing in front of the television, when sitting quietly reading, at social events, or while having a conversation or driving. The hypersomnias share a common feature in that they either shorten or fragment the major sleep period, or are a manifestation of central nervous system (CNS) dysfunction. This article discusses disorders including the hypersomnias that should be considered when evaluating individuals with excessive sleepiness (**Box 1**).

BISS

The normal average sleep duration in adults is about 7.5 to 8.0 hours. Banks and Dinges estimate about 30% of the adult US population sleep less than 7 hours per night and this prevalence seems to be increasing.[1] Excessive sleepiness as a result of a shortened sleep time is characteristic of individuals with BISS, who have less than their biologically determined sleep requirement. This disorder is classified by the *International Classification of*

a Neurology, Montefiore Medical Center, Albert Einstein College of Medicine, 111 East 210th Street, Bronx, NY 10467, USA; b Neurology Department, Sleep-Wake Disorders Center, 111 East 210th Street, Bronx, NY 10467, USA
* Corresponding author. Neurology Department, Sleep-Wake Disorders Center, 111 East 210th Street, Bronx, NY 10467.
E-mail address: iahmed@montefiore.org

Sleep Med Clin 7 (2012) 191–204
doi:10.1016/j.jsmc.2012.03.009
1556-407X/12/$ – see front matter © 2012 Published by Elsevier Inc

Box 1
Differential diagnosis of excessive sleepiness

Sleep-related breathing disorders
Obstructive sleep apnea (OSA)

Hypersomnias of central origin
Behaviorally induced insufficient sleep syndrome (BISS)
Idiopathic hypersomnia with long sleep time
Idiopathic hypersomnia without long sleep time
Narcolepsy with cataplexy
Narcolepsy without cataplexy
Narcolepsy caused by a medical disorder
Recurrent hypersomnia, Kleine-Levin syndrome (KLS)
Recurrent hypersomnia, menstrual-related hypersomnia
Hypersomnia caused by a medical condition
Hypersomnia caused by a drug or substance

Other
Long sleeper

Hypersomnia caused by a medical condition
Brain tumors (especially when involving hypothalamus)
Depression
Dementia
Genetic disorders (eg, Niemann-Pick type C disease, myotonic dystrophy)
Hypothyroidism
Infections (eg, infectious mononucleosis, Lyme disease, human immunodeficiency virus [HIV])
Parkinson disease
Posttraumatic hypersomnia
Toxic/metabolic (eg, hepatic encephalopathy, pancreatic insufficiency)

Hypersomnia caused by a drug or substance
Alcohol
Antidepressants
Antiepileptics
Antihistamines
Antihypertensives
Antipsychotics
Anxiolytics
Dopaminergic medications
Hypnotics
Pain medications

Sleep Disorders, Second Edition (ICSD-2) under the category of hypersomnias of central origin. BISS occurs when patients deprive themselves of sleep because of some personal or societal commitments. These patients tend to oversleep on weekends or days off when their commitments are less important. The diagnosis requires evidence for the presence of sleepiness that is present almost daily for at least 3 months. Polysomnography, although not necessary for the diagnosis, shows a reduced sleep latency (<10 minutes) and a sleep efficiency of at least 90%.

The sleep latency on the multiple sleep latency test (MSLT) should be less than 8 minutes, and sleep-onset rapid eye movement (REM) periods (SOREMPs) may or may not be present (**Box 2**). Insufficient sleep has been associated with higher risks of obesity and metabolic disorders as well as impairments in executive functioning.[2–4]

Epidemiology

BISS equally affects both males and females and may likely be more prevalent in the adolescent population.

Treatment

Patients with BISS should adhere to proper sleep hygiene and avoidance of sleep deprivation. The associated symptoms of BISS improve with return of the patient's normal sleep duration.

LONG SLEEPER

Long sleeper is not actually considered a hypersomnia; however, it is presented here as it can cause sleepiness, similar to BISS, if the total night's sleep needs are not met. It is a normal variant; characterized in adults who consistently sleep 10 or more hours. The sleep pattern is usually present since childhood (where the sleep duration is 2 hours longer than age-appropriate norms). If the individual's nightly sleep needs are

---

met, there is no complaint regarding quality of sleep, daytime sleepiness, abnormal mood, or daytime functioning.[5]

SLEEP-RELATED BREATHING DISORDERS

Sleep-related breathing disorders such as OSA or upper airway resistance syndrome (UARS) have been associated with EDS. OSA involves repetitive episodes of cessation of breathing (apneas) or partial upper airway obstruction (hypopneas) that last a minimum of 10 seconds.[6–8] These events are often associated with reduced blood oxygen saturation, snoring, and sleep disruption. Five or more respiratory events (apneas or hypopneas) per hour of sleep are required for diagnosis. UARS has been included by the ICSD-2 under the heading of obstructive sleep apnea (OSA) disorders. It usually presents with EDS but does not meet the standard criteria (in terms of desaturations, apneas, or hypopneas) for OSA syndrome (OSAS). Frequent arousals are noted in UARS, which are attributed to increased respiratory effort (respiratory effort-related arousals), and are best seen using esophageal balloon manometry.

One popular hypothesis for the association between EDS and OSA is the observation that sleep fragmentation can occur with these disorders. In a study of patients with OSA (evaluated with polysomnograms and MSLTs and compared with normal healthy individuals with no sleep complaints), the total number of arousals correlated significantly with the severity of sleepiness.[9] Oksenberg and colleagues[10] found a direct correlation with sleep fragmentation and excessive sleepiness in sleepy patients with OSA when compared with nonsleepy patients with OSA; however, this direct correlation is contradicted by another study.[11] Accordingly, it is likely that other factors, in addition to sleep fragmentation, play a role in the pathophysiology of the sleepiness seen in OSA and UARS. It has been suggested that inflammation, intermittent hypoxia, and comorbid medical conditions contribute to the EDS seen in patients with OSA.

Certain cytokines that cause sleepiness have been noted to be increased in patients with OSA. Vgontzas and colleagues[12] found increased levels of interleukin 6 and tumor necrosis factor α in sleepy patients with OSA. In addition, these investigators reported that certain cytokine antagonists improve sleepiness in these patients.

Patients with OSA or UARS often have associated oxygen desaturations that occur during sleep. Mediano and colleagues[13] showed the association between intermittent hypoxemia during sleep and daytime sleepiness. A possible explanation for this relationship is the probable

---

> **Box 2**
> **Diagnostic criteria for BISS**
>
> 1. Three months or more of almost daily sleepiness manifesting as either excessive daytime sleepiness (EDS) or behavioral abnormalities (more common in prepubertal children), suggesting sleepiness
>
> 2. The major sleep period is less than what is expected from age-adjusted normative data
>
> 3. The major sleep period is longer than usual when the patient is allowed to sleep without environmental interruptions or internal obligations to awaken
>
> 4. Nocturnal polysomnogram is not required; however, if performed, shows a sleep latency of less than 10 minutes with a sleep efficiency of greater than 90%
>
> 5. An MSLT is not required; however, if performed, it shows a mean sleep latency of less than 8 minutes. The SOREMPs are variable in number
>
> Adapted from the ICSD II with permission from the American Academy of Sleep Medicine, Darien, Illinois, USA. 2012.

hypoxic injury to the neurons responsible for wakefulness.

Many medical or psychiatric disorders (eg, depression or Parkinson disease) have been associated with excessive sleepiness. When these disorders are comorbid with OSA, the sleepiness is often more prominent. These disorders are discussed later in this article.

Epidemiology

The prevalence of OSA is estimated to be about 4% in men and about 2% in women when it is defined by an apnea-hypopnea index of greater than 5 that is associated with EDS.[5]

Treatment

With the understanding that there may be multiple pathophysiologies of the EDS seen in patients with OSA, it is logical to presume that treatment requires a multifaceted approach. The standard treatment of OSA includes continuous positive airway pressure (CPAP) or bilevel positive airway pressure therapy, oral appliance use, and upper airway surgery (eg, uvulopalatopharyngoplasty). Recently, Provent therapy, a pressure-limiting device that is inserted in the nares, has also shown efficacy in selected patients.[14] However, often some degree of sleepiness persists even after optimal treatment of OSA. These treatment options improve sleepiness either by eliminating or minimizing sleep fragmentation as well as improving cerebral oxygenation; however, other pathophysiologic mechanisms may play a prominent role in the residual EDS. Accordingly, treatment should also include treatment of comorbidities, exercise, and a weight loss regime. Wake-promoting medications such as modafinil and armodafinil have shown efficacy in treatment of this residual EDS[15] and are currently the only medications approved by the US Food and Drug Administration (FDA) for the treatment of residual EDS in patients with OSA, provided that patients are on CPAP treatment of their OSA and are not sleep deprived.

Disorders such as narcolepsy (with or without cataplexy), idiopathic hypersomnia (with and without long sleep time), and recurrent hypersomnia are associated with excessive sleepiness as a result of a suspected CNS abnormality.[16–19] Accordingly, these disorders are identified as the hypersomnias of central origin by the ICSD-2.

NARCOLEPSY

The ICSD-2 identifies 3 different subtypes of narcolepsy: narcolepsy with cataplexy, narcolepsy without cataplexy, and narcolepsy caused by a medical disorder. Each of these narcolepsy subtypes shares the symptom of excessive sleepiness and can also manifest symptoms of sleep paralysis, hypnagogic hallucinations, automatic behaviors, and fragmented or disrupted nighttime sleep. Cataplexy is present in all patients with narcolepsy with cataplexy and can be present in patients with narcolepsy caused by a medical disorder.

Sleep paralysis usually occurs during sleep-wake transitions and is characterized by brief loss of voluntary muscle control with an inability to move or speak, but with retention of awareness during the event. Unlike cataplexy, these episodes are not provoked by intense emotion or stress; however, they are often associated with fearful hypnopompic or hypnagogic hallucinations. Sleep paralysis episodes usually last about 1 to 10 minutes, terminating spontaneously or when someone touches the patient.[20]

Hypnagogic and hypnopompic hallucinations are prominent dreamlike states that occur when falling asleep (hypnagogic), or when awaking from sleep (hypnopompic).[21] These hallucinations can be either visual or auditory, and less often tactile or vestibular. They can vary widely in complexity from simple forms and sounds, such as basic geometric figures or the ringing of a telephone, to more complex images and tones, such as people or musical compositions.

Certain activities such as driving, walking, cooking a meal, or even talking on the phone can be performed automatically without continuous higher executive functioning. These simple or complex routine tasks performed by individuals who remain unaware of the activity are termed automatic behaviors. Automatic behaviors commonly occur in individuals with excessive sleepiness, including narcolepsy.

Narcolepsy with cataplexy[21,22] (**Box 3**) requires the presence of EDS for at least 3 months in conjunction with a definite history of cataplexy. Cataplexy is a sudden onset of muscle atonia or hypotonia that is typically provoked by emotion. Episodes can include jaw sagging, head drooping, garbled speech, upper or lower extremity weakness, or blurred vision; however, the diaphragm, middle ear, and ocular muscles are unaffected.[23] Diagnosis is often confirmed by many experts by nocturnal polysomnography followed by an MSLT, but these tests are not absolutely necessary to confirm the diagnosis.[23] The nocturnal polysomnogram should be performed to exclude other sleep disorders, such as OSA, and to document at least 6 hours of sleep. The MSLT, which can not only confirm the diagnosis but is helpful

---

Box 3
Diagnostic criteria for narcolepsy with cataplexy

1. Three months or more of almost daily EDS

2. Cataplexy is present

3. Polysomnography followed by MSLT is not necessary, but is useful for confirmation of diagnosis.

   a. The polysomnography shows the absence of other causes of sleepiness (eg, OSA) and at least 6 hours of sleep.

   b. The MSLT should show a sleep latency of less than or equal to 8 minutes with 2 or more SOREMPs

4. CSF studies are not necessary but are useful for confirmation of diagnosis; they should show a CSF hypocretin-1 level of less than or equal to 110 pg/mL or one-third of mean normal control values

Adapted from the *ICSD II* with permission from the American Academy of Sleep Medicine, Darien, Illinois, USA. 2012.

Box 4
Diagnostic criteria for narcolepsy without cataplexy

1. Three months or more of almost daily EDS

2. Cataplexy is not present or only atypical cataplexylike episodes are present

3. Polysomnography followed by MSLT is required for diagnosis.

   a. The polysomnography shows the absence of other causes of sleepiness (eg, OSA) and at least 6 hours of sleep.

   b. The MSLT should show a sleep latency of less than or equal to 8 minutes with 2 or more SOREMPs

4. CSF studies for evaluation of hypocretin levels are not applicable in these patients

Adapted from the *ICSD II* with permission from the American Academy of Sleep Medicine, Darien, Illinois, USA. 2012.

---

to show severity of the sleepiness, should show a mean sleep latency of less than or equal to 8 minutes with 2 or more SOREMPS. Cerebrospinal fluid (CSF) hypocretin-1 measurements of less than 110 pg/mL or one-third of mean normal control values can also help in confirming the diagnosis but are limited in availability and are usually performed for research purposes.

Narcolepsy without cataplexy is diagnosed when there is daytime sleepiness and possibly other associated features of narcolepsy, including sleep paralysis, hypnagogic hallucinations, and automatic behaviors; however, cataplexy is not present (**Box 4**). Nocturnal polysomnography with a positive MSLT is required for the diagnosis; CSF hypocretin levels are not useful, because they can often be normal. Narcolepsy caused by a medical condition is the diagnosis applied to a patient with sleepiness who has a significant neurologic or medical disorder (eg, tumor, neurosarcoidosis, Niemann-Pick type C) that accounts for the daytime sleepiness or cataplexy.

Epidemiology

Narcolepsy can begin at any age from infancy (rarely) to as late as old age, but it most commonly occurs within the first 2 decades of life. It affects both men and women equally, with an approximate prevalence of 1 in 2000 people (0.05%) in the United States.[24] In addition, there is an approximately 1% to 2% risk of a first-degree relative

developing narcolepsy with cataplexy.[25] The prevalence of narcolepsy without cataplexy or narcolepsy caused by a medical condition in the general population is not known; however, it is estimated that about 10% to 50% of the narcolepsy population has narcolepsy without cataplexy.[5]

Pathophysiology

It is suspected that patients with the HLA marker DQB1*0602 (and likely other currently unknown genetic links) may possess a genetic susceptibility for some event or trigger that leads to the development of narcolepsy. These triggers may include environmental factors such as infections, head trauma, or even a change in sleeping habits, all of which have been associated with the onset of narcolepsy.[25–28]

The excessive sleepiness in narcolepsy with cataplexy is related to the loss of hypocretin-containing neurons located in the perifornical and lateral hypothalamus, whereas cases of narcolepsy without cataplexy may be caused by a partial loss of these neurons.[29–31] An autoimmune process may be responsible for the loss of the hypocretin neurons; however, specific antibodies to hypocretin and hypocretin receptors have not been found.[32–35] On the other hand, antistreptococcal antibodies in patients with recent onset of narcolepsy have been reported, suggesting that infection may be an inciting event that initiates an autoimmune process.[27,36] Additional support to the autoimmune hypothesis came in 2010, when increased Tribbles homologue 2 (Trib2)-specific antibody levels were identified in patients with narcolepsy. Trib2 is an autoantigen that has been found in hypocretin neurons of a transgenic mouse model. Preliminary studies found that titers of Trib2-specific antibodies were highest in patients soon after narcolepsy onset, decreased within the first 3 years of the disorder, and then stabilized at levels higher than that of the control groups.[37] More work is still needed to establish a causal pathogenic role of these antigens and antibodies. In 2009, low CSF histamine levels were identified in patients with narcolepsy,[38] and they may have a role in the pathophysiology of narcolepsy.

Narcolepsy caused by a medical condition is the diagnosis applied to patients with sleepiness who have a significant neurologic or medical disorder that accounts for the daytime sleepiness or cataplexy. Some of these disorders involve the hypothalamus, including tumors, neurosarcoidosis, infarcts, or multiple sclerosis (MS) with hypothalamic plaques. Multiple system atrophy, Parkinson disease, and head trauma are also known to be responsible for narcolepsy in some patients. In addition, certain genetic disorders, such as Niemann-Pick type C disease or Coffin-Lowry syndrome, have been shown to cause narcolepsy in children (especially those less than 5 years of age). If definite cataplexy cannot be documented clinically, then a polysomnogram followed by an MSLT must show the absence of other causes of sleepiness, and show a mean sleep latency of less than 8 minutes and 2 or more SOREMPs. Other REM sleep phenomena, such as sleep paralysis and hypnagogic hallucinations, may or may not be present.

Treatment

The treatment of the hypersomnias of central origin is typically symptom directed, because there is no known cure for any of these disorders. Rarely, narcolepsy in CNS inflammatory disorders has responded to antiinflammatory treatment.

Nonpharmacologic management with proper sleep hygiene and avoiding sleep deprivation is the cornerstone of management; it should be encouraged in all patients with excessive sleepiness. In narcolepsy, strategic scheduling of 2 or 3 brief naps during the day may help alleviate some of the EDS.

Pharmacologic management of EDS is mainly with wake-promoting medications such as stimulants (eg, amphetamines and methylphenidate) and other agents, such as modafinil, armodafinil, or sodium oxybate. Cataplexy is often managed with medications, such as tricyclic antidepressants (TCAs) or norepinephrine reuptake inhibitors, which have REM sleep-suppressant properties or increase aminergic (especially by blocking the

norepinephrine transporter) activity.[39] Sodium oxybate is highly efficacious for the treatment of cataplexy in narcolepsy and is currently the only FDA-approved medication for its management.

Sodium oxybate has also been shown to improve the fragmented sleep seen in patients with narcolepsy by increasing slow wave sleep, decreasing light sleep (stage N1 sleep), and decreasing the number of arousals. Several other sleep-promoting medications have also been used to manage the fragmented sleep seen in patients with narcolepsy with varying success.

IDIOPATHIC HYPERSOMNIA

Idiopathic hypersomnia is characterized by constant daytime sleepiness despite adequate amount of total nocturnal sleep; it may be associated either with a long major sleep period (idiopathic hypersomnia with long sleep time) or without a long major sleep period (idiopathic hypersomnia without long sleep time). Sleep drunkenness (sleep inertia after awakening) may also occur after sleep periods[40] but usually patients report awakening from sleep unrefreshed. In addition, these patients often have an irresistible urge to take prolonged naps (up to 3 to 4 hours in duration) during the day, which are also typically unrefreshing, Some associated clinical features are similar to narcolepsy, including hypnagogic hallucinations, sleep paralysis, and automatic behaviors; however, cataplexy is not present. Some patients may also experience autonomic abnormalities. In 1997, Bassetti and Aldrich[41] identified symptoms of orthostatic hypotension, headaches, syncope, and Raynaud-type phenomenon in patients with idiopathic hypersomnia.[5] There is also a higher incidence of anxiety, depression, and generalized fatigued in these patients.[42]

Idiopathic hypersomnia (**Boxes 5** and **6**) is diagnosed by overnight polysomnography and MSLT performed to rule out other sleep disorders, and to confirm the diagnosis. Polysomnography generally rules out other causes of excessive sleepiness and shows a decreased sleep-onset latency, with a normal or increased total sleep duration. The percentage of slow wave sleep can also be increased and the sleep efficiency is generally greater than 85%. The MSLT, by definition, reveals a mean sleep latency of less than 8 minutes with less than 2 SOREMPs. However, a mean sleep latency of greater than 8 minutes should not necessarily preclude this diagnosis.[42] In patients with idiopathic hypersomnia with long sleep time, a 24-hour continuous polysomnogram without any induced arousals may help in documenting

Box 5
Diagnostic criteria for idiopathic hypersomnia with long sleep time

1. Three months or more of almost daily EDS
2. Major sleep period of greater than 10 hours
3. Difficulty awaking from major sleep period or from naps
4. Polysomnogram shows a short sleep latency with a sleep period of more than 10 hours in the absence of other causes of daytime sleepiness
5. If an MSLT is performed after polysomnogram, it should show a mean sleep latency of less than 8 minutes with less than 2 SOREMPs

Adapted from the *ICSD II* with permission from the American Academy of Sleep Medicine, Darien, Illinois, USA. 2012.

a prolonged major sleep episode as well as any daytime sleep episodes.

The formal diagnostic criteria of idiopathic hypersomnia require that complaints of EDS be present for at least 3 months and that other causes of excessive sleepiness, such as sleep deprivation, medications or substances, sleep-disordered breathing, periodic leg movement disorder, narcolepsy, and any underlying psychiatric or medical disorders, be ruled out. In idiopathic hypersomnia without long sleep time, there is a history of a nocturnal sleep period for more than 6 hours but less than 10 hours. In contrast, idiopathic hypersomnia with long sleep time has a prolonged sleep time of more than 10 hours, with a history of difficulty in awakening in the morning or from naps.

Box 6
Diagnostic criteria for idiopathic hypersomnia without long sleep time

1. Three months or more of almost daily EDS
2. Major sleep period of greater than 6 hours but less than 10 hours
3. Polysomnogram shows a normal sleep period of more than 6 hours, but less than 10 hours in the absence of other causes of daytime sleepiness
4. An MSLT should be performed after polysomnogram and show a mean sleep latency of less than 8 minutes with less than 2 SOREMPs

Adapted from the *ICSD II* with permission from the American Academy of Sleep Medicine, Darien, Illinois, USA. 2012.

Epidemiology

The prevalence of idiopathic hypersomnia was estimated to be about 0.005% of the population,[43] with an age of onset usually between the second and fourth decades of life. There is no sex predilection; however, a genetic predisposition is suggested, with a possible autosomal-dominant pattern of inheritance.[44,45] Although narcolepsy is associated with specific HLA haplotypes, recent studies have not found any association between idiopathic hypersomnia and specific HLA markers.[44,45]

Pathophysiology

The pathophysiology of idiopathic hypersomnia is not well understood, and thus far no animal models are available to explain the neurochemical basis of this condition. As in narcolepsy, CSF histamine levels are diminished, implicating a possible common pathway between the pathophysiology of these 2 disorders.[38]

Treatment

As in narcolepsy, there is no known cure for idiopathic hypersomnia; however, spontaneous recovery has been reported in some patients.[5,46] Wake-promoting medications, similar to narcolepsy, are used to treat the excessive sleepiness seen in these patients. Sodium oxybate has not been FDA approved for the treatment of excessive sleepiness in idiopathic hypersomnia nor has it been shown to be efficacious in these patients.

RECURRENT HYPERSOMNIAS

The recurrent hypersomnias consist of 2 disorders: KLS and menstrual-related hypersomnia. Both disorders result in recurrent episodes of EDS. The better characterized of the 2 is KLS. This disorder is distinguished by the presence of recurring episodes of excessive sleepiness with associated cognitive (impaired memory, attention, and concentration, as well as apathy and hallucinations) and behavioral (hyperphagia, hypersexuality, aggressiveness, delusions, and irritability) abnormalities that last up to several weeks at a time and recur at least once during the year (**Box 7**). The symptoms are typically triggered by an event such as a flu-like illness or other infection, sleep deprivation, alcohol consumption, anesthesia exposure, or head trauma. The excessive sleepiness is typically prevalent during the early part of an episode, whereas cognitive abnormalities and apathy are more prevalent toward the end of episodes. In between symptomatic periods, the patient has normal sleep, cognition, and behaviors. In most cases, KLS is self-limited and resolves after about 30 years of age.

The symptoms initially begin with a few hours of fatigue and headache and subsequently progress to periods involving excessive amounts of sleep lasting between 14 and 21 hours. These prolonged sleep periods can occur during either the night or the day, with no clear circadian pattern. Between sleep periods, patients typically experience behavioral and cognitive abnormalities. As these symptoms wane, the patient develops insomnia, which can last from 1 to several days.

Aside from the memory, attention, and concentration disturbances, other cognitive abnormalities experienced by patients with KLS include confusion, hallucinations, and feelings of unreality or apathy. Feelings of apathy often predominate over the other cognitive impairments. Patients occasionally indicate that they do not necessarily have difficulty performing tasks, but rather do not have any interest in performing them. With the feeling of unreality, patients often report that they do not know whether what they are experiencing is part of a dream or an actuality. In a series of 108 patients, Arnulf and colleagues[47] identified that this derealization occurred in every patient.

There are multiple behavioral abnormalities seen in patients with KLS; however, unlike the excessive sleepiness and cognitive abnormalities, the behavioral abnormalities are not present in all patients. Hypersexuality is more common in male patients and manifests as frequent masturbation and inappropriate sexual behaviors. Hyperphagia or binge eating on awakening from the long sleep periods is typically present in more than half the patients.[47] Irritability and aggressiveness can occur in some patients when they are aroused from the middle of their sleep episode. Other symptoms, including a depressed mood, anxiety, regressed behaviors, headache, photophobia, and phonophobia, can also be present to varying degrees.

Epidemiology

KLS is a rare disorder that has an age of onset that ranges from 9 years to older than 35 years, with a male/female ratio of about 4:1; it more commonly occurs during the teenage years. It also seems to be more prominent among people of Ashkenazi Jewish descent. However, the exact prevalence of KLS remains unknown.

Pathophysiology

The cause of KLS is unknown. Investigations to determine the pathophysiology of KLS have yielded inconsistent findings. Single-photon emission computed tomography studies have shown hypoperfusion of the thalamus, hypothalamus, temporal, or frontal areas in some patients.[48] In a European study, Dauvilliers and colleagues[49] suggested an association with the HLA genotypes DRB1*0301-DQB1*0201, and DRB1*0701-DQB1*0202; however, a larger American study did not confirm these findings.[47]

Menstrual-related hypersomnia is also classified as a recurrent hypersomnia. It is typified by cyclic episodes of excessive sleepiness that is by definition associated with the menstrual cycle. In contrast to KLS, it is not so well defined and studied; however, the sleepiness usually begins a few days before menses and lasts for about a week.[23] Some patients have been reported to sleep continuously for days, with minimal awakenings for micturition and eating. Behavioral changes, including irritability and aggressiveness, have been described to occur before the onset of the sleepiness in some patients.[23,50] The duration of this disorder is unknown.

Epidemiology

Menstrual-related hypersomnia is believed to be considerably less frequent than KLS; however, similar to KLS, the true prevalence is unknown. The disorder seems to affect mostly adolescents, although older patients have been identified.[50,51]

Pathophysiology

The pathophysiology of menstrual-related hypersomnia is unknown. However, it is believed that the excessive sleepiness seen in this condition is associated with ovulatory rather than anovulatory cycles.[50–52]

Treatment

Nonpharmacologic management with proper sleep hygiene is once again suggested. In addition, monitoring and regulating eating and drinking behaviors during symptomatic episodes of KLS is prudent. Pharmacologic management with wake-promoting medications, such as modafinil and armodafinil, have limited benefit in patients with KLS;

however, amphetamines and methylphenidate may be helpful. Amantadine, when taken at the onset of an attack, has been noted to abort the symptomatic period in KLS,[50,53] and the behavioral and cognitive abnormalities can respond to risperidone, benzodiazepines, or lithium.[50,53] For menstrual-related hypersomnia, use of oral contraceptives has been shown to result in remission in some patients.

HYPERSOMNIA CAUSED BY MEDICATIONS AND DRUGS

Many medications exist that can lead to hypersomnia, either when they are being used or when the user is in withdrawal. A thorough evaluation of the medications (both prescribed and over-the-counter) that a patient has used can help the clinician quickly spot a potential culprit for symptoms of hypersomnia. **Box 8** lists the ICSD-2 definition of hypersomnia due to drug or substance.

Hypnotics

Drugs that may be used to treat insomnia include benzodiazepine receptor agonists (BZRAs), melatonin receptor agonists, and histamine H_1 antagonists.

Box 8
Diagnostic criteria for hypersomnias due to drug or substance

Hypersomnia due to drug or substance (abuse; ICSD-2 definition)

a. The patient has a complaint of sleepiness or excessive sleep.

b. The complaint is believed to be secondary to current use, recent discontinuation, or previous prolonged use of drugs.

c. The hypersomnia is not better explained by another sleep disorder, medical or neurologic disorder, mental disorder, or medication use.

Hypersomnia due to drug or substance (medications; ICSD-2 definition)

a. The patient has a complaint of sleepiness or excessive sleep.

b. The complaint is associated with current use, recent discontinuation, or previous prolonged use of a prescribed medication

c. The hypersomnia is not better explained by another sleep disorder, medical or neurologic disorder, mental disorder, or substance use disorder.

Adapted from the *ICSD II* with permission from the American Academy of Sleep Medicine, Darien, Illinois, USA. 2012.

The sedating properties of these medications is helpful for the treatment of insomnia, but residual sedation during the morning and daytime hours can be seen with the use of some of these drugs. The severity of daytime sleepiness depends on the pharmacokinetic properties of the medication: BZRAs with long half-lives or BZRAs used in high doses result in more residual sleepiness. Although BZRAs with short half-lives do not affect daytime performance, zopiclone has shown daytime impairments upwards of 11 hours later,[54] and zolpidem has been shown to impair driving abilities when given 4 to 5 hours before driving.[55]

Antidepressants

TCAs (amitryptyline, doxepine, trazodone, mirtazapine, and trimipramine) seem to be the most sedating of the antidepressants prescribed. Sedation is a frequently reported side effect of TCAs, so they are commonly prescribed off-label in low doses as a treatment of insomnia. Although selective serotonin reuptake inhibitors and selective norpinephrine reuptake inhibitors are most often seen to produce insomnia as a side effect, some have reported sedation, sleep disruption, and REM sleep suppression.[56]

Anxiolytics

Medications commonly prescribed to treat anxiety include BZRAs, buspirone, and antidepressants. Antiepileptic drugs, β-antagonists, and atypical antipsychotics are also occasionally used. Although the pharmacologic profiles of anxiolytic benzodiazepines are similar to those used for insomnia, the half-lives of these medications are typically long, and when used during the daytime often lead to daytime sedation more frequently than with hypnotics. The risk of daytime sedation may lessen with repeated use and increased tolerance.[57,58]

Antipsychotics

Although no controlled studies exist that evaluate daytime sleepiness related to antipsychotics, medications with a strong antagonism of serotonin (5-HT$_2$), α_1, or H_1 receptors seem to be the most sedating. In the older class of antipsychotics (often labeled typical), thioridazine and chlorpromazine are seen to increase sleepiness more than haloperidol. In the newer atypical class, clozapine is believed to be most sedating, with olanzapine and quetiapine often being used off-label as hypnotics in patients with insomnia.

Antihistamines

Classic antihistamines have been divided into 2 groups (first-generation and second-generation) based on sedation. First-generation H_1 antihistamines include chlorpheniramine, diphenhydramine, cyprophetadine, doxylamine, hydroxyzine, meclizine, and promethazine. These H_1 antagonist medications cross the blood-brain barrier and affect 5-HT transmission. Most over-the-counter drugs marketed as hypnotics or analgesic-hypnotics contain diphenhydramine, with some using doxylamine. When used acutely, these medications have been shown to increase sedation. However, tolerance to these effects has been noticed after 4 days of consistent use.[59]

Compared with the first-generation antihistamines, the second-generation group (fexofenadine, desloratadine, cetirizine, levocetirizine, loratadine) are more selective on the H_1 receptor and do not penetrate the CNS so strongly. As a result, they generally do not cause sedation (with the exception of cetirizine).

Antiepileptics

Daytime sleepiness is common in this class of medications because they typically exert particular effects on γ-aminobutyric acid. The older antiepileptics seem to be more sedating than the newer ones, with phenobarbital, carbamazepine, and phenytoin seeming to create the most daytime sleepiness. Because of their complex mechanisms of action, the newer class of antiepileptic drugs are often used to treat disorders other than epilepsy, including bipolar disorder, restless legs syndrome, migraine, fibromyalgia, neuropathic pain, schizophrenia, anxiety, and insomnia. Fifteen percent to 25% of patients using gabapentin and pregabalin report symptoms of sedation,[60,61] with tiagabine and topiramate creating less overall sleepiness than others in the class.

Antihypertensive Drugs

This class of medication has both insomnia and sedation reported as side effects. Sedation is highly common in α_2 agonists, including clonidine and methyldopa, with tolerance often increasing over time. Carvedilol and labetolol (β-antagonists with vasodilating properties) and prazosin and terazosin (α_1 antagonists) have all been linked to sedation and fatigue.

Dopamine Agonists

Although daytime sleepiness is a common complaint in patients with Parkinson disease, sleepiness is likely a result of a combination of issues, including disease progression, comorbid sleep, and medical issues as well as medications. Levodopa/carbidopa and dopamine agonists are the most common treatments for Parkinson disease. Ergot agonists (pergolide, apomorphine) and nonergot agonists (pramipexole, ropinirole, rotigotine) seem to both be associated with daytime sleepiness and sleep attacks.[62,63]

Pain Medications

Hypersomnia is a common side effect of opioid medications, with the degree of sleepiness varying based on dosage, age, severity of underlying disease, and length of usage.[64] Central sleep apnea is commonly observed in patients with chronic opioid use, further increasing sleepiness. Used primarily in the treatment of acute migraine, triptans (especially eletriptan, rizatriptan, and zolmitriptan) are also linked to sedation. Most skeletal muscle relaxants lead to sedation as a result of their effects on the CNS, although the severity depends on the range of half-lives. No formal studies exist that research the effect of skeletal muscle relaxants on daytime alertness.

Alcohol

Alcohol presents with sedative or stimulant effects, depending on the quantity and time ingested. Alcohol is stimulating in low doses, but is sedating at high doses and after peak plasma concentration.[65] Alcohol is commonly used as a sleep aid, with lower doses creating faster sleep latencies. However, in the last two-thirds of the night, sleep becomes disrupted as a result of alcohol withdrawal. This disrupted, lighter sleep for the remainder of the night can lead to daytime sleepiness the next day. Hypersomnia is more pronounced when alcohol consumption is coupled with sleep deprivation or sleep restriction.

HYPERSOMNIA CAUSED BY MEDICAL CONDITION
Hypersomnia Secondary to Metabolic or Endocrine Disorders

Hypersomnia has been observed in patients with hepatic encephalopathy, hypothyroidism, hyperprolactinemia, Cushing syndrome, menopause, acromegaly, and diabetes (**Box 9**). Although sleep-related breathing disorders and periodic leg movement disorders are often seen in endocrine disorders, hypersomnia has occasionally been reported in endocrine disorders when another comorbid sleep disorder is not present. Changes in sleep architecture are often seen in these patients, with OSAS often being the primary culprit for daytime sleepiness. In all patients with endocrine disorders (or patients receiving hormone replacement therapy), the clinician should thoroughly evaluate for the presence of any sleep-related breathing disorders.

Patients with hypothyroidism are often seen with comorbid OSAS, although most patients with OSAS do not have hypothyroidism. These patients tend to report hypersomnia, attention/concentration problems, fatigue, snoring, and decreased sex drive. Sleepiness in obesity has gained significant attention because high rates of sleep-disordered breathing are commonly seen in overweight and obese individuals. Recently, however, daytime sleepiness has been observed in obese individuals without another primary sleep disorder. Sleepiness in this population can also be related to metabolic factors and depression in addition to sleep-disordered breathing.[66]

Hypersomnia Secondary to Infectious Disorders

Although limited research exists that examines the effect of infectious diseases on the CNS and sleep, some limited reports of hypersomnia secondary to infectious disease have been documented.[67,68]

HIV, Whipple disease, infectious mononucleosis, Guillain-Barré syndrome, Lyme disease, and neurocysticercosis (a parasitic infection of the CNS that develops by ingesting the eggs of a waterborne tapeworm and foods contaminated with feces) have all been associated with daytime sleepiness as a result of the infection itself or the medications used to treat them. Both viral and bacterial meningitis have been found to create disordered nocturnal sleep and associated daytime sleepiness as a result of cerebral edema or hydrocephalus. In many instances, hypersomnia may develop months after the initial infection. The effect of the Gambian form of human African trypanosomiasis on sleep architecture has been studied. In the meningoencephalitic phase of the virus, autoantibodies against nervous structures damage both sleep and wakefulness, creating circadian dysregulation and SOREMPs.[68] A careful history of patients presenting with daytime sleepiness and infectious disease aids in the determination of a proper differential diagnosis.

Hypersomnia Associated with Neurologic Causes

Intrinsic hypersomnia has been noted in patients with neurodegenerative disorders such as Parkinson disease or Alzheimer disease. Occasionally, daytime sleepiness may be caused by other factors such as medications, sleep-disordered breathing, and periodic leg movements.

Chronic sleepiness and insomnia have been reported in patients with acute stroke. Subthalamic, pontine, mesencephalic, and thalamic lesions are believed to disrupt the ascending reticular activating system, leading to symptoms of hypersomnia. Hemispheric strokes are associated with daytime sleepiness because of their ability to reduce total sleep time and sleep efficiency.[68] Hypothalamic strokes can lead to hypersomnia by disrupting the hypocretin-producing neurons. As a result, numerous strokes often have symptoms that appear to be narcolepsy.[69,70] In addition to intrinsic hypersomnia that is seen in stroke, studies have reported that upwards of two-thirds of these patients suffer from comorbid sleep-disordered breathing, another common cause for daytime sleepiness.[69,71]

Brain tumors, especially those affecting the thalamus, hypothalamus, and brainstem, have been linked to sleepiness. Craniopharyngioma, a benign tumor that develops near the pituitary gland, has been extensively studied for its symptoms of hypersomnia.[72,73] Other tumors that have been linked to hypersomnia include pilocytic astrocytoma, adenomas in the pituitary gland, hemispheric tumors, brainstem gliomas, subependymoma, and hemispheric tumors.

Hypersomnia has been reported in some patients with MS, particularly in those with lesions in the brainstem, ganglia, and thalamus. Hypersomnia in MS can also be related to several symptoms that are seen in nearly half of patients, including insomnia, fatigue, depression, periodic limb movements, and pain. Interferon, a common medication used to manage MS, has been seen to lead to disrupted nocturnal sleep and associated daytime sleepiness.

Conflicting data exist linking epilepsy to hypersomnia, with some reporting daytime sleepiness in nearly 25% of patients studied.[74,75] Many factors seem to influence the severity of hypersomnia in this population, with uncontrolled epilepsy and nocturnal frontal lobe epilepsy having the most impact. Other sleep-disrupting disorders such as insomnia, depression, and sleep-disordered breathing are all commonly seen in this population. As noted earlier, many antiepileptic medications can also lead to hypersomnia.

Several genetic disorders have been linked to hypersomnia. Arnold-Chiari malformations, Norrie disease, Niemann-Pick type C, myotonic dystrophy, and Prader-Willi syndrome have all been associated with hypersomnia, although in many instances, sleep-disordered breathing may be the main culprit.

SUMMARY

When evaluating a patient for excessive sleepiness, one should consider the various causes. Excessive sleepiness can occur with several disorders. It can be self-inflicted as in insufficient sleep syndrome; it can be secondary to sleep fragmentation as in OSA; it can have a central cause as in narcolepsy; it can be caused by a comorbid medical condition as in Parkinson's disease; or it can be caused by medications. Overnight polysomnography with or without an MSLT can be a useful adjunct to a thorough history in helping to arrive at the diagnosis. The treatment of these disorders usually requires stimulants or other wake-promoting agents; however, other symptoms associated with these disorders, such as cataplexy, may require additional medications. On the other hand, OSA is initially treated nonpharmaceutically (eg, CPAP or other device).

REFERENCES

1. Banks S, Dinges DF. Behavioral and physiological consequences of sleep restriction in humans. J Clin Sleep Med 2007;3:519–28.

2. Knutson KL, Spiegel K, Penev P, et al. The metabolic consequences of sleep deprivation. Sleep Med Rev 2007;11:163–78.

3. Brondel L, Romer MA, Nougues PM, et al. Acute partial sleep deprivation increases food intake in healthy men. Am J Clin Nutr 2010;91(6):1550–9.

4. Tucker AM, Whitney P, Belenky G, et al. Effects of sleep deprivation on dissociated components of executive functioning. Int J Neurosci 2010;120(5):328–34.

5. American Academy of Sleep Medicine. International classification of sleep disorders. In: Sateia MJ, editor. Diagnostic and coding manual. 2nd edition. Westchester (IL): American Academy of Sleep Medicine; 2005. p. 79–115, 198–200.

6. McNicholas WT, Ryan S. Obstructive sleep apnoea syndrome: translating science to clinical practice. Respirology 2006;11(2):136–44.

7. White DP. Sleep apnea. Proc Am Thorac Soc 2006; 3(1):124–8.

8. Ancoli-Israel S, Ayalon L. Diagnosis and treatment of sleep disorders in older adults. Am J Geriatr Psychiatry 2006;14(2):95–103.

9. Stepanski E, Lamphere J, Badia P, et al. Sleep fragmentation and daytime sleepiness. Sleep 1984;7(1): 18–26.

10. Oksenberg A, Arons E, Nasser K, et al. Severe obstructive sleep apnea: sleepy versus nonsleepy patients. Laryngoscope 2010;120(3):643–8.

11. Black JE, Hirshkowitz M. Modafinil for treatment of residual excessive sleepiness in nasal continuous positive airway pressure-treated obstructive sleep apnea/hypopnea syndrome. Sleep 2005;28:464–71.

12. Vgontzas AN, Zoumakis E, Bixler EO, et al. Adverse effects of modest sleep restriction on sleepiness, performance, and inflammatory cytokines. Clin Endocrinol Metab 2004;89:2119–26.

13. Mediano O, Barcelo A, de la Pena M, et al. Daytime sleepiness and polysomnographic variables in sleep apnoea patients. Eur Respir J 2007;30:110–3.

14. Berry RB, Kryger MH, Massie CA. A novel nasal expiratory positive airway pressure (EPAP) device for the treatment of obstructive sleep apnea: a randomized controlled trial. Sleep 2011;34(4):479–85.

15. Schwartz JR, Khan A, McCall WV, et al. Tolerability and efficacy of armodafinil in naïve patients with excessive sleepiness associated with obstructive sleep apnea, shift work disorder, or narcolepsy: a 12-month, open-label, flexible-dose study with an extension period. J Clin Sleep Med 2010;6(5):450–7.

16. Frenette E, Kushida CA. Primary hypersomnias of central origin. Semin Neurol 2009;29(4):354–67.

17. Bove A, Culebras A, Moore JT, et al. Relationship between sleep spindles and hypersomnia. Sleep 1994;17(5):449–55.

18. Sforza E, Gaudreau H, Petit D, et al. Homeostatic sleep regulation in patients with idiopathic hypersomnia. Clin Neurophysiol 2000;111(2):277–82.

19. Nishino S, Kanbayashi T. Symptomatic narcolepsy, cataplexy and hypersomnia, and their implications in the hypothalamic hypocretin/orexin system. Sleep Med Rev 2005;9(4):269–310.

20. Guilleminault C, Fromherz S. Narcolepsy: diagnosis and management. In: Kryger MH, Roth TA, Dement WC, editors. Principles and practice of sleep medicine. Philadelphia: WB Saunders; 2005. p. 780.

21. Dyken ME, Yamada T. Narcolepsy and disorders of excessive somnolence. Prim Care 2005;32(2):389–413.

22. Overeem S, Mignot E, van Dijk JG, et al. Narcolepsy: clinical features, new pathophysiologic insights, and future perspectives. J Clin Neurophysiol 2001;18(2):78–105.

23. Billiard M, Guilleminault C, Dement WC. A menstruation-linked periodic hypersomnia. Kleine-Levin syndrome or new clinical entity? Neurology 1975;25:436–43.

24. Ohayon MM, Ferini-Strambi L, Plazzi G, et al. Frequency of narcolepsy symptoms and other sleep disorders in narcoleptic patients and their first-degree relatives. J Sleep Res 2005;14(4):437–45.

25. Mignot E. Genetic and familial aspects of narcolepsy. Neurology 1998;50(2 Suppl 1):S16–22.

26. Aran A, Lin L, Nevsimalova S, et al. Elevated anti-streptococcal antibodies in patients with recent narcolepsy onset. Sleep 2009;32(8):979–83.

27. Picchioni D, Hope CR, Harsh JR. A case-control study of the environmental risk factors for narcolepsy. Neuroepidemiology 2007;29(3–4):185–92.

28. Castriotta RJ, Wilde MC, Lai JM, et al. Prevalence and consequences of sleep disorders in traumatic brain injury. J Clin Sleep Med 2007;3(4):349–56.

29. Thannickal TC, Moore RY, Niehus R, et al. Reduced number of hypocretin neurons in human narcolepsy. Neuron 2000;27:469–74.

30. Mignot E, Lammers GJ, Ripley B, et al. The role of cerebrospinal fluid hypocretin measurement in the diagnosis of narcolepsy and other hypersomnias. Arch Neurol 2002;59:1553–62.

31. Thannickal TC, Nienhuis R, Siegel JM. Localized loss of hypocretin (orexin) cells in narcolepsy without cataplexy. Sleep 2009;32(8):993–8.

32. Scammell TE. The frustrating and mostly fruitless search for an autoimmune cause of narcolepsy. Sleep 2006;29(5):601–2.

33. Black JL 3rd. Narcolepsy: a review of evidence for autoimmune diathesis. Int Rev Psychiatry 2005;17(6):461–9.

34. Dauvilliers Y, Tafti M. Molecular genetics and treatment of narcolepsy. Ann Med 2006;38(4):252–62.

35. Tanaka S, Honda Y, Inoue Y, et al. Detection of autoantibodies against hypocretin, hcrtrl, and hcrtr2 in narcolepsy: anti-Hcrt system antibody in narcolepsy. Sleep 2006;29(5):633–8.

36. Longstreth WT Jr, Ton TG, Koepsell TD. Narcolepsy and streptococcal infections. Sleep 2009;32(12):1548.

37. Cvetkovic V, Bayer L, Dorsaz S, et al. Tribbles homolog 2 as an autoantigen in human narcolepsy. J Clin Invest 2010;120:713–9.

38. Kanbayashi T, Kodama T, Kondo H, et al. CSF histamine contents in narcolepsy, idiopathic hypersomnia and obstructive sleep apnea syndrome. Sleep 2009;32(2):181–7.

39. Guilleminault C, Raynal D, Takahashi S, et al. Evaluation of short-term and long-term treatment of narcolepsy syndrome with clomipramine hydrochloride. Acta Neurol Scand 1976;54:71–87.

40. Roth B, Nevsimalova S, Rechtschaffen A. Hypersomnia with sleep "drunkenness". Arch Gen Psychiatry 1972;26:456–62.

41. Bassetti C, Aldrich MS. Idiopathic hypersomnia: a series of 42 patients. Brain 1997;120(8):1423–35.

42. Vernet C, Arnulf I. Idiopathic hypersomnia with and without long sleep time: a controlled series of 75 patients. Sleep 2009;32(6):753–9.

43. Billard M, Dauvilliers Y. Idiopathic hypersomnia. Sleep Med Rev 2001;5:349–58.

44. Roth B. Narcolepsy and hypersomnia. Basel (Switzerland): Karger; 1980.

45. Billiard M, Merle C, Carlander B, et al. Idiopathic hypersomnia. Psychiatry Clin Neurosci 1998;52:125–9.

46. Anderson KN, Pilsworth S, Sharples LD, et al. Idiopathic hypersomnia: a study of 77 cases. Sleep 2007;30:1274–81.

47. Arnulf I, Lin L, Gadoth N, et al. Kleine-Levin syndrome: a systematic study of 108 patients. Ann Neurol 2008;63:482–93.

48. Huang YS, Guilleminault C, Kao PF, et al. SPECT findings in the Kleine-Levin syndrome. Sleep 2005;28:955–60.

49. Dauvilliers Y, Mayer G, Lecendreux M, et al. Kleine-Levin syndrome: an autoimmune hypothesis based on clinical and genetic analysis. Neurology 2002;59:1739–45.

50. Sachs C, Persson HE, Hagenfeldt K. Menstruation-related periodic hypersomnia: a case study with successful treatment. Neurology 1982;32:1376–9.

51. Andreica B, Rauca I, Lazar C, et al. Recurrent hypersomnia–diagnostic difficulties. Eur Psychiatry 2008;23:S358.

52. Bamford CR. Menstrual-associated sleep disorder: an unusual hypersomniac variant associated with both menstruation and amenorrhea with a possible link to prolactin and metoclopramide. Sleep 1993;16:484–6.

53. Arnulf I, Zeitzer JM, File J, et al. Kleine-Levin syndrome: a systematic review of 186 cases in the literature. Brain 2005;128:2763–76.

54. Vermeeren A, Danjou PE, O'Hanlon JF. Residual effects of evening and middle of-the-night administration of zaleplon 10 and 20 mg on memory and actual driving performance. Hum Psychopharmacol 1998;13(Suppl 2):S98–107.

55. Zammig G, Corser B, Dohramji K, et al. Sleep and residual sedation after administration of zaleplon, zolpidem, and placebo during experimental middle-of-the-night awakening. J Clin Sleep Med 2006;2: 417–23.

56. DeMartinis NA, Winokur A. Effects of psychiatric medications on sleep and sleep disorders. CNS Neurol Disord Drug Targets 2007;6:17–29.

57. Neutel CI. Risk of traffic accident injury after a prescription for a benzodiazepine. Ann Epidemiol 1995;5:239–44.

58. Neutel CI. Benzodiazepine-related traffic accidents in young and elderly drivers. Hum Psychopharmacol 1998;13(Suppl 2):S115–23.

59. Verster JC, Volkerts ER. Antihistamines and driving ability: evidence from on-the-road driving studies during normal traffic. Ann Allergy Asthma Immunol 2004;92:294–303.

60. Guay DR. Pregabalin in neuropathic pain: a more "pharmaceutically elegant" gabapentin? Am J Geriatr Pharmacother 2005;3:274–87.

61. Arnold LM, Goldenberg DL, Stanford SB, et al. Gabapentin in the treatment of fibromyalgia: a randomized, double-blind, placebo-controlled multicenter trial. Arthritis Rheum 2007;56:1336–44.

62. Happe S, Berger K. The association of dopamine agonists with daytime sleepiness, sleep problems and quality of life in patients with Parkinson's disease–a prospective study. J Neurol 2001;248: 1062–7.

63. Etminan M, Samii A, Takkouche B, et al. Increased risk of somnolence with the new dopamine agonists in patients with Parkinson's disease: a meta-analysis of randomized controlled trials. Drug Saf 2001;24:863–8.

64. Nokolaus T, Zeyfang A. Pharmacological treatments for persistent non-malignant pain in older persons. Drugs Aging 2004;21:19–41.

65. Roehrs T, Roth T. Sleep, sleepiness, sleep disorders and alcohol use and abuse. Sleep Med Rev 2001;5: 287–97.

66. Bixler EO, Vgontzas AN, Lin HM, et al. Excessive daytime sleepiness in a general population sample: the role of sleep apnea, age, obesity, diabetes and depression. J Clin Endocrinol Metab 2005;90:4510–5.

67. Guilleminault C, Mondini S. Mononucleosis and chronic daytime sleepiness. A long-term follow-up study. Arch Intern Med 1986;146:1333–5.

68. Buguet A, Bourdon L, Bouteille B, et al. The duality of sleeping sickness: focusing on sleep. Sleep Med Rev 2001;5:139–53.

69. Guilleminault C, Quera-Salva MA, Goldberg MP. Pseudo-hypersomnia and pre-sleep behaviour with bilateral paramedian thalamic lesions. Brain 1993; 116:1549–63.

70. Autret A, Lucas B, Mondon K, et al. Sleep and brain lesions: a critical review of the literature and additional new cases. Neurophysiol Clin 2001;31:356–75.

71. Gibbs JW, Ciafaloni E, Radtke RA. Excessive daytime somnolence and increased rapid eye movement pressure in myotonic dystrophy. Sleep 2002;25:672–5.

72. Muller HL, Muller-Stover S, Gebhardt U, et al. Secondary narcolepsy may be a causative factor of increased daytime sleepiness in obese childhood craniopharyngioma patients. J Pediatr Endocrinol Metab 2006;19(Suppl 1):423–9.

73. Muller HL, Handwerker G, Gebhardt U, et al. Melatonin treatment in obese patients with childhood craniopharyngioma and increased daytime sleepiness. Cancer Causes Control 2006;17:583–9.

74. Malow BA, Bowes RJ, Lin X. Predictors of sleepiness in epilepsy patients. Sleep 1997;20:1105–10.

75. Piperidou C, Karlovasitou A, Triantafyllou N, et al. Influence of sleep disturbance on quality of life of patients with epilepsy. Seizure 2008;17:588–94.

Physical Examination of the Patient with Hypersomnia

Douglas B. Kirsch, MD[a,b,*], Maryann C. Deak, MD[a,b]

KEYWORDS

- Physical Examination • Hypersomnia • Obstructive sleep apnea • Narcolepsy • Sleepiness

KEY POINTS

- Hypersomnia is a common symptom of many medical disorders, including several sleep disorders.
- Although patients with hypersomnia may not always have examination abnormalities, certain sleep disorders have specific physical findings that an experienced clinician should be comfortable evaluating.
- In combination with an appropriate clinical-history taking, a sleep-specific physical examination will lead to more appropriate diagnostic testing and patient management.

As medical technology has evolved, many fields of medicine have placed less reliance on physical examination skills to aid in diagnosis. In this regard, some sleep medicine specialists pay little attention to physical examination findings, anecdotally claiming, "The examination won't change my testing or treatment recommendations." However, in some sleep patients, careful physical assessment may result in alteration of physician advice. This article reviews the physical examination findings linked with sleep disorders causing hypersomnia, aiding physicians in their ability to effectively manage their patients.

DEFINITION AND CAUSES OF HYPERSOMNIA

Hypersomnia, also commonly referred to as excessive daytime sleepiness (EDS), is defined as "the inability to stay awake and alert during the major waking episodes of the day, resulting in unintended lapses into drowsiness or sleep."[1] This symptom is commonly observed in the United States; polls performed by the National Sleep Foundation (NSF) have suggested that more than 30% of the surveyed population has daytime sleepiness that interferes with their quality of life.[2] Moreover, hypersomnia may have significant consequences, particularly when combined with operation of a motor vehicle. Unfortunately, drowsy driving is a common occurrence; 52% of polled subjects had driven while drowsy in a recent NSF poll.[3] Not all patients will use the words "daytime sleepiness" to describe their symptoms; some will use other terminology, such as "drowsiness," "tendency to fall asleep," and "decreased alertness."[4]

The most common reason for daytime sleepiness in the general population is behaviorally-induced insufficient sleep. According to the NSF's Sleep in America 2011 poll, 39% of subjects self-reported less than 7 hours per night on typical work or school days.[5] In a sleep clinic referral population, EDS is the most common presenting complaint; although, in contrast, obstructive sleep apnea (OSA) is the most common cause of hypersomnia.[6] Several other causes of hypersomnia exist; selected sleep disorders causing daytime sleepiness are listed in **Box 1**.

The authors have nothing to disclose.
a Division of Sleep Medicine, Harvard Medical School, Brighton, MA, USA; b Sleep HealthCenters, 1505 Commonwealth Avenue, 5th Floor, Brighton, MA 02135, USA
* Corresponding author. Sleep HealthCenters, 1505 Commonwealth Avenue, 5th Floor, Brighton, MA 02135.
E-mail address: Doug_Kirsch@sleephealth.com

Sleep Med Clin 7 (2012) 205–218
doi:10.1016/j.jsmc.2012.03.007
1556-407X/12/$ – see front matter © 2012 Elsevier Inc. All rights reserved.

Box 1
Selected sleep disorders causing hypersomnia

Idiopathic hypersomnias (with or without long sleep time)

Narcolepsy with or without cataplexy

Periodic limb movement disorder

Recurrent hypersomnias

Sleep-disordered breathing

Adjustment sleep disorder

Behaviorally induced insufficient sleep syndrome

Environmental sleep disorder

Advanced sleep type

Delayed sleep type

Irregular sleep-wake type

Jet lag type

Shift work type

THE PHYSICAL EXAMINATION
General

Across a broad range of patents with a complaint of hypersomnia, there are few specific examination abnormalities. As noted, many of these patients may not have an underlying medical condition and may solely suffer from insufficient sleep. However, there are several sleep disorders that may cause sleepiness, some of which have physical examination findings that are more specific to the condition. Patients with hypersomnia may fall asleep in the waiting room (**Fig. 1**) or may be visibly drowsy while speaking with a clinician (drooping eyelids, head nodding, difficulty in focusing).

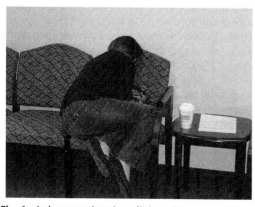

Fig. 1. A sleepy patient in a clinic waiting room. (*From* Kryger MH. Atlas of Clinical Sleep Medicine: Elsevier; 2009; with permission.)

OSA

Patients with OSA commonly have physical examination findings that signal the clinician to consider the diagnosis, particularly in combination with an appropriate clinical history. **Table 1** reviews the basic outline of the examination of a patient with OSA.

Demographics

The patient's sex, age, and race are often ascertained before they walk into the clinic. There is evidence that suggests men of all ages have a higher risk for OSA. Early studies pointed toward at least a fivefold risk increase in men compared with women. However, as research trials began to include more women, the risk increase for male gender dropped to a two to three times risk increase for men compared with women.[7,8] As women reach menopause with the resultant hormone shift, their risk for OSA seems to increase significantly.[9] Studies have demonstrated that prevalence of OSA does not seem dramatically different between racial groups; however, in Asian populations, obesity seems to be a less common risk factor for OSA than in non-Asian populations.[10]

Considering the vital signs

Typically, patients entering a medical office will have their vital signs checked. These may include height and weight (body mass index [BMI]), temperature, pulse rate, blood pressure, and oximetry. Of particular relevance to patients with OSA are the BMI and blood pressure.

The BMI is an estimate of body fat and defined by body weight in kilograms divided by the square of their height in meters. The classification by the World Health Organization categorizes a BMI of 25.0 to 29.9 as overweight, 30.0 to 34.9 as class I obesity, 35.0 to 39.9 as class II obesity, and greater than 40.0 as class III obesity.[11]

Obesity is one of the strongest predictive factors for a diagnosis of OSA. The adult population has been increasing in weight, particularly in developing countries (**Fig. 2**). Data from the Center for Disease Control demonstrates a vast worsening of obesity across the United States (**Fig. 3**, **Table 2**). One estimate suggested that 60% of the adult population in industrialized nations are overweight (BMI≥25 kg/m2) and 30% are obese (BMI≥30 kg/m2).[12]

Patients with obesity have a much higher risk of developing OSA. In one study, patients who were overweight or obese accounted for more than 70% of subjects with OSA.[13] Several large studies have suggested that approximately 25% of adults with a BMI between 25 kg/m2 and 28 kg/m2 have at least mild OSA (apnea-hypopnea index [AHI]

Table 1
Examination of OSA

Factor	Sampled Aspects to Consider
Demographics	Age, sex, race
Vital signs	Blood pressure, Body mass index
Neck	Neck circumference, thyroid abnormality
Nasal examination	Nasal polyps, septal abnormality
Oropharyngeal examination	Mallampati score, hard palate structure, palate length, uvula size, tonsil size
Dental examination	Overbite or overjet; gnathic status
Cardiopulmonary examination	Lung sounds, heart sounds, presence of edema
Neurologic examination	Muscle weakness, myotonia
Endoscopic evaluation	Retropalatal assessment
Imaging	Evaluation of airway size
Syndromes	Down syndrome, craniofacial syndromes

≥5).[14] The landmark paper by Young and colleagues[8] reviewed data from the Wisconsin Sleep Cohort and suggested that BMI was one of the largest risk factors for occurrence of OSA. Recent data from the pediatric literature demonstrates that children who are obese have a higher prevalence of OSA when compared with a control population in a general pediatric clinic.[15]

Thus, measurement of BMI is an essential part of the evaluation of the patient with hypersomnia, as it may suggest risk for OSA before the physician even sees the patient. Other obesity-related factors that have been measured and linked to OSA include waist circumference (measured at the narrowest point between the last costal arch and the iliac crest) and waist-to-hip ratio (hip circumference was measured as the greatest circumference at the level of the trochanters).[16]

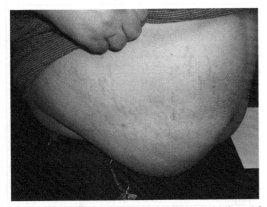

Fig. 2. Obese patients have a significantly higher risk of developing OSA. (*From* Kryger MH. Atlas of Clinical Sleep Medicine: Elsevier; 2009; with permission.)

Another essential vital sign in evaluation of the sleep apnea patient is blood pressure. As AHI increases, so does the risk for the presence of hypertension after 4 years, independent of other possible cofounders.[17] In addition, cross-sectional analysis of subjects included in the Sleep Heart Health Study (SHHS) suggested that those people with an AHI greater than or equal to 30 events per hour had 1.37-fold increased odds of hypertension compared with those without OSA (AHI<1.5 per hour) after adjusting for several confounders.[18] Although other recent data from the SHHS suggests a trend rather than clear statistical significance,[19] few clinicians would argue that there is a an association between OSA and hypertension.

Finally, although rarely abnormal in a general clinic population, respiratory rate and oximetry may provide valuable information. When abnormal, these respiratory vital signs may suggest hypoventilation (at times related to obesity) or underlying pulmonary conditions. OSA alone is unlikely to be a primary cause of these abnormalities.

Neck

Though more commonly part of the evaluation from a gentleman's tailor for appropriately fitting dress shirts, measurement of the neck circumference is a worthwhile part of the examination for OSA (**Fig. 4**).[20] Neck circumferences of more than 17 in in men and more than 16 in in women has been correlated with increased risk for a diagnosis of OSA.[21] A neck circumference greater than 40 cm seems predictive of OSA with a 61% sensitivity and 93% specificity regardless of gender.[22]

An adjusted neck circumference is an alternate method of assessing OSA risk. Adjusted neck circumference is defined as neck circumference

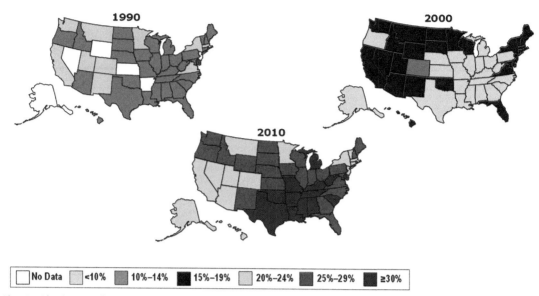

| No Data | <10% | 10%–14% | 15%–19% | 20%–24% | 25%–29% | ≥30% |

Fig. 3. Obesity trends among United States adults. (*From* Behavioral Risk Surveillance System. Atlanta (GA): Centers for Disease Control.)

(measured in centimeters) plus presence of hypertension (4 cm is added) plus habitual snoring (3 cm is added) plus reports of choking or gasping most nights (3 cm is added). Patients with an adjusted neck circumference of more than 48 cm have a 20-fold increased risk of having sleep apnea.[23]

Beyond circumferential measurement, palpation of the neck may occasionally provide clues to the diagnosis. Findings of an enlarged thyroid gland or swollen lymph nodes could potentially have an impact on airway patency. Goiters, which may be

related to euthyroid or hypothyroid state, may play a role in OSA.[24]

Nasal examination

As early as Hippocrates, nasal abnormalities (in association with other symptoms) were associated with restless sleep.[25] Abnormalities to nasal breathing may affect sleep because the nose contributes to approximately two-thirds of the total airflow resistance.[26] Participants in a population-based sample who reported nasal congestion

Table 2
2010 State obesity rates (obesity is defined by BMI ≥30 kg/m2)

State	%	State	%	State	%	State	%
Alabama	32.2	Illinois	28.2	Montana	23.0	Rhode Island	25.5
Alaska	24.5	Indiana	29.6	Nebraska	26.9	South Carolina	31.5
Arizona	24.3	Iowa	28.4	Nevada	22.4	South Dakota	27.3
Arkansas	30.1	Kansas	29.4	New Hampshire	25.0	Tennessee	30.8
California	24.0	Kentucky	31.3	New Jersey	23.8	Texas	31.0
Colorado	21.0	Louisiana	31.0	New Mexico	25.1	Utah	22.5
Connecticut	22.5	Maine	26.8	New York	23.9	Vermont	23.2
Delaware	28.0	Maryland	27.1	North Carolina	27.8	Virginia	26.0
District of Columbia	22.2	Massachusetts	23.0	North Dakota	27.2	Washington	25.5
Florida	26.6	Michigan	30.9	Ohio	29.2	West Virginia	32.5
Georgia	29.6	Minnesota	24.8	Oklahoma	30.4	Wisconsin	26.3
Hawaii	22.7	Mississippi	34.0	Oregon	26.8	Wyoming	25.1
Idaho	26.5	Missouri	30.5	Pennsylvania	28.6	—	

Data from Centers for Disease Control. Available at: http://www.cdc.gov/obesity/data/trends.html.

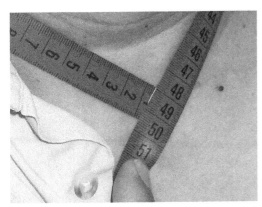

Fig. 4. Measurement of the neck circumference should be part of the physical examination for a patient with possible OSA. (*From* Kryger MH. Atlas of Clinical Sleep Medicine: Elsevier; 2009; with permission.)

Box 2
Some oropharyngeal findings in OSA

Nasal turbinate hypertrophy

Septal deviation

High and narrow hard palate

Elongated low-lying uvula

Redundant and low-lying soft palate

Crowding of the oropharynx with enlarged tonsils and adenoids

Prominent tonsillar pillars

Macroglossia

Narrow maxilla

Narrow mandible

Overjet and retrognathia

Crossbite

Dental malocclusion

Data from Guilleminault C, Abad V. Obstructive sleep apnea syndromes. Med Clin N Am 2004;88:611–30.

due to allergy were 1.8 times more likely to have moderate to severe sleep-disordered breathing than were those without nasal congestion due to allergy.[27] Therefore, an evaluation of the nasal airway is a valuable component of the physical examination of the patient with possible OSA.

Congestion of the nasal airway may have several causes: congenital, traumatic, infectious, or neoplastic. A simple method of assessing nasal congestion is the "sniff test." Asking the patient to manually occlude one side of the nose and then inhale through the other allows an audible assessment of nasal airflow that repeated on the alternate side. A brief internal evaluation with a nasal speculum may then identify obvious abnormalities on the fully or partially occluded side, such as a septal deviation or enlarged turbinates.

The internal nasal valve area is the narrowest portion of the nasal airway, thus assessment of this region is valuable. The Cottle test entails first assessing the collapsibility of the nasal passage via a sniff test. Next, the physician gently moves the patient's cheek near the nose laterally from the midline. If there is significant improvement in nasal airflow during the maneuver, at least partial obstruction of the nasal valve is likely occurring.[28]

Oropharyngeal examination

It is common sense that an evaluation the oropharyngeal space should lead to better understanding of the patient's risk of nocturnal airway closure. However, a single standardized metric for narrowing of the upper airway has not been fully determined. The size of the airway is determined by both bony and soft tissue structures and is likely related both to congenital or genetic and acquired factors. **Box 2** reviews some of the oropharyngeal findings in OSA.

Bony structures The hard palate may contribute to airway crowding if it is narrowed or if bony outgrowths, such as torus palatinus, are large. An increased pharyngeal narrowing ratio (the ratio between the airway cross section at the hard palate level and the narrowest cross section from the hard palate to the epiglottis) has been observed in patients with OSA.[29]

Soft tissues The soft palate and tonsils are particularly relevant to patency of the upper airway during sleep. Gauging the size of the oropharynx during sleep is difficult to predict while the patient is in the wake state. An anesthesiologist-designed assessment for the difficult-to-intubate airway, the Mallampati score, has been adopted by sleep specialists to help gauge risk for a patient having OSA.[30] The Mallampati score is determined by visually inspecting the oropharynx while the patient extends their tongue without phonating. Phonation may elevate the soft palate, leading to an underestimation of the Mallampati score.

The Mallampati score is defined as follows:

Class I soft palate, fauces, uvula, and posterior and anterior pillars are visible (**Fig. 5**)
Class II soft palate, fauces, and uvula are visible (**Fig. 6**)
Class III soft palate, fauces, and only base of uvula are visible (**Fig. 7**)
Class IV soft palate is not visible (**Fig. 8**).

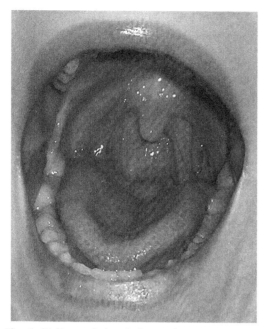

Fig. 5. Mallampati class I airway. (*From* Kryger MH. Atlas of Clinical Sleep Medicine: Elsevier; 2009; with permission.)

A higher Mallampati score has been associated with increased risk for OSA. On average, for every 1-point increase in the Mallampati score, the odds of having OSA (AHI≥5) increased more than twofold (odds ratio [per 1-point increase] = 2.5) and the AHI increased by more than 5 events per hour.[31]

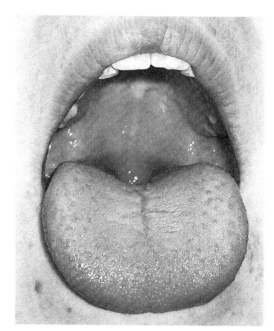

Fig. 7. Mallampati class III airway. (*From* Kryger MH. Atlas of Clinical Sleep Medicine: Elsevier; 2009; with permission.)

An alternate palate position scale was developed by Friedman and colleagues[32] that assessed the size of the upper airway and attempted to better model which surgical intervention for OSA would be most likely to be successful.

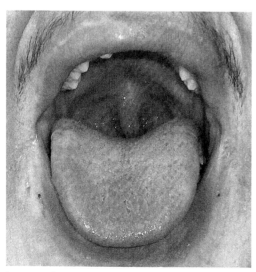

Fig. 6. Mallampati class II airway. (*From* Kryger MH. Atlas of Clinical Sleep Medicine: Elsevier; 2009; with permission.)

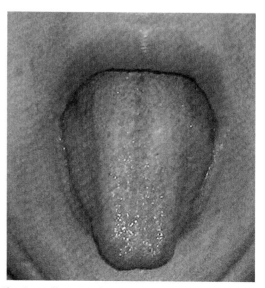

Fig. 8. Mallampati class IV airway. (*From* Kryger MH. Atlas of Clinical Sleep Medicine: Elsevier; 2009; with permission.)

"The Friedman Palate Position is based on visualization of structures in the mouth with the mouth open widely without protrusion of the tongue.

Palate grade I allows the observer to visualize the entire uvula and tonsils.

Grade II allows visualization of the uvula but not the tonsils.

Grade III allows visualization of the soft palate but not the uvula.

Grade IV allows visualization of the hard palate only."

The primary difference in the scales is that the tongue is not protruded in the Friedman palate assessment—a grading scale that has also been referred to as a Modified Mallampati Scale. In combining palate grade, tonsil size, and BMI, Friedman created a staging system in an attempt to determine best surgical practices for treating OSA. Lower staging on the Friedman system was demonstrated to predict successful treatment of OSA via uvulopalatopharyngoplasty only.[32]

The uvula may also inform the examiner about the upper airway. Swelling and/or erythema at the edge of the soft palate or affecting the uvula may suggest snoring. A long or wide uvula may also contribute to airway crowding and possible sleep apnea.

Size of the adenotonsillar tissue is another factor in assessment of the airway crowding. Particularly in children ages 2 to 8 years old, the tonsils and adenoids may be a large contributor to OSA.[33] However, although large tonsils may contribute to airway crowding in adults, soft tissue hypertrophy seems to play a less prominent role in the development of OSA. A standard grading of adenotonsillar tissue in children and adults is as follows:

Tonsil size 0 denotes surgically removed tonsils.
Tonsil size 1 implies tonsils hidden within the pillars (**Fig. 9**).
Tonsil size 2 implies the tonsils extending to the pillars (see **Fig. 9**).
Tonsil size 3 tonsils are beyond the pillars but not to the midline (**Fig. 10**).
Tonsil size 4 implies tonsils extend to the midline (**Fig. 11**).[32]

Tongue volume and position likely affect airway patency and they have been correlated with OSA in cephalometric studies.[24] Gradation of tongue size has not been well described, although tongue "scalloping" (in which the impressions of the teeth of the mandible are easily visible when the tongue

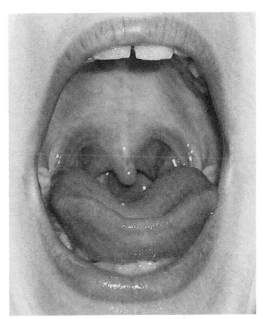

Fig. 9. A patient with a tonsil classification 1 on the right side and 2 on the left side. (*From* Kryger MH. Atlas of Clinical Sleep Medicine: Elsevier; 2009; with permission.)

is extended) implies that either the tongue is large or the lower jaw is small.

Dental examination

Evaluation of dental and jaw structure is not a skill typically used by many physicians; however, certain aspects of this practice should be commonplace for physicians performing a sleep assessment.

The finding of retrognathia (posteriorly positioned jaw) (**Fig. 12**) or micrognathia (undersized jaw) may have a large impact on the physician's

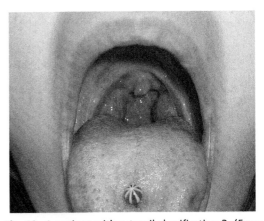

Fig. 10. A patient with a tonsil classification 3. (*From* Kryger MH. Atlas of Clinical Sleep Medicine: Elsevier; 2009; with permission.)

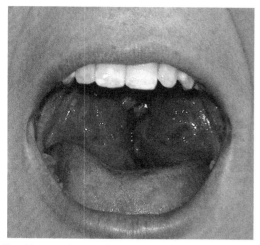

Fig. 11. A patient with a tonsil classification 4. (*From* Kryger MH. Atlas of Clinical Sleep Medicine: Elsevier; 2009; with permission.)

assessment of risk for OSA. Many non-sleep physicians assume that OSA is a disease solely related to obesity; however, these jaw findings are a common cause of significant sleep-disordered breathing in patients without an elevated BMI. Assessment of jaw position is best performed looking at the patient's face from the side while the patient is looking straight ahead in the natural head posture (the upright position of the head of a standing or sitting patient, while it is balanced by the postcervical and masticatory-suprahyoid-infrahyoid muscle groups, with the eyes directed forward so that the visual axis is parallel to the floor).[34] Men may grow facial hair (beards or goatees) to mask recessed or small jaws. Jaw structure variants shift the patient's tongue superiorly and posteriorly and, therefore, likely lead to airway impingement. Frequency of

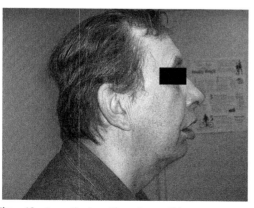

Fig. 12. A patient with retrognathia, a common anatomic jaw finding in OSA. (*From* Kryger MH. Atlas of Clinical Sleep Medicine: Elsevier; 2009; with permission.)

abnormal mandibular position may have a racial or ethnic relationship. In some Asian populations, retrognathia or micrognathia may be one of the most significant risk factors for OSA.[24]

Teeth location may be a clue to the position of the jaw. Increased levels of overbite and overjet may guide the physician to a suspicion of a retroposi-tioned mandible. Overbite presents as the vertical overlap of the maxillary central incisors over the mandibular central incisors. Overjet is the horizontal displacement between the maxillary central incisors and the mandibular central incisors.[35] Teeth crowding, particularly on the mandible may also point toward a small lower-jaw structure.

Cardiopulmonary examination

Evaluation of the heart and lungs are unlikely to help predict the presence of OSA. However, findings related to asthma or chronic obstructive pulmonary disease may be relevant to a patient's nocturnal breathing. In asthma, patient examination finding may include wheezing, increased respiratory rate, prolonged expiratory phase, use of accessory muscles, and cyanosis.[36] Signs related to chronic obstructive pulmonary disease consist of a barrel chest with increased anterior-posterior diameter, increased respiratory rate, accessory respiratory muscle use, diminished breath sounds, crackles and wheezes, and/or cyanosis in severe cases.[37]

OSA over the long term may have many effects on the heart. Also, poor heart function may affect nocturnal breathing. For instance, congestive heart failure may be linked to both OSA and central sleep apnea.[38] Findings linked with congestive heart failure may include rales, S3 gallop, hypotension, peripheral edema (**Fig. 13**), jugular venous distension, and a positive hepatojugular reflex,[39,40] Pulmonary hypertension, a possible effect of OSA, may cause: increased second heart sound (P2 portion) intensity, murmurs from pulmonary and tricuspid insufficiency, distended neck veins, pulsatile liver, peripheral edema, pleural effusion and ascites.[41]

Neurologic examination

On face value, the neurologic examination may not seem to be valuable in the OSA evaluation. However, in some cases, the findings of neurologic disease may be germane to a diagnosis of sleep-disordered breathing. Patients with strokes have a higher prevalence of nocturnal apnea (central or obstructive), so findings of prior strokes (eg, muscle weakness, sensory changes, and language difficulties) may be useful.[42] Neuromuscular syndromes, such as post-poliomyelitis, amyotrophic lateral sclerosis, or muscular dystrophies have been

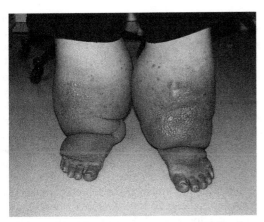

Fig. 13. Ankle edema may suggest poor cardiac function, which may also correlate with sleep-disordered breathing. (*From* Kryger MH. Atlas of Clinical Sleep Medicine: Elsevier; 2009; with permission.)

associated with sleep-disordered breathing. Therefore, testing of the bulbar muscles, chest wall muscles, and skeletal muscles may lead toward a better assessment of risk for OSA and hypoventilation.[24] Patients with myotonic dystrophy may have both obstructive and central apneas during the night, but also have an increased risk for daytime sleepiness including sleep-onset rapid eye movement (REM) periods on multiple sleep latency testing.[43] Physical signs of myotonic dystrophy may include myotonia, muscle wasting and weakness, dysarthria, ptosis, and cataracts.[44]

Nasopharyngeal endoscopy

Although many noninvasive sleep physicians do not use this form of assessment, otolaryngologists perform it frequently on patients referred to them for an evaluation of snoring and possible OSA. Nasal endoscopy has ostensibly been used to predict surgical outcomes for OSA; however, the data regarding its utility in that regard has been mixed.[45]

This procedure snakes a thin fiberoptic tube down the nose to observe the retropharyngeal and hypopharyngeal spaces as well as evaluating possible abnormalities of the nose (septal deviation, polyps, and narrowing with inspiratory collapse at the level of the nasal valve).[45] Typically, this procedure is performed while the patient is awake and alert in the seated position, although in a few centers, the patients are sedated to better assess the airway while the patient is "sleeping."[46] In theory, determining the potential sites of airway collapse (palatal, retrolingual, both palatal and retrolingual), could determine the best options for intervention, particularly from a surgical viewpoint. However, visualization of the airway alone has not been highly predictive of surgical success, even

with the addition of simulated snoring.[47] Use of the Müeller maneuver (inspiration at end-expiration against a closed nasal-oral airway) during nasal endoscopy was initially thought to be predictive of site of collapse during sleep; however, the maneuver has not reliably reflected location of obstruction.[47] Part of the variability may be because of the subjective assessment of the airway and the effect of patient effort on the Müeller maneuver.

Imaging

Cephalometric radiographs Cephalometric radiographs are the simplest form of imaging the upper airway. However, because the view is only two-dimensional, there are some limitations in understanding the true airway size. A standard cephalometric radiograph will evaluate primarily the skeletal anatomy, although some aspects of the soft tissue are also visible. Typically, the radiograph is performed in a standardized position with the subject seated, teeth opposed, eyes directed forward and at end expiration. Skeletal landmarks and their associated plane angles can give a more in-depth understanding of determinants of the upper airway size.[45]

There are a variety of findings that have been reported in cephalometric studies, in different races, genders, and weight groups. Some reported differences are observed in **Box 3**.

CT and MRI scanning CT scanning and MRI have also been used to evaluate the airway. The advantage to CT scanning is the ability to obtain images quickly and quietly. However, the CT scan is limited in resolution quality, which can limit detailed observation of the airway. When comparing apneic patients to control patients with a CT scan, the upper airway tends to be smaller, particularly in the retropalatal region.[48]

Box 3
Selected cephalometric findings in patients with OSA

Longer soft palate

Reduced minimum palatal airway widths

Increased thickness of the soft palate

Increased pharyngeal length

A retroposition of the mandible or the maxilla

Micrognathia

An increased midfacial height

Differences in hyoid bone position

Data from Stuck BA, Maurer JT. Airway evaluation in obstructive sleep apnea. Sleep Med Rev 2008; 12:411–36.

MRI scans are much more detailed in quality, although the loud noise of the machine and prolonged imaging time challenges researchers attempting to evaluate the sleeping patient. In comparing awake patients to controls with volumetric MRI, the greatest odds ratios for the development of sleep apnea were associated with increased volume of the lateral pharyngeal walls, tongue, and total soft tissue.[49]

Specific syndromes

Down syndrome is one of the more common chromosomal conditions to be associated with sleep-disordered breathing (**Fig. 14**). Depending on the study, the prevalence of sleep disordered breathing in patient's with Down syndrome is between 57% and 100%.[50] This finding can be explained by several observable factors: obesity, midfacial and mandibular hypoplasia, an abnormally small upper airway with superficially positioned tonsils and relative tonsillar and adenoidal encroachment, an increased incidence of lower respiratory tract anomalies, and generalized hypotonia with resultant collapse of the airway during inspiration.[51]

Other diagnoses that may be related to OSA with resultant specific findings include Prader-Willi syndrome, neuromuscular disorders (such as Duchenne muscular dystrophy), and Chiari malformations. Craniofacial anomalies, such as in achondroplasia, craniofacial dystoses, and Pierre Robin sequence also have a high prevalence of OSA.[50]

Narcolepsy and Other Central Hypersomnias

A diagnosis of narcolepsy is based on clinical features elicited from a patient's history, such as sleepiness, cataplexy, sleep paralysis, hypnagogic or hypnopompic hallucinations, and disturbed nighttime sleep, in combination with objective testing with either polysomnography followed by mean sleep latency testing or hypocretin-1 levels in cerebrospinal fluid.[1] Physical examination, including neurologic examination, is often unremarkable in patients with narcolepsy. However, an understanding of physical examination features that may be present remains an important element of diagnosis of narcolepsy.

Certain general physical examination features are common in narcolepsy but are not specific for the disorder. General signs of sleepiness may be present on examination such as yawning, ptosis, reduced activity, lapses in attention, and head nodding.[52] Narcolepsy generally manifests in the teens and twenties, and patients are commonly in this age range at first presentation.[53] However, narcolepsy can develop in young childhood or after age 40. Patients with narcolepsy have an increased incidence of obesity[54] and non-insulin dependent diabetes mellitus.[55]

The presence of cataplexy is characteristic of narcolepsy associated with hypocretin deficiency and can help distinguish narcolepsy from other causes of EDS.[56] Cataplexy is a sudden loss of muscle strength that occurs in response to emotion, mostly commonly laughter or anger.[53] Cataplexy has a wide range of clinical manifestations. Most commonly, episodes are mild and may consist of brief episodes of knee buckling, mild neck or jaw weakness, or arms falling to the side (**Fig. 15**).[56] In more severe cases, episodes may consist of generalized weakness and last several minutes. Patients maintain consciousness, although sleep may occur during prolonged episodes. Muscle function of the respiratory and extraocular muscles is preserved, although ptosis and blurred vision have been described. Rarely, prolonged episodes (ie, status cataplecticus) can occur, often associated with abrupt withdrawal from anticataplectic medications.

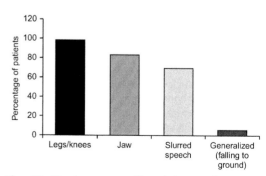

Fig. 15. Muscle groups affected in cataplexy. Most patients experience partial episodes consisting of unbuckling at the knees or legs. It is rare that episodes generalize to compromise posture and cause the patient to fall. (*Data from* Anic-Labat S, Guilleminault C, Kraemer HC, et al. Validation of a cataplexy questionnaire in 983 sleep-disordered patients. Sleep 1999;22(1):77. *From* Kryger MH. Atlas of clinical sleep medicine. Philadelphia: Elsevier; 2010.)

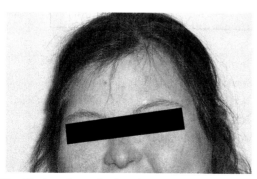

Fig. 14. A patient who has the typical facial findings of Down syndrome. (*From* Kryger MH. Atlas of Clinical Sleep Medicine: Elsevier; 2009; with permission.)

Although cataplexy may not be seen during physical examination of a patient with narcolepsy, clinicians must be able to recognize cataplexy and may consider trying to elicit it when considering the diagnosis (telling a joke, startling the patient).

Although the presence of cataplexy is a useful diagnostic tool because it occurs almost exclusively in narcolepsy, only about 60% of patients with narcolepsy have cataplexy.[53] In narcolepsy without cataplexy and idiopathic hypersomnia, there are no pathognomonic features that can potentially manifest on physical examination.

Recurrent Hypersomnia

Kleine-Levin syndrome
Kleine-Levin syndrome (KLS) is an uncommon disorder that is associated with periodic episodes of hypersomnia, as well as cognitive and behavioral disturbances such as hyperphagia and hypersexuality. On clinical presentation, over 80% of KLS patients are in the second decade of life, and the mean age of onset is 17 years.[57] Additionally, almost 70% of patients are male. Physical examination abnormalities can be seen in KLS during episodes of hypersomnia. However, in between episodes of hypersomnia, physical and neurologic examinations are normal, without evidence of behavioral or cognitive abnormalities.[58]

Although neurologic examination does not reveal evidence of focal abnormality in KLS, cognitive and behavioral abnormalities are seen during episodes of hypersomnia.[58] Possible cognitive abnormalities seen on examination may include speech difficulties, such as incoherent speech or use of short sentences with limited vocabulary, and confusion.[57] On psychiatric examination, depressive symptoms are common. Hallucinations, delusions, and feelings of derealization have also been described. Behaviorally, these patients spend an average of 18 hours per day asleep. Patients are irritable and sometimes aggressive if awakened from sleep. Increased food intake occurs in 75% of the patients, sometimes causing significant weight gain.[57] Increased sexual drive occurs in almost half of patients. Medical examination is generally normal during episodes of hypersomnia, with rare signs of autonomic dysfunction.

Sleep-Related Movement Disorders

Restless legs syndrome
Restless legs syndrome (RLS) can be associated with fatigue and, in some cases, hypersomnia.[59] Diagnosis of RLS is based on four essential diagnostic criteria elicited from a patient's history.[60] In idiopathic RLS, there are no specific physical examination findings. Physical examination findings in secondary RLS can represent the underlying cause of the disorder such as uremia, neuropathy, or pregnancy. In patients with possible neuropathy symptoms, a brief sensory screen may be performed via testing of the distal and proximal areas of the legs using light touch, pinprick, and vibration.

Though used primarily for research, the suggested immobilization test objectively evaluates limb movements while the patient has their legs outstretched and attempts to keep still. Periodic limb movements of wakefulness are measured over the course of 60 minutes via electromyography of the anterior tibialis muscles of both legs. Patients with RLS typically have more leg movements than controls.[61]

Periodic limb movement disorder
Diagnosis of periodic limb movement disorder is based on finding it on a sleep study, in conjunction with the presence of insomnia or symptoms of fatigue or hypersomnia.[1] There are generally no specific examination findings in periodic limb movement disorder.

Parasomnias

Parasomnias may cause sleep disruption, although these disorders are rarely a cause of hypersomnia. Non-REM parasomnias are not associated with particular physical examination findings. REM Behavior Disorder (RBD) may be associated with abnormalities on neurologic examination.

RBD
A diagnosis of RBD is based on the presence of REM sleep without atonia on polysomnography, in conjunction with a history or polysomnographic documentation of dream enactment behavior.[1] RBD is frequently a manifestation of α-synucleinopathies such as Parkinson disease or Lewy body dementia, although RBD may be idiopathic. RBD often precedes the development of the associated neurodegenerative disorder by an average of 10 years, although intervals of up to 50 years have been described.[62] As a result, physical examination and neurologic examination may be unremarkable in RBD on presentation. However, even before clear manifestation of motor, cognitive, or autonomic dysfunction that may accompany α-synucleinopathies, subtle abnormalities have been seen on detailed neurologic testing.[63] Patients with idiopathic RBD may display evidence of early Parkinson disease, including abnormalities in color vision and olfactory discrimination, as well as subtle deficits in motor and gait speed.[63]

Circadian Rhythm Disorders

There are no specific physical examination findings in circadian rhythm disorders. The diagnosis of these disorders is based on a patient's history and it may involve sleep diaries, actigraphy, or salivary or urinary melatonin levels. In some cases, blindness may lead to circadian rhythm disturbance, including symptoms of daytime sleepiness.

Secondary Hypersomnia

In any evaluation of a patient with hypersomnia, it is important to consider that hypersomnia may be secondary to a medical or neurologic condition. A wide range of disorders can result in sleepiness, including head trauma, stroke, hypothalamic disorders, toxic-metabolic disorders such as hepatic encephalopathy, endocrine disorders such as hypothyroidism, and genetic disorders such

as myotonic dystrophy. Evidence of an underlying disorder may be apparent on comprehensive physical examination. **Box 4** lists selected medical causes of EDS.

SUMMARY

Hypersomnia is a common symptom of many medical disorders, including several sleep disorders. Although patients with hypersomnia may not always have examination abnormalities, certain sleep disorders have specific physical findings that an experienced clinician should be comfortable evaluating. In combination with an appropriate clinical history taking, a sleep-specific physical examination will lead to more appropriate diagnostic testing and patient management.

Box 4
Selected medical causes of EDS

Cancer

Cardiac disease:

   Congestive heart failure

Central nervous system disorders:

   Hydrocephalus

   Lesions (tumors, abscess, infection, sarcoidosis)

   Multiple sclerosis

   Parkinsonism

   Stroke

Endocrine disorders:

   Growth hormone deficiency

   Hypothyroidism

Genetic disorders:

   Fragile X syndrome

   Myotonic dystrophy

   Niemann-Pick type C

   Prader-Willi

Hypersomnia due to drug or substance

Posttraumatic hypersomnia

Pulmonary disorders

   Chronic obstructive pulmonary disease

   Sleep-related asthma

Sleeping sickness (protozoan infection)

Toxic-metabolic disorders:

   Adrenal insufficiency

   Chronic renal insufficiency

   Hepatic encephalopathy

   Toxic exposure

REFERENCES

1. AASM. The international classification of sleep disorders. In: Diagnostic and coding manual. 2nd edition. Westchester (IL): American Academy of Sleep Medicine; 2005. p. 79.
2. National Sleep Foundation poll, 2009, Slide 34. Available at: http://www.sleepfoundation.org/article/sleep-america-polls/2009-health-and-safety. Accessed October 15, 2011.
3. National Sleep Foundation poll, 2011, Slide 13. Available at: http://www.sleepfoundation.org/article/sleep-america-polls/2011-communications-technology-use-and-sleep. Accessed October 15, 2011.
4. Pigeon W, Sateia M, Ferguson R. Distinguishing between excessive daytime sleepiness and fatigue: toward improved detection and treatment. J Psychosom Res 2003;54(1):61–9.
5. National Sleep Foundation poll, 2011, Slide 41. Available at: http://www.sleepfoundation.org/article/sleep-america-polls/2011-communications-technology-use-and-sleep. Accessed October 1, 2011.
6. National Commission on Sleep Disorders Research. Wake up America: a national sleep alert. Executive Summary and Executive Report, Report of the National Commission on Sleep Disorders Research. Washington, DC: National Institutes of Health, US Government Printing Office; 1993. p. 45.
7. Bixler EO, Vgontzas AN, Lin HM, et al. Prevalence of sleep-disordered breathing in women: effects of gender. Am J Respir Crit Care Med 2001;163(3 Pt 1): 608–13.
8. Young T, Palta M, Dempsey J, et al. The occurrence of sleep-disordered breathing among middle-aged adults. N Engl J Med 1993;328(17):1230–5.
9. Kapsimalis F, Kryger MH. Gender and obstructive sleep apnea syndrome, part 2: mechanisms. Sleep 2002;25(5):499–506.

10. Punjabi NM. The epidemiology of adult obstructive sleep apnea. Proc Am Thorac Soc 2008;5(2):136–43.

11. Available at: http://apps.who.int/bmi/index.jsp?introPage=intro_3.html. Accessed October 29, 2011.

12. Ogden CL, Carroll MD, Curtin LR, et al. Prevalence of overweight and obesity in the United States, 1999-2004. JAMA 2006;295(13):1549–55.

13. Resta O, Foschino-Barbaro MP, Legari G, et al. Sleep-related breathing disorders, loud snoring and excessive daytime sleepiness in obese subjects. Int J Obes Relat Metab Disord 2001;25(5):669–75.

14. Romero-Corral A, Caples SM, Lopez-Jimenez F, et al. Interactions between obesity and obstructive sleep apnea: implications for treatment. Chest 2010;137(3):711–9.

15. Rudnick EF, Walsh JS, Hampton MC, et al. Prevalence and ethnicity of sleep-disordered breathing and obesity in children. Otolaryngol Head Neck Surg 2007;137(6):878–82.

16. Martinez-Rivera C, Abad J, Fiz JA, et al. Usefulness of truncal obesity indices as predictive factors for obstructive sleep apnea syndrome. Obesity (Silver Spring) 2008;16(1):113–8.

17. Peppard PE, Young T, Palta M, et al. Prospective study of the association between sleep-disordered breathing and hypertension. N Engl J Med 2000; 342(19):1378–84.

18. Nieto FJ, Young TB, Lind BK, et al. Association of sleep-disordered breathing, sleep apnea, and hypertension in a large community-based study. Sleep Heart Health Study. JAMA 2000;283(14): 1829–36.

19. O'Connor GT, Caffo B, Newman AB, et al. Prospective study of sleep-disordered breathing and hypertension: the Sleep Heart Health Study. Am J Respir Crit Care Med 2009;179(12):1159–64.

20. Davies RJ, Stradling JR. The relationship between neck circumference, radiographic pharyngeal anatomy, and obstructive sleep apnea syndrome. Eur Respir J 1990;3(5):509–14.

21. Epstein LJ, Kristo D, Strollo PJ, et al. Clinical guideline for the evaluation, management and long-term care of obstructive sleep apnea in adults. J Clin Sleep Med 2009;5(3):263–76.

22. Kushida CA, Efron B, Guilleminault C. A predictive morphometric model for the obstructive sleep apnea syndrome. Ann Intern Med 1997;127(8 Pt 1): 581–7.

23. Flemons WW. Clinical practice: obstructive sleep apnea. N Engl J Med 2002;347(7):498–504.

24. Avidan A, Malow B. Physical examination in sleep medicine. In: Kryger MH, Roth T, Dement WC, editors. Principles and practice of sleep medicine. 5th edition. St Louis (MO): Saunders Elsevier; 2011.

25. Available at: http://www.perseus.tufts.edu/hopper/text?doc=Perseus:abo:tlg,006:1:4&lang=original, 607. Accessed September 1, 2011.

26. Ferris B, Mead J, Opie L. Partitioning of respiratory flow resistance in man. J Appl Physiol 1964;19: 653–8.

27. Young T, Finn L, Kim H. Nasal obstruction as a risk factor for sleep-disordered breathing. The University of Wisconsin Sleep and Respiratory Research Group. J Allergy Clin Immunol 1997;99:S757–62.

28. Available at: http://www.sports-anatomy-research.com/sports-anatomy-research/cottle-s-test-and-sign-associated-history-and-clinical-anatomy-of-the-nasal-valve. Accessed October 18, 2011.

29. Koren A, Groselj LD, Fajdiga I. CT comparison of primary snoring and obstructive sleep apnea syndrome: role of pharyngeal narrowing ratio and soft palate-tongue contact in awake patient. Eur Arch Otorhinolaryngol 2009;266:727–34.

30. Mallampati SR, Gatt SP, Gugino LD, et al. A clinical sign to predict difficult tracheal intubation: a prospective study. Can Anaesth Soc J 1985;32: 429–34.

31. Nuckton TJ, Glidden DV, Browner WS, et al. Physical examination: Mallampati score as an independent predictor of obstructive sleep apnea. Sleep 2006; 29(7):903–8.

32. Friedman M, Ibrahim H, Joseph NJ. Staging of obstructive sleep apnea/hypopnea syndrome: a guide to appropriate treatment. Laryngoscope 2004;114: 454–9.

33. Hoban TF. Sleep disorders in children. Ann N Y Acad Sci 2010;1184:1–14.

34. Ozbek MM, Miyamoto K, Lowe AA, et al. Natural head posture, upper airway morphology and obstructive sleep apnoea severity in adults. Eur J Orthod 1998;20(2):133–43.

35. Hoffstein V. Review of oral appliances for treatment of sleep-disordered breathing. Sleep Breath 2007; 11(1):1–22.

36. Kaplan AG, Balter MS, Bell AD, et al. Diagnosis of asthma in adults. CMAJ 2009;181(10):E210–20.

37. Anthonisen N. Chronic obstructive pulmonary disease. In: Goldman L, Ausiello D, editors. Cecil medicine. 23rd edition. Philadelphia: Saunders Elsevier; 2008. Available at: www.expertconsult.com. Accessed March 9, 2012.

38. Naughton MT, Bradley TD. Sleep apnea in congestive heart failure. Clin Chest Med 1998;19(1): 99–113.

39. Badgett RG, Lucey CR, Mulrow CD. Can the clinical examination diagnose left-sided heart failure in adults? JAMA 1997;277(21):1712–9.

40. Butman SM, Ewy GA, Standen JR, et al. Bedside cardiovascular examination in patients with severe chronic heart failure: importance of rest or inducible jugular venous distension. J Am Coll Cardiol 1993; 22(4):968–74.

41. Barst RJ. Pulmonary hypertension. In: Goldman L, Ausiello D, editors. Cecil medicine. 23rd edition.

Philadelphia (PA): Saunders Elsevier; 2008. Available at: www.expertconsult.com. Accessed March 9, 2012.

42. Ramar K, Surani S. The relationship between sleep disorders and stroke. Postgrad Med 2010;122(6): 145–53.

43. Yu H, Laberge L, Jaussent I, et al. Daytime sleepiness and REM sleep characteristics in myotonic dystrophy: a case-control study. Sleep 2011;34(2): 165–70.

44. Available at: http://depts.washington.edu/neurogen/downloads/myotonic.pdf. Accessed October 18, 2011.

45. Shepard JW, Gefter WB, Guilleminault C, et al. Evaluation of the upper airway in patients with obstructive sleep apnea. Sleep 1991;14(4):361–71.

46. Kotecha BT, Hannan SA, Khalil HM, et al. Sleep nasendoscopy: a 10-year retrospective audit study. Eur Arch Otorhinolaryngol 2007;264:1361–7.

47. Stuck BA, Maurer JT. Airway evaluation in obstructive sleep apnea. Sleep Med Rev 2008;12:411–36.

48. Schwab RJ, Gupta KB, Gefter WB, et al. Upper airway soft tissue anatomy in normals and patients with sleep disordered breathing: significance of the lateral pharyngeal walls. Am J Respir Crit Care Med 1995;152:1673–89.

49. Schwab RJ, Pasirstein M, Pierson R, et al. Identification of upper airway anatomic risk factors for obstructive sleep apnea with volumetric magnetic resonance imaging. Am J Respir Crit Care Med 2003;168(5):522–30.

50. Aurora RN, Zak RS, Karippot A, et al. Practice parameters for the respiratory indications for polysomnography in children. Sleep 2011;34(3):379–88.

51. Marcus CL, Keens TG, Bautista DB, et al. Obstructive sleep apnea in children with Down syndrome. Pediatrics 1991;88(1):132–9.

52. Roehrs T, Carskadon M, Dement W. Daytime sleepiness and alertness. In: Kryger M, Roth T, Dement W, editors. Principles and practice of sleep medicine. 5th edition. Phildelphia (PA): W.B. Saunders; 2011.

53. Scammell TE. The neurobiology, diagnosis, and treatment of narcolepsy. Ann Neurol 2003;53(2):154–66.

54. Schuld A, Hebebrand J, Geller F, et al. Increased body-mass index in patients with narcolepsy. Lancet 2000;355(9211):1274–5.

55. Honda Y, Doi Y, Ninomiya R, et al. Increased frequency of non-insulin-dependent diabetes mellitus among narcoleptic patients. Sleep 1986;9(1 Pt 2): 254–9.

56. Nishino S. Clinical and neurobiological aspects of narcolepsy. Sleep Med 2007;8(4):373–99.

57. Arnulf I, Zeitzer JM, File J, et al. Kleine-Levin syndrome: a systematic review of 186 cases in the literature. Brain 2005;128(Pt 12):2763–76.

58. Gadoth N, Kesler A, Vainstein G, et al. Clinical and polysomnographic characteristics of 34 patients with Kleine-Levin syndrome. J Sleep Res 2001; 10(4):337–41.

59. Hening W, Walters AS, Allen RP, et al. Impact, diagnosis and treatment of restless legs syndrome (RLS) in a primary care population: the REST (RLS epidemiology, symptoms, and treatment) primary care study. Sleep Med 2004;5(3):237–46.

60. Allen RP, Picchietti D, Hening WA, et al. Restless legs syndrome: diagnostic criteria, special considerations, and epidemiology. A report from the restless legs syndrome diagnosis and epidemiology workshop at the National Institutes of Health. Sleep Med 2003;4(2):101–19.

61. Montplaisir J, Boucher S, Nicholas A, et al. Immobilization tests and periodic leg movements in sleep for the diagnosis of restless legs syndrome. Mov Disord 1998;13:324–9.

62. Claassen DO, Josephs KA, Ahlskog JE, et al. REM sleep behavior disorder preceding other aspects of synucleinopathies by up to half a century. Neurology 2010;75(6):494–9.

63. Postuma RB, Lang AE, Massicotte-Marquez J, et al. Potential early markers of Parkinson disease in idiopathic REM sleep behavior disorder. Neurology 2006;66(6):845–51.

Objective and Subjective Measurement of Excessive Sleepiness

Neil Freedman, MD*

KEYWORDS

- Multiple sleep latency test (MSLT) • Maintenance of wakefulness test (MWT)
- Epworth sleepiness scale • Stanford sleepiness scale • Hypersomnia • Narcolepsy

KEY POINTS

- There is much debate concerning which of many objective and subjective tests of daytime sleepiness is best for use in clinical practice.
- Objective and subjective tests likely assess different dimensions of sleepiness, and aside from using the multiple sleep latency test (MSLT), which is indicated as part of the evaluation of patients with suspected narcolepsy or idiopathic hypersomnia, the best test for a given situation remains to be defined.
- Typically, a combination of subjective and objective testing with clinical history is necessary to best determine the degree and clinical significance of a given patient's daytime sleepiness.

Symptoms of daytime sleepiness are common in normal individuals as well as in those with various sleep disorders. Several formal objective and subjective measures of daytime sleepiness have been devised to quantify the degree of an individual's sleepiness, help differentiate normal states from abnormal states, and monitor the response to various interventions. This article reviews several commonly used and referenced instruments including

- Multiple sleep latency test (MSLT),
- Maintenance of wakefulness test (MWT),
- Epworth sleepiness scale (ESS), and
- Stanford sleepiness scale (SSS).

Other alternative modalities used to assess sleepiness, including the Oxford sleep resistance (OSLER) test, the Karolinska sleepiness scale (KSS), and psychomotor vigilance test (PVT) are also discussed in this article.

MULTIPLE SLEEP LATENCY TEST

MSLT is the most commonly used and experimentally validated objective test of daytime sleepiness and is currently the standard for objectively quantifying sleepiness.[1–4] It is a sensitive test of daytime sleepiness in different types of sleep deprivation (partial, complete, acute, and chronic) and in a variety of pathologic conditions.[5–9] This test is also used to document the presence or absence of sleep-onset rapid eye movement sleep periods (SOREMPs), which is helpful in supporting the diagnosis of narcolepsy or idiopathic hypersomnia in the proper clinical setting.[3,10]

The standard MSLT protocol uses 4 to 5 20-minute nap opportunities that occur at 2-hour intervals throughout the day in a sleep-inducing environment.[3] Patients are instructed to try and fall asleep during each trial and are kept awake in between nap trials. Several parameters are monitored during the study, including electroencephalography

Disclosures: The author has nothing to disclose.
Division of Pulmonary and Critical Care Medicine, Department of Medicine, NorthShore University Healthcare System, 265 Ridge Avenue, Evanston, IL 60201, USA
* 33944 Wooded Glen Drive, Grayslake, IL 60030.
E-mail address: Neilfreedman@comcast.net

Sleep Med Clin 7 (2012) 219–232
doi:10.1016/j.jsmc.2012.03.003
1556-407X/12/$ – see front matter © 2012 Elsevier Inc. All rights reserved.

(EEG) (central and occipital leads), right and left electrooculography, chin electromyography, and electrocardiography (**Fig. 1**). Because the MSLT results may be affected by influences that increase homeostatic and REM sleep drives, an overnight sleep study is required on the night before the MSLT to objectively document the amount of sleep on the preceding night as well as to assess for causes that might result in sleep fragmentation.

The timing of when the MSLT should be performed must take into account the patient's usual sleep schedule, with the first nap typically beginning 1.5 to 3 hours after the patient's habitual wake up time. The sleep latency of each nap is calculated as the time from lights out at beginning of each nap session to the first 30-second epoch of any stage of sleep, including stage N1 sleep. The REM latency is defined as the time from the beginning of the first epoch scored as sleep to the first epoch of REM sleep.[1,3,4] If non-rapid eye movement (NREM) sleep occurs during the initial 20-minute period of a given session, the nap trial is allowed to continue for an additional 15 minutes of clock time to allow for the onset of REM sleep. Each nap session is terminated if one of the following events occurs: (1) No sleep is observed after 20 minutes or (2) 15 minutes after the onset of NREM sleep. The mean sleep latency (MSL) is

calculated by averaging the sleep latencies across all nap sessions.[3,11]

Under proper testing conditions, the MSLT is a reliable test for both the MSL and documentation of SOREMPs.[12] The MSLT has a high test-retest reliability for the MSL (correlation coefficient [r] = 0.97) in normal individuals, a high inter-rater and intra-rater reliability for both the MSL (r = 0.85–0.90) and SOREMPs (r = 0.91) in normal and clinical populations, and the test results tend not to be affected by testing interval or degree of sleepiness.[2,4,11] The five nap protocol is the recommended standard. The protocol may be reduced to four sessions if two of more sleep onset REM periods occur during the first four nap sessions. A minimum of 4 nap sessions must be performed because there is a significant reduction in the test-retest reliability for the MSL when less than 4 nap sessions are performed.[13]

Stringent adherence to the proper MSLT protocol and procedures must be followed to ensure accurate results.[3] A subject's baseline sleep-wake schedule must be taken into account, because the sleep latency and propensity to go into REM sleep vary depending on the phase of the subject's circadian clock.[6,14,15] Medications such as stimulants, depressants, antidepressants, and other REM suppressants should be strictly avoided for at least 2 weeks before testing

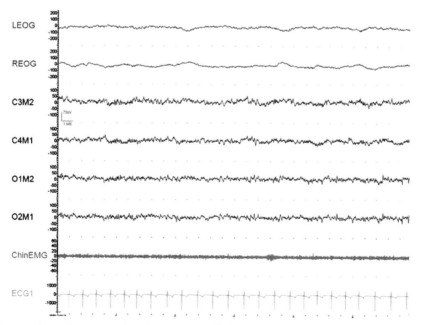

Fig. 1. Thirty second epoch representing the recommended MSLT montage. As defined by the AASM practice parameters, the standard MSLT montage should include central and occipital leads, right and left electrooculography (EOG) leads, chin electromyography (EMG) and electrocardiography (ECG). (*Data from* Littner MR, Kushida C, Wise M, et al. Practice parameters for clinical use of the multiple sleep latency test and the maintenance of wakefulness test. Sleep 2005;28(1):113–21.)

because these compounds may influence the ability to fall asleep as well as attain REM sleep. Depending on a particular patient's motivation (ie, disability from or ability to continue in a specific occupation), spot drug screening may be required to ensure valid results.

Strict adherence to the proper MSLT protocol is also critical as changes in the state of physiologic arousal may significantly affect MSLT results. As an example, Bonnet and Arand studied a group of normal subjects who underwent the MSLT after either a 5-minute walk or a 15-minute period of resting in bed and watching television before each nap session.[16] Sleep latencies were significantly increased in the group of patients who walked before the MSLT in both sleep-deprived and non-sleep-deprived conditions, despite similar homeostatic and circadian influences. These data imply that measured sleepiness is influenced by a combination of sleep drive and physiologic arousal, which may act independently of each other. These results and the results of other tests emphasize the importance of adhering to the proper MSLT protocol because factors other than sleepiness (eg, the level of physiologic arousal and sleep/wake state pathophysiology) may influence the MSLT results.[17,18]

Finally, a patient's underlying sleep complaint must also be taken into account when interpreting MSLT results. Several studies have demonstrated that patients with primary insomnia have significantly longer MSL values on the MSLT than those of matched normal controls.[19–22] Because the MSL is affected by factors that increase homeostatic sleep drive, these findings are somewhat paradoxic in that patients with insomnia tend to sleep for fewer hours per night than normal individuals. It is likely that patients with primary insomnia have increased levels of physiologic arousal that impair their ability to initiate sleep, resulting in longer sleep latencies. Thus, in this patient population, the increased MSL compared with that of normal individuals reflects a combination of both their drive for sleep as well as their increased level of physiologic arousal.

With regard to the assessment of objective sleepiness, the concept of MSLT is relatively straight forward. In the absence of confounding influences, the sleepier the subject, the faster he or she will fall asleep as reflected in a shorter MSL. A central question that needs to be addressed is what defines a normal MSL on the MSLT? The mean sleep latency on the MSLT was previously interpreted as normal if the mean sleep latency was greater than 10 minutes, consistent with pathologic sleepiness if the value was less than 5 minutes, and in a gray zone if the value

was between 5 and 10 minutes.[1,23] These recommendations were based on results from normal individuals measured at baseline and those measured after total sleep deprivation.

Information gathered from the 2005 American Academy of Sleep Medicine (AASM) practice parameters literature review regarding the clinical use of the MSLT, as well as more recent population based data, have changed the way MSLT results are interpreted with regard to the assessment of objective sleepiness.[3,24] Normative data demonstrate that there is a wide spectrum of normal values for the MSL on both the 4 and 5 nap protocols, with MSL values for the 4 nap protocol being 10.4 ± 4.3 minutes and the 5 nap protocol being 11.6 ± 5.2 minutes. Based on these data, normal MSL values on the 4 and 5 nap protocols range from 1.8 to 19 minutes and 1.2 to 20 minutes, respectively. There is also significant overlap between normal and pathologic states, such as narcolepsy and idiopathic hypersomnia, such that the MSL value does not adequately discriminate between normal and abnormal sleepiness (**Fig. 2**). While most of the narcolepsy patients (about 90%) have an MSL of less than 8 minutes on the MSLT, 30% of the general population also has an MSL value of less than 8 minutes and 16% of normal individuals have an MSL value of less than 5 minutes (**Fig. 3**).[24] Finally, 39% to 42% of all patients with idiopathic hypersomnia have an MSL of greater than 8 minutes.[25,26] Given these results, the AASM practice parameters recommend that the MSL should not be the sole criteria for determining the presence or absence of excessive sleepiness, thus certifying a diagnosis or a response to treatment.

In patients with idiopathic hypersomnia, the International Classification for Sleep Disorders Second Edition defines a threshold MSL value of less than or equal to 8 minutes as one of the criteria for the diagnosis of both idiopathic hypersomnia with long sleep time and idiopathic hypersomnia without long sleep time.[27] As noted previously, studies of patients with these disorders would suggest that many of these patients have MSL values above this threshold. As a group, the MSL is 6.2 ± 3 minutes.[3] More recent studies of patients with idiopathic hypersomnia demonstrate that approximately 40% of all patients have an MSL of greater than 8 minutes.[25,26] In those individuals with idiopathic hypersomnia with long sleep time, 71% have MSL values greater than 8 minutes and 54% have values greater than 10 minutes.[25] These data call into question the application of the 8-minute MSL threshold as a strict diagnostic criterion in this patient population, because using this threshold may result in a missed diagnosis in many patients with the disease.

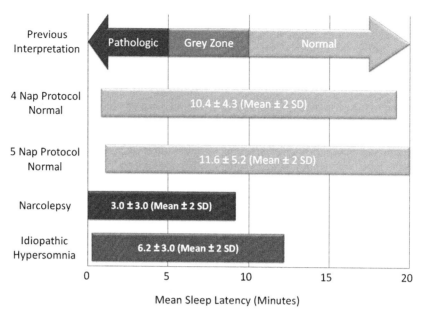

Fig. 2. Comparison of normal mean sleep latency (MSL) values for the 4 and 5 nap MSLT protocols with pathologic states (narcolepsy and idiopathic hypersomnia) and prior definitions of normal and abnormal MSL values. There is a wide spectrum of normal values for the MSL in both the 4 and 5 nap protocols and significant overlap between normal individuals and pathologic states. The data demonstrate that the MSL on the MSLT does not discriminate normal from abnormal well. The data also show that and our previous threshold definition of normal (ie, MSL >10 minutes) was not valid. (*Data from* Littner MR, Kushida C, Wise M, et al. Practice parameters for clinical use of the multiple sleep latency test and the maintenance of wakefulness test. Sleep 2005;28(1):113–21.)

Finally, several studies assessing driving risk using both actual driving and driving simulators have demonstrated a poor correlation between MSL values on the MSLT and risk of accidents in real world settings. As noted previously, the MSL on the MSLT should not be used to predict safety in real world settings, because the data do not support using the MSLT for this purpose.[3] In

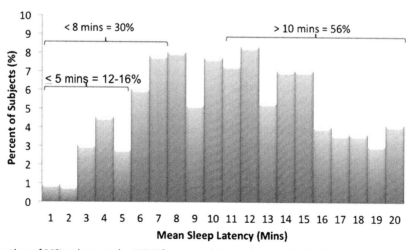

Fig. 3. Distribution of MSL values on the MSLT for a population of normal individuals. The graph represents data from 618 middle aged normal individuals from southeastern Michigan who had no sleep complaints and had normal overnight polysomnograms. Fifty six percent of normal individuals had MSL values of >10 minutes and thirty percent had MSL values of <8 minutes. These data are consistent with other studies demonstrating a wide spectrum of MSL values in normal individuals and significant overlap with pathologic states, such as narcolepsy, which are in part defined by MSL values of less than 8 minutes. (*Data from* Drake C, Roehrs T, Breslau N, et al. The 10-year risk of verified motor vehicle crashes in relation to physiologic sleepiness. Sleep 2010;33(6):745–52.)

general, there are no subjective or objective tests that accurately predict a sleepy individual's ability to safely operate a motor vehicle. A combination of clinical judgment and close follow-up is recommended to reduce the risk of future problems.

Given the wide spectrum of normal values in the MSL and significant overlap between normal individuals and pathologic sleepiness states such as narcolepsy and idiopathic hypersomnia, the utility of the MSLT in the diagnosis of narcolepsy is not only based on the MSL but also on the presence of SOREMPs. SOREMPs are common in patients with narcolepsy, with most patients having at least 2 SOREMPs during the MSLT (**Fig. 4**). In patients with narcolepsy, the sensitivity and specificity for 2 or more SOREMPs is 0.78 and 0.93, respectively.[3,12] Many patients with narcolepsy who have a false-negative result with less than 2 SOREMPs on initial testing will have more than or equal to 2 SOREMPs on repeat testing.[28] The presence and or absence of SOREMPs is helpful in differentiating narcolepsy without cataplexy from idiopathic hypersomnia, because SOREMPs are common in patients with narcolepsy and uncommon in patients with idiopathic hypersomnia. In fact, SOREMPs during a standard MSLT are typically absent in most patients (92%) with idiopathic hypersomnia.[25,26]

The presence of 2 or more SOREMPs only support a diagnosis of narcolepsy in the proper clinical setting, as SOREMPs are not specific to this patient population (**Box 1**). In fact, population-based studies have demonstrated that 3% to 17% of the general population and up to 25% of patients with untreated severe obstructive sleep apnea (OSA) may also demonstrate 2 or more SOREMPs on a standard MSLT.[29–32] These data highlight the importance of following the prescribed MSLT protocol, knowing your patient population, and interpreting the results in the context of the entire clinical presentation.

Given the limitations of the MSL value on the MSLT and the high prevalence of SOREMPs in patients with narcolepsy, the MSLT is only indicated as part of the evaluation of patients with suspected narcolepsy or idiopathic hypersomnia.[3] It is not indicated for the assessment of other patient populations or for predicting safety in real world situations. A key point is that the MSLT is not diagnostic of anything by itself, but only supports a diagnosis of narcolepsy or idiopathic hypersomnia in the proper clinical context. Its main utility in the assessment of patients with excessive daytime sleepiness in the absence of cataplexy is differentiating patients with narcolepsy without cataplexy from those with idiopathic hypersomnia, as the presence of 2 or more SOREMPs is common in patients with narcolepsy and uncommon in patients with idiopathic hypersomnia.

MAINTENANCE OF WAKEFULNESS TEST

The MWT is a daytime polysomnographic procedure that objectively measures the ability of a subject to remain awake. This test is used in association with the clinical history to assess an individual's ability to maintain wakefulness for a defined period of time. It has questionable utility in clinical practice as its results do not consistently predict an individual's safety while driving or in the work place in real world situations.[3]

The MWT protocol has several differences from the MSLT protocol. Unlike the MSLT, which has a well-defined standard protocol, the MWT has several described protocols, none of which are universally accepted.[3,33,34] In clinical practice, the AASM practice parameters recommend that the

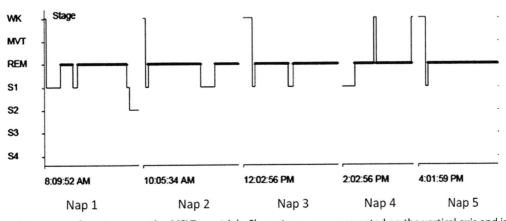

Fig. 4. Hypnogram from 5 consecutive MSLT nap trials. Sleep stages are represented on the vertical axis and individual MSLT naps and start times are represented on the horizontal axis. Multiple sleep onset REM periods (SOREMPs) are demonstrated throughout the protocol with SOREMPs being observed on each of the 5 nap trials.

Box 1
Differential diagnosis of sleep onset REM periods

Narcolepsy

Sleep deprivation

Untreated obstructive sleep apnea

Rebound from REM suppressing agents

Delayed sleep phase syndrome

Normal variant (3% to 17% of population)

40-minute 4 trial protocol be performed in clinical practice. The 40-minute protocol is recommended to avoid a ceiling effect that may be present in normal individuals using protocols of lesser duration. Twenty-minute protocols have been described and may be used in a research setting at the discretion of the investigator.[33] Each test consists of 4 discrete 40-minute trials conducted at 2-hour intervals, commencing 1.5 to 3 hours after awakening from a night of sleep. During the MWT, the subject is placed in a semirecumbent position with a dim light behind their head and instructed to remain awake, as opposed to the MSLT in which the subject is lying flat and instructed to fall asleep. Performing polysomnography on the night before the MWT is optional, as is the use of certain medications that may affect the ability to fall asleep or remain awake. Finally, the definition of trial termination on the MWT differs from the MSLT. A given MWT trial is terminated after 40 minutes of no sleep or after unequivocal sleep occurs, which is defined by 3 consecutive epochs of stage N1 sleep or 1 epoch of any other stage of sleep.

Similar to the MSLT, the sleep latency on the MWT is calculated for each trial, and an MSL is calculated for all 4 trials at the end of the day. So what is a normal MSL on the MWT? Using limited pooled normative data from 5 studies for the 40-minute protocol, normal individuals demonstrate an MSL of 30.4 ± 11.2 minutes. These data are not normally distributed, with 43% of normal individuals being able to remain awake for 40 minutes on all 4 trials. Using 2 standard deviations from the mean, an MSL of less than 8 minutes is considered abnormal. Values between 8 and 40 minutes are considered to be of uncertain significance, and being able to remain awake for 40 minutes on all 4 tests is considered to be most representative of normal.[3] There are limited normative data using other protocols of shorter duration. Using a 20-minute protocol, normal individuals demonstrate an MSL of 18.1 ± 3.6 minutes, with a lower limit of normal being 10.8 minutes.[35,36]

Untreated patients with narcolepsy demonstrate an MSL of 6.0 ± 4.8 minutes using the 20-minute protocol.[34] Fifteen percent of the patients with narcolepsy have an MSL of more than 12 minutes, but unlike normal individuals, only 1.5% of narcoleptics are able to remain awake for 20 minutes on all 4 trials. Little normative data are available for other clinical patient populations.

Although the MWT is indicated to assess an individual's ability to remain awake for a defined period of time and assess a response to a given therapy, it has questionable use in clinical practice. There is no established threshold MSL value or magnitude of change among sequential tests that has been demonstrated to be clinically significant or consistently predict safety in the work place or while driving.[3] Studies in patients with narcolepsy assessing the effects of various stimulants on wakefulness have demonstrated improvements in the MSL ranging from 2 to 10 minutes.[37-40] Studies evaluating the use of modafinil and armodafinil in patients with OSA with residual daytime sleepiness despite the use of continuous positive airway pressure (CPAP) have demonstrated objective improvements in the MSL on the MWT, ranging from 1.1 to 1.9 minutes compared with baseline.[41,42] These results demonstrate that the range of improvement in various clinical populations is relatively small. The relevance of these findings remains unclear as mentioned previously, as there is no threshold value of improvement that has been determined to be clinically significant.

The MSL on the MWT demonstrates consistently greater values at baseline when compared with the MSL on the MSLT in normal individuals and in various clinical populations.[43,44] These results highlight the importance of understanding the concept that the tendency to fall asleep as measured by the MSLT and the ability to stay awake as measured by the MWT represent 2 distinct physiologic processes.[44] These differences may in part be secondary to the directions given before each test.[45] Before performing the MSLT, subjects are instructed to try to fall asleep, whereas before the MWT, subjects are instructed to try to stay awake. Thus, patient motivation and expectations can influence test results.

Responses to interventions meant to improve alertness are also consistently different when comparing the MWT with the MSLT. Under similar testing conditions, the MSL on the MWT consistently demonstrates statistically significant improvements in response to interventions meant to improve alertness as opposed to the MSL on the MSLT, which tends to show little change with similar interventions.[44,46] This difference in response to interventions that are meant to improve alertness between the MWT and MSLT is related to the different physiologic processes that each test is measuring. The consistent improvement in MSL values on the MWT to various interventions focused on improving wakefulness make the MWT the more commonly used measurement assay in research protocols.

As is the case with the MSL on the MSLT, the predictive value of the MSL from the MWT in real world situations is not established. The MSL on the MWT shows little correlation with the severity of OSA as defined by the respiratory disturbance index.[47] Most patients with severe OSA are able to remain awake for 40 minutes on all 4 trials. The ability of the MSL on the MWT to predict safety in the work place or while driving under research and real world conditions has not been consistently established.[3,48,49] Given that normal values and clinically significant threshold values for change for the MSL on the MWT are not well defined, the MSL on the MWT should not be used to determine the presence or severity of excessive sleepiness, response to treatment, or ability to predict safety in real world situations.

In clinical practice, the MWT has little utility as the MSL on the MWT has little correlation with driving safety, and like the MSL on the MSLT, the predictive value of the MSL on the MWT in real world situations has not been established.[3] Its utility in research lies in its ability to measure different physiologic tendencies from the MSLT. Specifically, the MWT consistently demonstrates more robust improvements to interventions that increase alertness when compared with the MSLT. The utility of the MWT in research has its limitations because normal values and threshold values that define clinically significant improvement are not clear.

OSLER TEST

The Oxford Sleep Resistance (OSLER) test is a simplified version of the MWT.[50] Similar to the MWT, subjects are asked to lie in a semirecumbent position in a quiet and darkened room for a maximum testing time of 40 minutes per session. A total of 4 sessions are conducted at 2-hour intervals. Instead of determining the onset of sleep by EEG criteria, the presence of sleep is assessed behaviorally. Subjects sit in front of a light emitting diode screen that flashes a light regularly at 3-second intervals. The subjects are instructed to touch a button every time they see the light flash. The test is terminated after 7 consecutive flashes (21 seconds) without a response. The 21-second threshold was chosen because it corresponds to the minimal sleep duration generally used to score 1 epoch of sleep when using standard sleep scoring rules.[51] Priest and colleagues[51]

demonstrated that the OSLER test has a sensitivity and specificity of 85% and 94%, respectively, for detecting sleep of more than 3 seconds in duration. An MSL is calculated in a fashion similar to that of the MWT. The MSLs on the MWT and OSLER test are highly correlated in both normal individuals and in clinical populations, although most studies evaluating the OSLER test have been performed in relatively small samples.[52,53]

Compared to the MWT, the OSLER test offers the advantages of simplicity, lower cost, automatic reading, and lower technical requirements for personnel. One disadvantage is the inability to detect the presence of REM sleep during daytime naps. This is not a significant disadvantage; as similar to the MWT, the main purpose of the OSLER test is to assess an individual's ability to remain awake for a defined period of time, and it is not used as part of the evaluation for suspected narcolepsy. The OSLER test is currently not widely used in clinical medicine, although it is increasingly being used in research protocols given its ease of use and excellent correlation with the MWT.[54–57] Further testing in larger samples of normal subjects and different disease populations are required to confirm its validity and reliability.

PSYCHOMOTOR VIGILANCE TESTING

PVT has become one of the most widely used measures of behavioral alertness in research protocols.[58–60] The PVT assesses sustained or vigilant attention by measuring response times to visual or auditory stimuli that occur at random intervals. Subjects sit in front of a screen for 10-minute testing periods and are instructed to respond to stimuli that occur at random intervals. Response times to stimuli are calculated within trials and across testing periods that occur throughout the day. The PVT has been shown to be a valid and sensitive measure of both acute and chronic sleep loss. Studies have demonstrated that varying degrees of sleep deprivation result in reliable changes in PVT performance, with a high test-retest reliability that is consistently above 0.8.[58] Ongoing total and chronic partial sleep deprivation result in an overall slowing of responses. In response to sleep deprivation there is a steady increase in errors of omission, characterized by lapses of attention with absent or late responses to stimuli and a modest increase in errors of commission, characterized by "false starts" or responses that occur without stimuli.

EPWORTH SLEEPINESS SCALE

The ESS was first published in 1991 and was designed to measure subjective sleep propensity as it occurs in ordinary life situations.[61] It is currently the most-used subjective test of daytime sleepiness in clinical practice. The questionnaire describes 8 situations as follows:

- Sitting and reading,
- Watching television,
- Sitting inactively in a public place,
- Riding as a passenger in a car for 1 hour without a break,
- Lying down to rest in the afternoon when circumstances permit,
- Sitting and talking with someone,
- Sitting quietly after lunch without alcohol, and
- Sitting in a car as the driver while stopped for a few minutes in traffic.

The participant scores the likelihood of falling asleep in each situation on a scale of 0 to 3:

- 0 = would never doze,
- 1 = slight chance of dozing,
- 2 = moderate chance of dozing, and
- 3 = high chance of dozing.

The total ESS score can range from 0 through 24, with higher scores correlating with increasing degrees of subjective sleepiness (**Fig. 5**).

What value defines the threshold of normal and abnormal on the ESS? In its original description, a score of greater than 10 was determined to be consistent with excessive daytime sleepiness. This cutoff between normal and abnormal subjective sleepiness was derived from the original study's control group data, which demonstrated a mean ESS score of 5.9 ± 2.2.[61] In the original description, individual ESS scores of greater than 16 were seen only in individuals with narcolepsy, idiopathic hypersomnia, and in patients with moderate to severe OSA. Primary snorers, patients with insomnia, and patients with periodic limb movements demonstrated ESS scores that were not significantly different from that of controls.[61]

ESS results may be affected by several factors other than sleep duration and underlying sleep disorder. Gander and colleagues[62] demonstrated that Epworth values of greater than 10 were independently associated with male gender, lower socioeconomic status, and greater body mass index in certain populations. Data from the Sleep Heart Health Study (SHHS) have shown that while men have higher Epworth scores than age-matched women, younger age (age ≤65 years) has been associated with significantly lower scores.[63] Ethnicity may also affect Epworth results, with African Americans demonstrating higher scores when compared with age-matched Caucasians.[64] In a follow-up report by Johns[65] evaluating the reproducibility of the ESS in normal individuals (87 healthy medical students), the mean ESS score was 7.4 ± 3.9. In the SHHS that evaluated 1824 subjects with a mean age of

Epworth Sleepiness Scale (ESS)

How likely are you to doze off or fall asleep in the following situations, in contrast to feeling just tired? This refers to your usual way of life in recent times.

0 = would *never* doze
1 = *slight* chance of dozing
2 = *moderate* chance of dozing
3 = *high* chance of dozing

Situation	Chance of dozing
1) Sitting and Reading	_____
2) Watching TV	_____
3) Sitting, inactive in a public place (e.g. a theater or a meeting)	_____
4) As a passenger in a car for an hour without a break	_____
5) Lying down to rest in the afternoon when circumstances permit	_____
6) Sitting and talking to someone	_____
7) Sitting quietly after a lunch without alcohol	_____
8) In a car, while stopped for a few minutes in the traffic	_____

Fig. 5. Epworth sleepiness scale. (*Data from* Johns M. A new method of measuring daytime sleepiness: the Epworth sleepiness scale. Sleep 1991;14(6):540–5.)

65 ± 11 years, the mean ESS in patients without OSA (respiratory disturbance index [RDI] <5) was 7.2 ± 4.3. Using 2 standard deviations above the mean, the upper limits of normal in these patient groups would range from 15.2 to 15.8, respectively.[63] Thus, defining normal depends on several factors and using a cutoff threshold of 10 for everyone may not be valid.

It should be emphasized that there is significant controversy as to the validity of the ESS.[66–68] Although in its original descriptions[61,69] the ESS demonstrated a strong correlation (−0.514; $P<.01$) with results of the mean sleep latency test, subsequent studies have demonstrated that the ESS has little or no correlation to MSL values on the MSLT.[67,68,70] One group demonstrated that the sleep propensity as measured by the MSLT was significantly related to only 3 of the 8 items (sitting inactive in a public place, sitting quietly after lunch, and sitting in a car stopped for a few minutes in the traffic) on the ESS.[69] Using these 3 items from the ESS, the correlation between the MSLT and ESS was significant, with an $r = 0.64$. Further research has also demonstrated weak correlations with considerable discordant results between the MWT and the ESS in patients with sleep apnea and narcolepsy.[71,72] The reasons for the lack of strong association between the ESS and sleep latency on the MSLT and MWT are unclear, but it is likely that these tests measure different, but complimentary aspects of sleepiness.

One of the main reasons for this discrepancy between the ESS and objective measures of sleepiness was the lack of large scale population-based studies assessing the relationship between the ESS and the results of the MSLT. Punjabi and colleagues[73] used a population-based sample from the Wisconsin Sleep Cohort Study to better assess this question. They demonstrated that individuals with intermediate (6–11) and high (>12) ESS scores had a 30% and 69% increased risk for sleep onset during the 4 naps of the MSLT, respectively. They concluded that the ESS was moderately associated with objective sleep tendency. These findings help to confirm the validity of the ESS as a measure of sleep propensity.

Most of the studies assessing the reliability of the ESS have been done in normal individuals who have normal ESS scores (≤10) at baseline.[65,69] These studies in normal individuals have demonstrated that the results are reproducible over durations of up to 5 months and across various cultures. Data evaluating the reliability in patients with untreated OSA have demonstrated conflicting results. Nguyen and colleagues[74] evaluated a large group of patients with untreated OSA who had Epworth testing at their initial evaluation and an average of 75 days later. Although the mean difference for the entire group between testing periods was only 0.08, the Bland-Altman analysis demonstrated significant individual variability in results across the spectrum of Epworth scores that was not associated with the severity of disease as defined by the RDI. Forty percent of the patients demonstrated discrepancies in results of greater than or equal to 3 and 23% demonstrated discrepancies in results of greater than or equal to 5 between testing periods. Other data in patients with untreated OSA have demonstrated variability in the Epworth results depending on the method of test administration.[75] Specifically, administration of the test by a physician resulted in values that were significantly lower than those obtained during self-administration. Because many studies in various clinical populations use changes in Epworth scores as a primary outcome measurement, results from Nguyen, Kaminska, and others call in to question the reproducibility of the Epworth value, as well as what may represent clinically and statistically significant changes after a given intervention.

The utility of the ESS in clinical practice, especially in patients with OSA, is also of questionable value. Data from the SHHS have consistently demonstrated that although there is a dose-dependent increase in ESS values with increasing severity of OSA, the minority of patients with OSA demonstrate subjective sleepiness as defined by an ESS score of greater than 10.[63] Only 35% of patients with severe OSA, as defined by an RDI of greater than 30, have Epworth scores of greater than 10. Even when subjective sleepiness is defined more broadly as having an Epworth score greater than 10 or feeling sleepy or unrested, most patients with untreated OSA do not demonstrate significant subjective sleepiness across the spectrum of disease severity.[76] Thus, the ESS is not a reliable screening tool for OSA because it is neither sensitive nor specific for the diagnosis. In patients with OSA, responses to treatment with CPAP that are based on the Epworth score may also show individual variability that is not necessarily dependent of nightly CPAP compliance.[77,78] Although these studies have demonstrated a dose-dependent improvement in subjective sleepiness in association with greater nightly CPAP compliance, a substantial minority of patients show improvement with little nightly CPAP use (≤2 hours) and a significant proportion of patients who use their CPAP for 7 hours or greater per night continue to demonstrate abnormal subjective sleepiness as defined by the Epworth scale.

Stanford Sleepiness Scale (SSS)

Circle the <u>one</u> number that best describes your level of alertness or sleepiness right now:

1) Feeling active, vital, alert, wide awake.
2) Functioning at a high level but not at peak, able to concentrate.
3) Relaxed, awake but not fully alert, responsive.
4) A little foggy, let down.
5) Foggy, beginning to lose track, difficulty in staying awake.
6) Sleep, prefer to lie down, woozy.
7) Almost in reverie, cannot stay awake, sleep onset appears imminent.

Fig. 6. Stanford sleepiness scale. (*Data from* Hoddes E, Zarcone V, Smythe H, et al. Quantification of sleepiness: a new approach. Psychophysiology 1973;10:431–6.)

STANFORD SLEEPINESS SCALE

Among the subjective measures of sleepiness, the SSS is the best validated.[79] Respondents choose 1 of 7 statements that best describe their current state of sleepiness (**Fig. 6**). The list of statements includes the following:

- Feeling active and vital, alert, wide awake;
- Functioning at a high level, but not at peak, able to concentrate;
- Relaxed, awake, not at full alertness, responsive;
- A little foggy, not at peak, let down;
- Fogginess, beginning to lose interest in remaining awake, slowed down;
- Sleepiness, prefer to be lying down, fighting sleep, woozy;
- Almost in reverie, sleep onset soon, losing struggle to remain awake.

The advantages of the SSS are that it (1) can be administered at multiple times throughout the day and night, (2) correlates with standard measures of performance, and (3) reflects the effect of sleep loss.

Although the SSS is the best-validated subjective measure of sleepiness, its utility in clinical practice is limited. Although the SSS has been demonstrated to be a valid measure of subjective sleepiness in individuals undergoing acute total sleep deprivation, its ability to accurately measure changes that occur with chronic partial sleep deprivation has been called in to question. Van Dongen and colleagues[60] demonstrated that although chronic partial sleep restriction over a 14-day period resulted in cumulative dose-dependent deficits in neurocognitive performance, subjective sleepiness ratings as assessed by the SSS showed little change over time, suggesting that subjects were largely unaware of these increasing deficits. Other disadvantages of the SSS include the absence of normal reference values, a response spectrum that may not be linear to a given degree of sleep loss, and its inability to differentiate sleep-deprived normal subjects from those individuals with sleep disorders. Finally, SSS has limited utility in clinical practice because it only conveys information about a patient's state of sleepiness at single points in time.

KAROLINSKA SLEEPINESS SCALE

The KSS developed at the Karolinska Institute in Sweden, is a subjective measure of sleepiness that is somewhat similar to the SSS.[80] Respondents choose 1 of 9 statements that best describe their current state of sleepiness from 1 = "very alert" to 9 = "very sleepy, great effort to stay awake". The KSS has been validated against EEG, and behavioral parameters and scores of greater than or euqal to 7 are considered pathologic.[80,81] Studies have demonstrated that its sensitivity to sleepiness is similar to the SSS. The KSS has similar limitations to the SSS and thus has limited utility in clinical practice.

SUMMARY

There is much debate concerning which of many objective and subjective tests of daytime sleepiness is best for use in clinical practice. The following is an overview of the tests reviewed in this article, their limitations, and potential indications in clinical practice and research settings:

- The MSLT is indicated to help support a diagnosis of narcolepsy or idiopathic hypersomnia in the proper clinical setting, although the utility of this test is mainly based on the presence of SOREMPs and not the MSL. It is not indicated in the evaluation of other patient populations nor do the results predict safety in real world situations.
- The utility of the MWT is limited in clinical practice; as like the MSLT, its results do not predict safety in real world situations. Its utility in research lies in its ability to measure different physiologic tendencies from the MSLT. Specifically, the MWT consistently demonstrates more robust improvements to interventions that increase alertness when compared with the MSLT. The utility of the MWT in research has its limitations, as normal values and threshold values that define clinically significant improvement are not clear.
- The OSLER test is a modified version of the MWT that measures the sleep onset via behavioral outcomes. The MSL results correlate highly with the MWT in normal individuals and clinical populations. Given its ease of use and lower cost, it is being used more frequently in clinical research. Further testing in larger samples of normal subjects and different disease populations is required to confirm its validity and reliability. Like the MWT, its utility is limited in clinical practice.
- PVT assesses sustained or vigilant attention by measuring response times to visual or auditory stimuli that occur at random intervals. The PVT has been shown to be a valid and reliable measure of both acute and chronic sleep loss. Its use is mainly limited to research settings.
- The ESS measures subjective sleepiness as it applies to everyday life, and it is currently the most used subjective test of daytime sleepiness in clinical practice. Its utility in clinical practice has limitations, as normal values may vary by population, and its results may be affected by several factors. Its utility in the diagnosis and management of patients with OSA is also limited, as it is neither sensitive nor specific for the diagnosis, with most patients across the spectrum of disease severity having Epworth values of less than 10.

- The SSS is the best-validated subjective measure of sleepiness, especially in individuals subjected to acute total sleep deprivation. It has limited use in clinical practice as it only conveys information about a patient's state of sleepiness at a single point in time. Other limitations include the absence of normal reference values, a response spectrum that may not be linear to a given degree of sleep loss, questionable validity in the measurement of the effects of chronic partial sleep deprivation, and its inability to differentiate sleep-deprived normal subjects from those individuals with true sleep disorders.
- The KSS demonstrates a sensitivity to subjective sleepiness that is similar to the SSS. The KSS has similar limitations to the SSS and thus has limited utility in clinical practice.
- None of the described tests accurately predict safety in real world situations, and they do not accurately differentiate sleepiness in normal individuals from sleepiness in patients with various sleep disorders.
- The correlation of results between objective and subjective tests of sleepiness is in many cases inconsistent. The discrepancies in results may be because of several confounding factors, including individual responses and perceptions.
- Objective and subjective tests likely assess different dimensions of sleepiness, and aside from using the MSLT, which is indicated as part of the evaluation of patients with suspected narcolepsy or idiopathic hypersomnia, the best test for a given situation remains to be defined.
- Typically, a combination of subjective and objective testing in combination with the clinical history is necessary to best determine the degree and clinical significance of a given patient's daytime sleepiness.

REFERENCES

1. Carskadon M, Dement W, Mitler M, et al. Guidelines for the multiple sleep latency test (MSLT): a standard measure of sleepiness. Sleep 1986;9:519–24.
2. Zwyghuizen-Doorenbos A, Roehrs T, Schaefer M, et al. Test-retest reliability of the MSLT. Sleep 1988; 11(6):562–5.
3. Littner MR, Kushida C, Wise M, et al. Practice parameters for clinical use of the multiple sleep latency test and the maintenance of wakefulness test. Sleep 2005;28(1):113–21.
4. Thorpy MJ. The clinical use of the Multiple Sleep Latency Test. The Standards of Practice Committee

of the American Sleep Disorders Association. Sleep 1992;15(3):268–76.

5. Lumley M, Roehrs T, Asker D, et al. Ethanol and caffeine effects on daytime sleepiness/alertness. Sleep 1987;19:306–12.

6. Carskadon M, Dement W. Multiple sleep latency test during the constant routine. Sleep 1992;15(5):396–9.

7. Levine B, Roehrs T, Stepanski E, et al. Fragmenting sleep diminishes its recuperative value. Sleep 1987; 10:590–9.

8. Carskadon M, Dement W. Nocturnal determinants of daytime sleepiness. Sleep 1982;5(Suppl 2): S73–81.

9. Richardson G, Carskadon M, Orav E, et al. Circadian variation of sleep tendency in elderly and young adult subjects. Sleep 1982;5:S82–94.

10. Aldrich M, Chervin R, Malow B. Value of the multiple sleep latency test (MSLT) for the diagnosis of narcolepsy. Sleep 1997;20(8):620–9.

11. Benbadis SR, Perry MC, Wolgamuth BR, et al. The multiple sleep latency test: comparison of sleep onset criteria. Sleep 1996;19(8):632–6.

12. Drake CL, Rice MF, Roehrs TA, et al. Scoring reliability of the multiple sleep latency test in a clinical population. Sleep 2000;23(7):911–3.

13. Golish JA, Sarodia BD, Blanchard AR, et al. Prediction of the final MSLT result from the results of the first three naps. Sleep Med 2002;3(3):249–53.

14. Clodore M, Benoit O, Foret J, et al. The Multiple Sleep Latency Test: individual variability and time of day effect in normal young adults. Sleep 1990; 13(5):385–94.

15. Czeisler C, Zimmerman J, Ronda J, et al. Timing of REM sleep coupled to the circadian rhythm of body temperature in man. Sleep 1980;2:329–46.

16. Bonnet M, Arand D. Sleepiness as measured by the MSLT varies as a function of preceding activity. Sleep 1998;21:477–83.

17. Bonnet MH, Arand DL. Arousal components which differentiate the MWT from the MSLT. Sleep 2001; 24(4):441–7.

18. Bonnet MH. ACNS clinical controversy: MSLT and MWT have limited clinical utility. J Clin Neurophysiol 2006;23(1):50–8.

19. Bonnet M, Arand D. Activity, arousal and the MSLT in patients with insomnia. Sleep 2000;23(2):205–12.

20. Stepanski E, Zorick F, Roehrs T, et al. Effects of sleep deprivation on daytime sleepiness in primary insomnia. Sleep 2000;23(2):215–9.

21. Stepanski E, Zorick F, Roehrs T, et al. Daytime alertness in patients with chronic insomnia compared with asymptomatic control subjects. Sleep 1988; 11:54–60.

22. Schneider-Helmert D. Twenty-four-hour sleep-wake function and personality patterns in chronic insomniacs and healthy controls. Sleep 1987;10: 452–62.

23. Carskadon M, Dement W. Cumulative effects of sleep restriction on daytime sleepiness. Psychophysiology 1981;18:107–13.

24. Drake C, Roehrs T, Breslau N, et al. The 10-year risk of verified motor vehicle crashes in relation to physiologic sleepiness. Sleep 2010;33(6): 745–52.

25. Vernet C, Arnulf I. Idiopathic hypersomnia with and without long sleep time: a controlled series of 75 patients. Sleep 2009;32(6):753–9.

26. Anderson KN, Pilsworth S, Sharples LD, et al. Idiopathic hypersomnia: a study of 77 cases. Sleep 2007;30(10):1274–81.

27. American Academy of Sleep Medicine. The international classification of sleep disorders: diagnostic and coding manual. 2nd edition. Westchester (IL): American Academy of Sleep Medicine; 2005.

28. Coelho FM, Georgsson H, Murray BJ. Benefit of repeat multiple sleep latency testing in confirming a possible narcolepsy diagnosis. J Clin Neurophysiol 2011;28(4):412–4.

29. Chervin RD, Aldrich MS. Sleep onset REM periods during multiple sleep latency tests in patients evaluated for sleep apnea. Am J Respir Crit Care Med 2000;161(2 Pt 1):426–31.

30. Bishop C, Rosenthal L, Helmus T, et al. The frequency of multiple sleep onset REM periods among subjects with no excessive daytime sleepiness. Sleep 1996;19(9):727–30.

31. Singh M, Drake CL, Roth T. The prevalence of multiple sleep-onset REM periods in a population-based sample. Sleep 2006;29(7):890–5.

32. Mignot E, Lin L, Finn L, et al. Correlates of sleep-onset REM periods during the Multiple Sleep Latency Test in community adults. Brain 2006; 129(Pt 6):1609–23.

33. Mitler MM, Gujavarty KS, Browman CP. Maintenance of wakefulness test: a polysomnographic technique for evaluation treatment efficacy in patients with excessive somnolence. Electroencephalogr Clin Neurophysiol 1982;53(6):658–61.

34. Mitler MM, Walsleben J, Sangal RB, et al. Sleep latency on the maintenance of wakefulness test (MWT) for 530 patients with narcolepsy while free of psychoactive drugs. Electroencephalogr Clin Neurophysiol 1998;107(1):33–8.

35. Doghramji K, Mitler MM, Sangal RB, et al. A normative study of the maintenance of wakefulness test (MWT). Electroencephalogr Clin Neurophysiol 1997;103(5):554–62.

36. Mitler MM, Doghramji K, Shapiro C. The maintenance of wakefulness test: normative data by age. J Psychosom Res 2000;49(5):363–5.

37. Schwartz JR, Feldman NT, Bogan RK, et al. Dosing regimen effects of modafinil for improving daytime wakefulness in patients with narcolepsy. Clin Neuropharmacol 2003;26(5):252–7.

38. Moldofsky H, Broughton RJ, Hill JD. A randomized trial of the long-term, continued efficacy and safety of modafinil in narcolepsy. Sleep Med 2000;1(2): 109–16.

39. Broughton RJ, Fleming JA, George CF, et al. Randomized, double-blind, placebo-controlled crossover trial of modafinil in the treatment of excessive daytime sleepiness in narcolepsy. Neurology 1997;49(2):444–51.

40. Black J, Houghton WC. Sodium oxybate improves excessive daytime sleepiness in narcolepsy. Sleep 2006;29(7):939–46.

41. Black JE, Hirshkowitz M. Modafinil for treatment of residual excessive sleepiness in nasal continuous positive airway pressure-treated obstructive sleep apnea/hypopnea syndrome. Sleep 2005;28(4): 464–71.

42. Roth T, White D, Schmidt-Nowara W, et al. Effects of armodafinil in the treatment of residual excessive sleepiness associated with obstructive sleep apnea/hypopnea syndrome: a 12-week, multicenter, double-blind, randomized, placebo-controlled study in nCPAP-adherent adults. Clin Ther 2006;28(5): 689–706.

43. Sangal RB, Thomas L, Mitler MM. Maintenance of wakefulness test and multiple sleep latency test. Measurement of different abilities in patients with sleep disorders. Chest 1992;101(4): 898–902.

44. Sangal R, Thomas L, Milter M. Disorders of excessive sleepiness. Treatment improves ability to stay awake but does not reduce sleepiness. Chest 1992;102:699–703.

45. Hartse K, Roth T, Zorick F. Daytime sleepiness and daytime wakefulness: the effect of instruction. Sleep 1982;5:S107–18.

46. Patel SR, White DP, Malhotra A, et al. Continuous positive airway pressure therapy for treating sleepiness in a diverse population with obstructive sleep apnea: results of a meta-analysis. Arch Intern Med 2003;163(5):565–71.

47. Arzi L, Shreter R, El-Ad B, et al. Forty- versus 20-minute trials of the maintenance of wakefulness test regimen for licensing of drivers. J Clin Sleep Med 2009;5(1):57–62.

48. Philip P, Sagaspe P, Taillard J, et al. Maintenance of Wakefulness Test, obstructive sleep apnea syndrome, and driving risk. Ann Neurol 2008;64(4):410–6.

49. Sagaspe P, Taillard J, Chaumet G, et al. Maintenance of wakefulness test as a predictor of driving performance in patients with untreated obstructive sleep apnea. Sleep 2007;30(3):327–30.

50. Bennett LS, Stradling JR, Davies RJ. A behavioural test to assess daytime sleepiness in obstructive sleep apnoea. J Sleep Res 1997;6(2):142–5.

51. Priest B, Brichard C, Aubert G, et al. Microsleep during a simplified maintenance of wakefulness test. A validation study of the OSLER test. Am J Respir Crit Care Med 2001;163(7):1619–25.

52. Mazza S, Pepin JL, Deschaux C, et al. Analysis of error profiles occurring during the OSLER test: a sensitive mean of detecting fluctuations in vigilance in patients with obstructive sleep apnea syndrome. Am J Respir Crit Care Med 2002; 166(4):474–8.

53. Krieger AC, Ayappa I, Norman RG, et al. Comparison of the maintenance of wakefulness test (MWT) to a modified behavioral test (OSLER) in the evaluation of daytime sleepiness. J Sleep Res 2004;13(4): 407–11.

54. Cross MD, Vennelle M, Engleman HM, et al. Comparison of CPAP titration at home or the sleep laboratory in the sleep apnea hypopnea syndrome. Sleep 2006;29(11):1451–5.

55. West SD, Jones DR, Stradling JR. Comparison of three ways to determine and deliver pressure during nasal CPAP therapy for obstructive sleep apnea. Thorax 2006;61(3):226–31.

56. Nussbaumer Y, Bloch KE, Genser T, et al. Equivalence of autoadjusted and constant continuous positive airway pressure in home treatment of sleep apnea. Chest 2006;129(3):638–43.

57. Vennelle M, White S, Riha RL, et al. Randomized controlled trial of variable-pressure versus fixed-pressure continuous positive airway pressure (CPAP) treatment for patients with obstructive sleep apnea/hypopnea syndrome (OSAHS). Sleep 2010; 33(2):267–71.

58. Basner M, Dinges DF. Maximizing sensitivity of the psychomotor vigilance test (PVT) to sleep loss. Sleep 2011;34(5):581–91.

59. Dinges DF, Pack F, Williams K, et al. Cumulative sleepiness, mood disturbance, and psychomotor vigilance performance decrements during a week of sleep restricted to 4-5 hours per night. Sleep 1997;20(4):267–77.

60. Van Dongen HP, Maislin G, Mullington JM, et al. The cumulative cost of additional wakefulness: dose-response effects on neurobehavioral functions and sleep physiology from chronic sleep restriction and total sleep deprivation. Sleep 2003; 26(2):117–26.

61. Johns M. A new method of measuring daytime sleepiness: the Epworth Sleepiness Scale. Sleep 1991;14(6):540–5.

62. Gander PH, Marshall NS, Harris R, et al. The Epworth Sleepiness Scale: influence of age, ethnicity, and socioeconomic deprivation. Epworth Sleepiness scores of adults in New Zealand. Sleep 2005; 28(2):249–53.

63. Gottlieb DJ, Whitney CW, Bonekat WH, et al. Relation of sleepiness to respiratory disturbance index: the Sleep Heart Health Study. Am J Respir Crit Care Med 1999;159(2):502–7.

64. Whitney CW, Enright PL, Newman AB, et al. Correlates of daytime sleepiness in 4578 elderly persons: the Cardiovascular Health Study. Sleep 1998;21(1):27–36.

65. Johns MW. Reliability and factor analysis of the Epworth Sleepiness Scale. Sleep 1992;15(4):376–81.

66. Johns M. Sensitivity and specificity of the multiple sleep latency test (MSLT), the maintenance of wakefulness test and the epworth sleepiness scale: failure of the MSLT as the gold standard. J Sleep Res 2000;9(1):5–11.

67. Chervin RD, Aldrich MS. The Epworth Sleepiness Scale may not reflect objective measures of sleepiness or sleep apnea. Neurology 1999;52(1):125–31.

68. Chervin RD, Aldrich MS, Pickett R, et al. Comparison of the results of the Epworth Sleepiness Scale and the Multiple Sleep Latency Test. J Psychosom Res 1997;42(2):145–55.

69. Johns M. Sleepiness in different situations measured by the Epworth Sleepiness Scale. Sleep 1994;17(8):703–10.

70. Benbadis SR, Mascha E, Perry MC, et al. Association between the Epworth sleepiness scale and the multiple sleep latency test in a clinical population. Ann Intern Med 1999;130(4 Pt 1):289–92.

71. Sangal R, Sangal J, Belisle C. Subjective and objective indices of sleepiness (ESS and MWT) are not equally useful in patients with sleep apnea. Clin Electroencephalogr 1999;30(2):73–5.

72. Sangal RB, Mitler MM, Sangal JM. Subjective sleepiness ratings (Epworth sleepiness scale) do not reflect the same parameter of sleepiness as objective sleepiness (maintenance of wakefulness test) in patients with narcolepsy. Clin Neurophysio 1999;110(12):2131–5.

73. Punjabi NM, Bandeen-Roche K, Young T. Predictors of objective sleep tendency in the general population. Sleep 2003;26(6):678–83.

74. Nguyen AT, Baltzan MA, Small D, et al. Clinical reproducibility of the Epworth Sleepiness Scale. J Clin Sleep Med 2006;2(2):170–4.

75. Kaminska M, Jobin V, Mayer P, et al. The Epworth Sleepiness Scale: self-administration versus administration by the physician, and validation of a French version. Can Respir J 2010;17(2):e27–34.

76. Kapur VK, Baldwin CM, Resnick HE, et al. Sleepiness in patients with moderate to severe sleep-disordered breathing. Sleep 2005;28(4):472–7.

77. Weaver TE, Maislin G, Dinges DF, et al. Relationship between hours of CPAP use and achieving normal levels of sleepiness and daily functioning. Sleep 2007;30(6):711–9.

78. Antic NA, Catcheside P, Buchan C, et al. The effect of CPAP in normalizing daytime sleepiness, quality of life, and neurocognitive function in patients with moderate to severe OSA. Sleep 2011;34(1):111–9.

79. Hoddes E, Zarcone V, Smythe H, et al. Quantification of sleepiness: a new approach. Psychophysiology 1973;10:431–6.

80. Kaida K, Takahashi M, Akerstedt T, et al. Validation of the Karolinska sleepiness scale against performance and EEG variables. Clin Neurophysiol 2006;117(7):1574–81.

81. van den Berg J, Neely G, Nilsson L, et al. Electroencephalography and subjective ratings of sleep deprivation. Sleep Med 2005;6(3):231–40.

Neurochemistry and Biomarkers of Narcolepsy and Other Primary and Secondary Hypersomnias

Seiji Nishino, MD, PhD[a],*, Carl Deguzman[a],
Wataru Yamadera, MD, PhD[a], Shintaro Chiba, MD, PhD[a],
Takashi Kanbayashi, MD, PhD[b]

KEYWORDS

- Narcolepsy • Biomarkers • Hypocretin/orexin • EDS • Idiopathic hypersomnia • Histamine • CSF

KEY POINTS

- The recent progress for understanding the pathophysiology of EDS owes itself to the discovery of hypocretin ligand deficiency in human narcolepsy.
- The hypocretin deficiency can be clinically detected by CSF hypocretin-1 measures, and low CSF hypocretin-1 levels have been included in the 2nd revision of the International Classifications of Sleep Disorder as a positive diagnosis for narcolepsy-cataplexy.
- The pathophysiology of symptomatic EDS likely overlaps with that of primary hypersomnia, including recently identifying MS/NMO cases with bilateral symmetric hypothalamic damage.
- The pathophysiology of idiopathic hypersominia is largely unknown, but hypocretin deficiency is not likely be involved in this condition.
- Decreased histaminergic neurotransmission is observed in narcolepsy and idiopathic hypersomnia, regardless of hypocretin-deficient status.
- Although much progress was made regarding the pathophysiology of EDS, the new knowledge is not yet incorporated for the development of new treatments.

INTRODUCTION

This article discusses the neurochemistry and biomarkers of hypersomnia (or excessive daytime sleepiness [EDS]). Although no systematic epidemiologic study has been conducted, available data suggest that hypersomnia (both primary and secondary) is common but underdiagnosed; both types of hypersomnia significantly reduce the quality of life of the subjects. Narcolepsy-cataplexy, narcolepsy without cataplexy, and idiopathic hypersomnia (a primary hypersomnia not associated with rapid eye movement [REM] sleep abnormalities) are 3 major primary hypersomnias,[1] but substantial clinical overlap among these disorders has been noted, because each disorder is currently diagnosed mostly by sleep phenotypes and not by biologic/pathophysiologic tests. Similarly, secondary hypersomnia is a heterogeneous disease entity and the biologic/pathophysiologic mechanisms underlying the secondary hypersomnia are mostly unknown.

[a] Stanford University Sleep and Circadian Neurobiology Laboratory, Department of Psychiatry and Behavioral Sciences, Stanford University School of Medicine, 3165 Porter Drive, Room 1195, Palo Alto, CA 94304, USA; [b] Department of Neuropsychiatry, Akita University Graduate School of Medicine, 1-1-1 Hondo, Akita, 010-8543, Japan
* Corresponding author.
E-mail address: nishino@stanford.edu

Sleep Med Clin 7 (2012) 233–248
doi:10.1016/j.jsmc.2012.03.015
1556-407X/12/$ – see front matter © 2012 Published by Elsevier Inc.

Recent progress in understanding the pathophysiology of EDS has stemmed from the discovery of narcolepsy genes (ie, hypocretin receptor and peptide genes) in animals in 1999 and the subsequent discovery (in 2000) of hypocretin ligand deficiency (ie, loss of hypocretin neurons in the brain) in idiopathic cases of human narcolepsy-cataplexy. The hypocretin deficiency can be clinically detected by cerebrospinal fluid (CSF) hypocretin-1 measures; low CSF hypocretin-1 levels are seen in more than 90% of patients with narcolepsy-cataplexy. Because the specificity of the CSF finding is also high (no hypocretin deficiency was seen in patients with idiopathic hypersomnia), low CSF hypocretin-1 levels have been included in the second revision of the International Classifications of Sleep Disorder (ICSD) as a positive diagnosis for narcolepsy-cataplexy.

Narcolepsy-cataplexy is tightly associated with human leukocyte antigen (HLA) DQB1*0602. Hypocretin deficiency in narcolepsy-cataplexy is also tightly associated with HLA positivity, suggesting an involvement of immune-mediated mechanisms for the loss of hypocretin neurons. However, the specificity of HLA positivity for narcolepsy-cataplexy is lower than that of low CSF hypocretin-1 levels, because up to 30% of the general population shares this HLA haplotype. Therefore, low CSF hypocretin-1 level is the first biomarker established for a prototypical hypersomnia, narcolepsy-cataplexy.

The prevalence of primary hypersomnia, such as narcolepsy and idiopathic hypersomnia, is not high (0.05% and 0.005%, respectively), but the prevalence of symptomatic (secondary) hypersomnia may be much higher. For example, several million subjects in the United States suffer from chronic brain injury, 75% of those people have sleep problems, and about half claim sleepiness.[2] Symptomatic narcolepsy has also been reported, but the prevalence of symptomatic narcolepsy is smaller, and only about 120 cases of symptomatic narcolepsy have been reported in the literature in the past 30 years. The meta-analysis of these symptomatic cases indicates that hypocretin deficiency may also partially explain the neurochemical mechanisms of EDS associated with symptomatic cases of narcolepsy and EDS.[3]

Anatomic and functional studies show that the hypocretin systems integrate and coordinate the multiple wake-promoting systems, such as monoamine and acetylcholine systems, to keep people fully alert,[4] suggesting that an understanding of the roles of hypocretin peptidergic systems in sleep regulation in normal and pathologic conditions is important, because alternations of these systems may also be responsible for narcolepsy and for other less defined hypersomnia.

Histamine is one of these wake-active monoamines, and low CSF histamine levels are also found in narcolepsy with hypocretin deficiency.[5,6] Because hypocretin neurons project and excite histamine neurons in the posterior hypothalamus, it is conceivable that impaired histamine neurotransmission may mediate sleep abnormalities in hypocretin-deficient narcolepsy. However, low CSF histamine levels were also observed in narcolepsy with normal hypocretin levels, and, in idiopathic hypersomnia, decreased histamine neurotransmission may be involved in a broader category of EDS than in hypocretin-deficient narcolepsy.[6] Because CSF histamine levels are normalized in patients with EDS treated with wake-promoting compounds, low CSF histamine levels may be a new state marker for the hypersomnia of central origin, and functional significances of this finding should be studied further.[6]

Greater knowledge about the neurochemistry and biomarkers of EDS will likely lead to the development of new diagnostic tests as well as new treatments and management of patients with hypersomnia of various causes.

NEUROBIOLOGY OF WAKEFULNESS

To help in the understanding of the neurochemistry of hypersomnia, this article discusses current understanding of the neurobiology of wakefulness. Sleep/wake is a complex physiology regulated by brain activity, and multiple neurotransmitter systems such as monoamines, acetylcholine, excitatory and inhibitory amino acids, peptides, purines, and neuronal and nonneuronal humoral modulators (ie, cytokines and prostaglandins)[7] are likely to be involved. Monoamines are perhaps the first neurotransmitters recognized to be involved in wakefulness,[8] and the monoaminergic systems have been the most common pharmacologic targets for wake-promoting compounds in the past years. Nevertheless, most hypnotics target the γ-aminobutyric acid (GABA)–ergic system, a main inhibitory neurotransmitter system in the brain.[9]

Cholinergic neurons also play critical roles in cortical activation during wakefulness (and during REM sleep).[7] Brainstem cholinergic neurons originating from the laterodorsal and pedunculopontine tegmental nuclei activate thalamocortical signaling, and cortex activation is further reinforced by direct cholinergic projections from the basal forebrain. However, currently no cholinergic compounds are used in sleep medicine, perhaps because of the complex nature of the systems and prominent peripheral side effects.

Monoamine neurons, such as norepinephrine (NE)-containing locus coeruleus neurons, serotonin (5-HT)-containing raphe neurons, and histamine-containing tuberomammillary neurons (TMN) are wake-active and act directly on cortical and subcortical regions to promote wakefulness.[7] In contrast with the focus on these wake-active monoaminergic systems, researchers have often underestimated the importance of dopamine (DA) in promoting wakefulness. Most likely, this is because the firing rates of midbrain DA-producing neurons (ventral tegmental area [VTA] and substantia nigra) do not have an obvious variation according to behavioral states.[10] In addition, DA is produced by many different cell groups,[11] and which of these promote wakefulness remains undetermined. Nevertheless, DA release is greatest during wakefulness,[12] and DA neurons increase discharge and tend to fire bursts of action potentials in association with significant sensory stimulation, purposive movement, or behavioral arousal.[13] Lesions that include the dopaminergic neurons of the VTA reduce behavioral arousal.[14] Recent work has also identified a small wake-active population of DA-producing neurons in the ventral periaqueductal gray that project to other arousal regions.[15] People with DA deficiency from Parkinson disease are often sleepy,[16] and DA antagonists (or small doses of DA autoreceptor [D2/3] agonists) are frequently sedating. These physiologic and clinical findings show that DA also plays a role in wakefulness.

Wakefulness (and various physiologies associated with wakefulness) is essential for the survival of creatures and thus is likely to be regulated by multiple systems, each having a distinct role. Some arousal systems may have essential roles for cortical activation, attention, cognition, or neuroplasticity during wakefulness, whereas others may only be active during specific times to promote particular aspects of wakefulness. Some of the examples may be motivated-behavioral wakefulness or wakefulness in emergency states. Wakefulness may thus likely be maintained by many systems with differential but coordinated roles. Similarly, the wake-promoting mechanism of some drugs may not explained by a single neurotransmitter system.

BASIC SLEEP PHYSIOLOGY AND SYMPTOMS OF NARCOLEPSY

To help understanding the neurochemistry of hypersomnia, basic sleep physiology and symptoms of narcolepsy are briefly discussed. Because narcolepsy is a prototypical EDS disorder and because the major pathophysiology of narcolepsy

(ie, deficient in hypocretin neurotransmission) has recently been revealed, a discussion of neurochemical aspects of narcolepsy contributes to a general understandings of neurochemistry in EDS.

Patients with narcolepsy manifest symptoms specifically related to dysregulation of REM sleep.[7] In the structured, cyclic process of normal sleep, 2 distinct states (REM and 4 stages using the previously standardized Rechtschaffen and Kales sleep stages: S1, S2, S3, S4 of non-REM [NREM] sleep) alternate sequentially every 90 minutes in a cycle repeating 4 to 5 times per night.[8] As electroencephalogram signals in humans indicate, NREM sleep, characterized by slow oscillation of thalamocortical neurons (detected as cortical slow waves) and muscle tonus reduction, precedes REM sleep, when complete muscle atonia occurs. Slow wave NREM predominates during the early phase of normal sleep, followed by a predominance of REM during the later phase.[8]

Sleep and wake are highly fragmented in narcolepsy, and affected individuals cannot maintain long bouts of wake and sleep. Normal sleep physiology is currently understood as dependent on coordination of the interactions of facilitating sleep centers and inhibiting arousal centers in the brain, such that stable sleep and wake states are maintained for specific durations.[8] An ascending arousal pathway, running from the rostral pons and through the midbrain reticular formation, promotes wakefulness.[8,9] As discussed earlier, this arousal pathway may be composed of neurotransmitters (acetylcholine, NE, DA, excitatory amino acids), produced by brainstem and hypothalamic neurons (hypocretin/orexin and histamine), and also linked to muscle tonus control during sleep.[8,9] Although full alertness and cortical activation require coordination of these arousal networks, effective sleep requires suppression of arousal by the hypothalamus.[9] Patients with narcolepsy may experience major neurologic malfunction of this control system.

Narcoleptics exhibit a phenomenon, termed short REM sleep latency or sleep onset REM period (SOREMP), in which REM sleep is entered more immediately on falling asleep than is normal.[7] In some cases, NREM sleep is completely bypassed and the transition to REM sleep occurs instantly.[7] SOREMPs are not observed in idiopathic hypersomnia.

Moreover, intrusion of REM sleep into wakefulness may explain the cataplexy, sleep paralysis, and hypnogogic hallucinations that are symptomatic of narcolepsy. However, although sleep paralysis and hypnogogic hallucinations manifest in other sleep disorders (sleep apnea syndromes and disturbed sleep patterns in normal populations),[10] cataplexy is pathognomic for narcolepsy.[7] As such, identifying the unique pathophysiologic mechanism of cataplexy emerged as potentially crucial to describing the mechanisms underlying narcolepsy overall.

DISCOVERY OF HYPOCRETIN DEFICIENCY AND POSTNATAL CELL DEATH OF HYPOCRETIN NEURONS

The significant roles, first of hypocretin deficiency, and, subsequently, of postnatal cell death of hypocretin neurons as the major pathophysiologic processes underlying narcolepsy with cataplexy emerged from a decade of investigation, using both animal and human models. In 1998, the simultaneous discovery by 2 independent research groups of a novel hypothalamic peptide neurotransmitter (variously named hypocretin and orexin) proved pivotal.[11,12] These neurotransmitters are produced exclusively by thousands of neurons that are localized in the lateral hypothalamus (LHT) and project broadly to specific cerebral regions and, more densely, to others.[13]

Within a year, Stanford researchers, using positional cloning of a naturally occurring familial canine narcolepsy model, identified an autosomal recessive mutation of hypocretin receptor (Hcrtr)

2, responsible for canine narcolepsy, characterized by cataplexy, reduced sleep latency, and SOREMPs.[14] This finding coincided with the simultaneous observation of the narcolepsy phenotype, characterized by cataplectic behavior and sleep fragmentation, in hypocretin ligand–deficient mice (prepro-orexin gene knockout mice).[15] Together, these findings confirmed hypocretins as principal sleep-modulating neurotransmitters and prompted investigation of the involvement of the hypocretin system in human narcolepsy.

Although screening of patients with cataplexy failed to implicate hypocretin-related gene mutation as a major cause of human narcolepsy, narcoleptic patients did exhibit low CSF hypocretin-1 levels (**Fig. 1**).[16] Postmortem brain tissue of narcoleptic patients, assessed through immunochemistry, radioimmunologic peptide assays, and in situ hybridization, revealed hypocretin peptides loss and undetectable levels of hypocretin peptides or preprohypocretin RNA (see **Fig. 1**). Melanin-concentrating hormone neurons, normal to the same brain region,[17] were observed intact, thus indicating that damage to hypocretin neurons and production is selective in narcolepsy, rather than being caused by generalized neuronal degeneration.

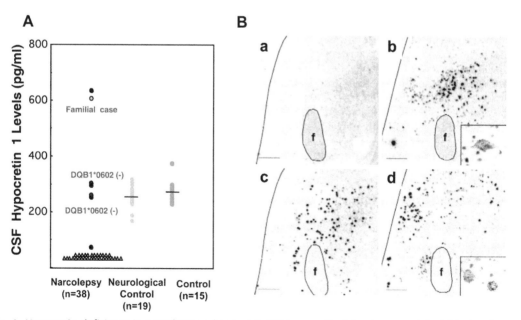

Fig. 1. Hypocretin deficiency in narcoleptic subjects. (*A*) CSF hypocretin-1 levels are undetectably low in most narcoleptic subjects (84.2%). Note that 2 HLA DQB1*0602-negative and 1 familial case have normal or high CSF hypocretin levels. (*B*) Preprohypocretin transcripts are detected in the hypothalamus of control (b) but not in narcoleptic subjects (a). Melanin-concentrating hormone (MCH) transcripts are detected in the same region in both control (d) and narcoleptic (c) sections. f and fx, fornix. Scale bar represents 10 mm (a–d). (*Data from* Peyron C, Faraco J, Rogers W, et al. A mutation in a case of early onset narcolepsy and a generalized absence of hypocretin peptides in human narcoleptic brains. Nat Med 2000;6(9):991–7.)

As a result of these findings, a diagnostic test for narcolepsy, based on clinical measurement of CSF hypocretin-1 levels for detecting hypocretin ligand deficiency, is now available.[1] Although CSF hypocretin-1 concentrations of more than 200 pg/mL almost always occur in controls and patients with other sleep and neurologic disorders, concentrations less than 110 pg/mL are 94% predictive of narcolepsy with cataplexy (**Fig. 2**).[18] Because this represents a more specific assessment than the multiple sleep latency test (MSLT), CSF hypocretin-1 levels less than 110 pg/mL are indicated in the International Classification of Sleep Disorders, second edition (ICSD-2), as diagnostic of narcolepsy with cataplexy.[1]

Moreover, separate coding of narcolepsy with cataplexy and narcolepsy without cataplexy in the ICSD-2 underscores how discovery of specific diagnostic criteria now informs understanding of the nosology of narcolepsy; narcolepsy with cataplexy, as indicated by low CSF hypocretin-1, seems etiologically homogenous and distinct from most patients with narcolepsy without cataplexy, exhibiting normal hypocretin levels.[18] Moreover, the potential of hypocretin receptor agonists (or cell transplantation) in narcolepsy treatment is currently being explored for the hypocretin ligand deficient narcolepsy, and CSF hypocretin-1 measures may be useful in identifying appropriate patients for a novel therapeutic option, namely hypocretin replacement therapy.

Soon after the discovery of human hypocretin deficiency, researchers identified specific substances and genes, such as dynorphin and neuronal activity-regulated pentraxin (NARP),[19] and, most recently, insulinlike growth factor binding protein 3 (IGFBP3),[20] which colocalize in neurons containing hypocretin. These findings underscored

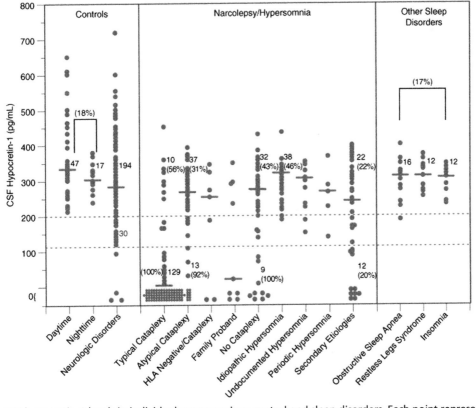

Fig. 2. CSF hypocretin-1 levels in individuals across various control and sleep disorders. Each point represents the crude concentration of hypocretin-1 in a single person. The cutoffs for normal (>200 pg/mL) and low (<110 pg/mL) hypocretin-1 concentrations are shown. Also noted is the total number of subjects in each range, and the percentage HLA-DQB1*0602 positivity for a given group in a given range is parenthetically noted for certain disorders. Note that control carrier frequencies for DQB1*0602 are 17% to 22% in healthy control subjects and secondary narcolepsy, consistent with control values reported in white people. In other patient groups, values are higher, with almost all hypocretin-deficient narcolepsy being HLA DQB1*0602 positive. The median value in each group is shown as a horizontal bar. (*Data from* Mignot E, Lammers GJ, Ripley B, et al. The role of cerebrospinal fluid hypocretin measurement in the diagnosis of narcolepsy and other hypersomnias. Arch Neurol 2002;59(10):1553–62.)

selective hypocretin cell death as the cause of hy-pocretin deficiency (as opposed to transcription/biosynthesis or hypocretin peptide processing problems) because these substances are also defi-cient in postmortem brain LHT of hypocretin-deficient narcoleptic patients.[19,20] In view of the generally late onsets of sporadic narcolepsy compared with those of familial cases, these find-ings suggest that postnatal cell death of hypocretin neurons constitutes the major pathophysiologic process in human narcolepsy with cataplexy.

Because neurons containing dynorphin, NARP, and IGFBP3, are also located outside the LHT (and colocalize with other neurotransmitters), it is unlikely that measurements of these substances can be used for biomarkers for narcolepsy.[21]

CONSIDERATIONS FOR THE PATHOPHYSIOLOGY OF NARCOLEPSY WITH NORMAL HYPOCRETIN LEVELS

There are debates about the pathophysiology of narcolepsy with normal hypocretin levels. More than 90% patients with narcolepsy without cata-plexy show normal CSF hypocretin levels, but they show apparent REM sleep abnormalities (ie, SOREMPs). Furthermore, even if the strict criteria for narcolepsy-cataplexy are applied, up to 10% of patients with narcolepsy-cataplexy show normal CSF hypocretin levels. Considering that occurrence of cataplexy is tightly associated with hypocretin deficiency, impaired hypocretin neurotransmission is still likely involved in narcolepsy with normal CSF hypocretin levels. Conceptually, there are 2 possibilities to explain these mechanisms: specific impairment of hypocretin receptors and their down-stream pathway and partial/localized loss of hypo-cretin ligand (but still exhibit normal CSF levels). A good example for the first is Hcrtr 2 mutated narco-leptic dogs, which exhibit normal CSF hypocretin-1 levels,[22] but have narcolepsy. Thannickal and colleagues[23] recently reported on a patient with narcolepsy without cataplexy (HLA typing was unknown) who had an overall loss of 33% of hypo-cretin cells compared with normal, with maximal cell loss in the posterior hypothalamus. This result favors the second hypothesis, but studies with more cases are needed.

IDIOPATHIC HYPERSOMNIA, HYPOCRETIN NONDEFICIENT PRIMARY HYPERSOMNIA

With the clear definition of narcolepsy (cataplexy and dissociated manifestations of REM sleep), it became apparent that some patients with hyper-somnia suffer from a different disorder. Bedrich Roth[24] was the first in the late 1950s and early 1960s to describe a syndrome characterized by EDS, prolonged sleep, and sleep drunkenness, and the absence of sleep attacks, cataplexy, sleep paralysis, and hallucinations. The terms indepen-dent sleep drunkenness and hypersomnia with sleep drunkenness were initially suggested,[24] but they are now categorized as idiopathic hypersom-nia with and without long sleep time.[1] Idiopathic hypersomnia should not be considered synony-mous with hypersomnia of unknown origin.

In the absence of systematic studies, the preva-lence of idiopathic hypersomnia is unknown. Noso-logic uncertainty causes difficulty in determining the epidemiology of the disorder. Recent reports from large sleep centers reported the ratio of idio-pathic hypersomnia to narcolepsy to be 1:10.[25] The age of onset of symptoms varies, but it is frequently between 10 and 30 years. The condition usually develops progressively over several weeks or months. Once established, symptoms are generally stable and long lasting, but spontaneous improvement in EDS may be observed in up to one-quarter of patients.[25]

The pathogenesis of idiopathic hypersomnia is unknown. Hypersomnia usually starts insidiously. EDS is occasionally first experienced after tran-sient insomnia, abrupt changes in sleep-wake habits, overexertion, general anesthesia, viral ill-ness, or mild head trauma.[25] Despite reports of an increase in HLA DQ1, 11 DR5, and Cw2, and DQ3, and of a decrease of Cw3, no consistent findings have emerged.[25]

The most recent attempts to understand the pathophysiology of idiopathic hypersomnia relate to the potential role of the hypocretins. However, most studies suggest normal CSF levels of hypo-cretin-1 in idiopathic hypersomnia.[18,26]

NOSOLOGIC AND DIAGNOSTIC CONSIDERATIONS OF MAJOR PRIMARY HYPERSOMNIAS

Narcolepsy-cataplexy, narcolepsy without cata-plexy, and idiopathic hypersomnia are diagnosed mostly by sleep phenotypes, especially by occur-rences of cataplexy and SOREMPs (Fig. 3). Discovery of hypocretin deficiency in narcolepsy-cataplexy was a breakthrough but also brought a new nosologic and diagnostic uncertainty of the primary hypersomnias. Up to 10% of patients with narcolepsy-cataplexy show normal CSF hy-pocretin-1 levels (see Fig. 3). As discussed earlier, altered hypocretin neurotransmissions may still be involved in some of these cases. However, up to 10% of patients with narcolepsy without cataplexy instead show low CSF hypocretin-1 levels, sug-gesting a substantial pathophysiologic overlap

MAJOR HYPERSOMNIAS OF CENTRAL ORIGIN
Cataplexy and MSLT findings

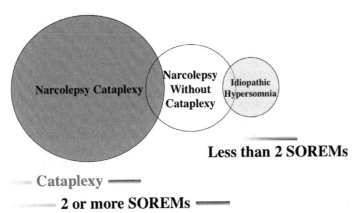

Fig. 3. Nosologic and diagnostic considerations of major primary hypersomnias. Narcolepsy-cataplexy, narcolepsy without cataplexy, and idiopathic hypersomnia are diagnosed by occurrences of cataplexy and sleep onset REM period (SOREMP). Pathophysiology-based marker, low CSF hypocretin levels are included in the ICSD-2 for the positive diagnosis for narcolepsy-cataplexy. However, up to 10% of patients with narcolepsy-cataplexy show normal CSF hypocretin levels. In contrast, up to 10% of patients with narcolepsy without cataplexy show low CSF hypocretin-1 levels. These results suggest a substantial pathophysiologic overlap between narcolepsy-cataplexy and narcolepsy without cataplexy. Similarly, a substantial overlap likely exist between narcolepsy without cataplexy and idiopathic hypersomnia, because these disorders are diagnosed by the occurrences of SOR-EMP (2 or more). However, test-retest reliability of detecting number of SOREMPs in these conditions has not been systematically evaluated.

between narcolepsy-cataplexy and narcolepsy without cataplexy, and the hypocretin-deficient status (measured in CSF) does not completely separate these 2 disease conditions (see **Fig. 3**). Similarly, concerns about the nosology of narcolepsy without cataplexy and idiopathic hypersomnia should also be addressed. Because patients with typical cases of idiopathic hypersomnia exhibit unique symptoms, such as long hours of sleep, no refreshment from naps, and general resistance to stimulant medications, the pathophysiology of idiopathic hypersomnia may be distinct from that of narcolepsy without cataplexy. However, current diagnostic criteria are not specific enough to diagnose these disorders, especially because the test-retest reliability of numbers of SOREMPs during MSLT have not been systematically evaluated.

HOW DOES HYPOCRETIN LIGAND DEFICIENCY CAUSE THE NARCOLEPSY PHENOTYPE?

Because hypocretin deficiency is a major pathophysiologic mechanism for narcolepsy-cataplexy,

this article includes a discussion of how the hypocretin ligand deficiency can cause the narcolepsy phenotype.

Hypocretin/Orexin System and Sleep Regulation

Hypocretins/orexins were discovered by 2 independent research groups in 1998. One group called the peptides hypocretin because of their primary hypothalamic localization and similarities with the hormone secretin.[12] The other group called the molecules orexin after observing that central administration of these peptides increased appetite in rats.[11]

Hypocretins/orexins (hypocretin-1 and hypocretin-2/orexin A and orexin B) are cleaved from a precursor preprohypocretin (prepro-orexin) peptide).[11,12,27] Hypocretin-1 with 33 residues contains 4 cysteine residues forming 2 disulfide bonds. Hypocretin-2 consists of 28 amino acids and shares similar sequence homology, especially at the C-terminal side, but has no disulfide bonds (a linear peptide).[11] There are 2 G-protein–coupled hypocretin receptors, Hcrtr 1 and Hcrtr 2, also called orexin receptor 1 and 2 (OX$_1$R and OX$_2$R), and distinct distribution of these receptors in the brain is known. Hcrtr 1 is abundant in the locus coeruleus (LC), whereas Hcrtr 2 is found in the TMN and basal forebrain. Both receptor types are found in the midbrain raphe nuclei and mesopontine reticular formation.[4]

Hypocretin-1 and hypocretin-2 are produced exclusively by a well-defined group of neurons localized in the LHT. The neurons project to the olfactory bulb, cerebral cortex, thalamus, hypothalamus, and brainstem, particularly the LC, raphe nucleus, and to the cholinergic nuclei (the laterodorsal tegmental and pedunculopontine tegmental nuclei) and cholinoceptive sites (such as pontine reticular formation) thought to be important for sleep regulation.[13,27]

A series of recent studies have now shown that the hypocretin system is a major excitatory system that affects the activity of monoaminergic (DA, NE, 5-HT, and histamine) and cholinergic systems with major effects on vigilance states.[27,28] It is thus likely that a deficiency in hypocretin neurotransmission induces an imbalance between these classic neurotransmitter systems, with primary effects on sleep-state organization and vigilance.

Many measurable activities (brain and body) and compounds manifest rhythmical fluctuations over a 24-hour period. Whether or not hypocretin tone changes with zeitgeber time was assessed by measuring extracellular hypocretin-1 levels in the rat brain CSF across 24-hour periods, using in vivo dialysis.[29] The results show the involvement of a slow diurnal pattern of hypocretin neurotransmission regulation (as in the homeostatic and/or circadian regulation of sleep). Hypocretin levels increase during, and are highest at the end of, the active periods, and the levels decline with the onset of sleep. Furthermore, sleep deprivation increases hypocretin levels.[29]

Recent electrophysiologic studies have shown that hypocretin neurons are active during wakefulness and reduce the activity during slow wave.[30] The neuronal activity during REM sleep is the lowest, but intermittent increases in the activity associated with body movements or phasic REM activity are observed.[30] In addition to this short-term change, the results of microdialysis experiments also suggest that basic hypocretin neurotransmission fluctuates across the 24-hour period and slowly builds up toward the end of the active period. Adrenergic LC neurons are typical wake-active neurons involved in vigilance control, and it has recently been shown that basic firing activity of wake-active LC neurons also significantly fluctuates across various circadian times.[31]

Several acute manipulations such as exercise, low glucose use in the brain, and forced wakefulness increase hypocretin levels.[28,29] It is therefore hypothesized that a buildup/acute increase of hypocretin levels may counteract the homeostatic sleep propensity that typically increases during the daytime and during forced wakefulness.[32]

Hypocretin/Orexin Deficiency and Narcoleptic Phenotype

Human studies have shown that the occurrence of cataplexy is closely associated with hypocretin deficiency.[18] Furthermore, the hypocretin deficiency was already observed at early stages of the disease (just after the onset of EDS), even before the occurrences of clear cataplexy. Occurrences of cataplexy are rare in acute symptomatic cases of EDS associated with a significant hypocretin deficiency[3]; it seems that a chronic and selective deficit of hypocretin neurotransmission may be required for the occurrence of cataplexy. The possibility of involvement of a secondary neurochemical change for the occurrence of cataplexy cannot be ruled out. If some of these changes are irreversible, hypocretin supplement therapy may only have limited effects on cataplexy.

Sleepiness in narcolepsy is most likely caused by the difficulty in maintaining wakefulness as normal people do. The sleep pattern of narcoleptics is also fragmented; they exhibit insomnia (frequent wakening) at night. This fragmentation occurs across 24 hours, and, thus, the loss of hypocretin signaling is likely to play a role in this vigilance stage stability,[33] but other mechanisms may also be involved in EDS in narcoleptics. One of the most important characteristics of EDS in narcolepsy is that sleepiness is reduced, and patients feel refreshed after a short nap, but this does not last long and they become sleepy within a short period of time. Hypocretin-1 levels in the extracellular space and in the CSF of rats significantly fluctuate across 24 hours, and build up toward the end of the active periods.[32] Several manipulations (such as sleep deprivation, exercise, and long-term food deprivation) are also known to increase hypocretin tonus.[29,32] Thus, the lack of this hypocretin buildup (or increase) caused by circadian time and by various alerting stimulations may also play a role for EDS associated with hypocretin-deficient narcolepsy.

Mechanisms for cataplexy and REM sleep abnormalities associated with impaired hypocretin neurotransmission have been studied. Because hypocretin strongly inhibits REM sleep and local application of hypocretin activates both brainstem

REM-inactive LC and raphe neurons and REM-active cholinergic neurons, as well as local GABAergic neurons, disfacilitation of (REM-inactive) monoaminergic neurons and disinhibition of (REM-active) cholinergic neurons mediated through disfacilitation of inhibitory GABAergic inter neurons associated with impaired hypocretin neurotransmission are proposed for abnormal manifestations of REM sleep.

NEUROCHEMISTRY IN SYMPTOMATIC NARCOLEPSY AND EDS: HYPOCRETIN INVOLVEMENTS

Narcolepsy symptoms can also occur during the course of other neurologic conditions (eg, symptomatic narcolepsy), and discovery of hypocretin ligand deficiency in idiopathic narcolepsy has led to new insights into the pathophysiology of symptomatic (or secondary) narcolepsy and EDS. In a recent meta-analysis, 116 symptomatic narcolepsy cases reported in the literature were analyzed.[3] As several investigators have previously reported, inherited disorder (n = 38), tumors (n = 33), and head trauma (n = 19) are the 3 most frequent causes for symptomatic narcolepsy. Of the 116 cases, 10 were associated with multiple sclerosis (MS), 1 with acute disseminated encephalomyelitis, and few with vascular disorders (n = 6), encephalitis (n = 4), degeneration (n = 1), and heterodegenerative disorder (autosomal dominant cerebrospinal ataxia with deafness, 3 cases in 1 family). Although it is difficult to rule out the comorbidity of idiopathic narcolepsy in some cases, literature review reveals numerous unquestionable cases of symptomatic narcolepsy.[3] These include HLA-negative and/or late-onset cases and cases in which occurrence of narcoleptic symptoms parallels the progress of the causative disease. The review of these cases (particularly those with brain tumors) clearly shows that the hypothalamus is most often involved.[3]

In addition, many EDS cases without cataplexy or REM sleep abnormalities (defined as symptomatic cases) are associated with these neurologic conditions.[3] Although the same review lists about 70 symptomatic EDS cases, prevalence of symptomatic EDS is likely much higher. For example, several million people in the United States suffered chronic brain injury, 75% experienced sleep problems, and about 50% reported sleepiness.[2] Thus, symptomatic EDS may have significant clinical relevance.

CSF hypocretin-1 measurement was also conducted in these symptomatic narcolepsy and EDS cases, and reduced CSF hypocretin-1 levels were noted in most, with various causes.[3] EDS in these cases is sometimes reversible with an improvement of the causative neurologic disorder or hypocretin-deficient status, thus suggesting a functional link between hypocretin deficiency and sleep symptoms in these patients.

Low CSF hypocretin-1 concentrations were also found in some immune-mediated neurologic conditions, namely subsets of Guillain-Barre syndrome,[34] Ma2-positive paraneoplastic syndrome[35] and MS,[3] and EDS are often associated with patients with low CSF hypocretin-1 levels.

Kanbayashi and colleagues[36] recently reported 7 cases of EDS occurring in the course of MS in patients initially diagnosed with symmetric hypothalamic inflammatory lesions together with hypocretin ligand deficiency that contrasts with the characteristics of classic MS (**Fig. 4**).

Symptomatic narcolepsy in patients with MS was reported several decades ago. Because both MS and narcolepsy are associated with the HLA-DR2 positivity, an autoimmune target on the same brain structures has been proposed to be a common cause for both diseases.[37] However, the discovery of the selective loss of hypothalamic hypocretin neurons in narcolepsy indicates that narcolepsy coincidently occurs in patients with MS when MS plaques appear in the hypothalamic area and secondarily damage the hypocretin/orexin neurons. In favor of this interpretation, the hypocretin system is not impaired in patients with MS who do not exhibit narcolepsy.[38] Nevertheless, a subset of patients with MS predominantly shows EDS and REM sleep abnormalities, and it is likely that specific immune-mediated mechanisms may be involved in these cases.

CSF hypocretin measures revealed that marked (≤110 pg/mL, n = 3) or moderate (110–200 pg/mL, n = 4) hypocretin deficiency was observed in all 7 cases.[36] Therefore, 4 cases met with ICSD-2 criteria[1] for narcolepsy caused by a medical condition, and 3 cases met criteria for hypersomnia caused by a medical condition. Four of them had either optic neuritis and spinal cord lesions, or both, sharing the clinical characteristics of neuromyelitis optica (NMO). HLA was evaluated in only 2 cases (case 2 and case 4) and was negative for DQB1*0602. Repeated evaluations of the hypocretin status were performed in 6 cases, and CSF hypocretin-1 levels returned to normal or significantly increased with marked improvements of EDS and hypothalamic lesions in all 6 cases. Because 4 of them showed clinical characterization of NMO, anti-AQP4 antibody was evaluated and 3 out of 7 cases were anti-AQP4 antibody positive, and were thus diagnosed as having an NMO-related disorder.[36]

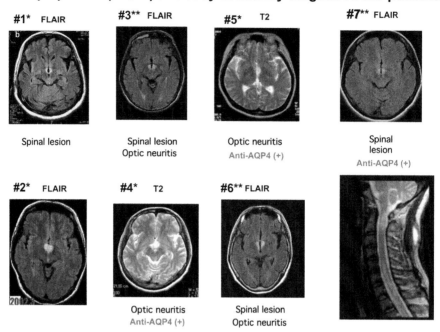

Fig. 4. Magnetic resonance imaging (MRI) findings (fluid-attenuated inversion recovery or T2) of patients with MS/neuromyelitis optica (NMO) with hypocretin deficiency and EDS. A typical horizontal slice including the hypothalamic periventricular area from each case is presented. All cases were female. *, met with ICSD-2 criteria for narcolepsy caused by a medical condition; **, met with ICSD-2 criteria for hypersomnia caused by a medical condition. All cases were initially diagnosed as MS. Cases 3 to 7 had optic neuritis and/or spinal cord lesions and cases 4, 5, and 7 are seropositive for anti-AQP4 antibody and thus were diagnosed as NMO. (*Data from* Kanbayashi T, Shimohata T, Nakashima I, et al. Symptomatic narcolepsy in MS and NMO patients; new neurochemical and immunologic implications. Arch Neurol 2009;66:1563–6.)

AQP4, a member of the AQP superfamily, is an integral membrane protein that forms pores in the membrane of biologic cells.[39] Aquaporins selectively conduct water molecules in and out of the cell while preventing the passage of ions and other solutes, and are known as water channels. AQP4 is expressed throughout the central nervous system, especially in periaqueductal and periventricular regions,[39,40] and is found in nonneuronal structures such as astrocytes and ependymocytes, but is absent from neurons. Recently, NMO-IgG, which can be detected in the serum of patients with NMO, has been shown to selectively bind to AQP4.[41]

Because AQP4 is enriched in periventricular regions in the hypothalamus, where hypocretin-containing neurons are primarily located, symmetric hypothalamic lesions associated with reduced CSF hypocretin-1 levels in our 3 NMO cases with anti-AQP4 antibody might be caused by the immunoattack to the AQP4, and this may secondarily affect the hypocretin neurons.

However, the other 4 MS cases with EDS and hypocretin deficiency were anti-AQP4 antibody negative at the time of blood testing, which leaves a possibility that other antibody-mediated mechanisms are additionally responsible for the bilateral symmetric hypothalamic damage causing EDS in the MS/NMO subjects. There is also a possibility that the 4 MS cases whose anti-AQP4 antibody was negative could be NMO, because anti-AQP4 antibody was tested only once for each subject during the course of the disease and the assay was not standardized among the institutes.[36] It is thus essential to further determine the immunologic mechanisms that cause the bilateral hypothalamic lesions with hypocretin deficiency and EDS, and their association with NMO and AQP4. This effort may lead to establishment of a new clinical entity, and the knowledge is essential to prevent and treat EDS associated with MS and its related disorders. None of these cases had cataplexy, contrary to the 9 out of 10 symptomatic narcoleptic MS cases reported in the past.[3] Early therapeutic intervention with steroids and other immunosuppressants may thus prevent irreversible damage of hypocretin neurons and prevent chronic sleep-related symptoms.

CHANGES IN OTHER NEUROTRANSMITTER SYSTEMS IN NARCOLEPSY AND IDIOPATHIC HYPERSOMNIA

Narcolepsy in Dogs and Humans

Studies in humans with narcolepsy have shown a decrease in dopamine concentration in the CSF.[42] Studies on Hcrtr 2 mutated narcoleptic dogs performed before and after probenecid administration showed an increased turnover of monoamines with significantly less free homovanillic acid (HVA), dihydroxyphenylacetic acid (DOPAC), 3-methoxy-4-hydroxyphenylglycol (MHPG), and 5-hydroxyindoleacetic acid (5-HIAA).[43]

The lower concentration of 5-HIAA in the CSF of narcoleptic dogs suggests a decreased concentration of the parent amine 5-HT, a decreased turnover of 5-HT in the brain, or both. Similarly, the lower steady-state CSF of 5-HIAA and HVA, as well as the reduced accumulation of 5-HIAA and HVA after probenecid, suggests decreased dopamine concentration, decreased turnover, or both. In addition, the lower concentration of MHPG after probenecid administration suggests decreased NE activity.

Analyses of both human and animal narcoleptic brain tissue also suggest dopaminergic dysfunction. In postmortem human autoradiographic studies, striatal DA D2 receptor binding was increased in narcolepsy, more so than for D1 receptors.[44] However, most in vivo studies with single-photon emission computed tomography[45] and positron emission tomography[46] found no increase in striatal D2 receptor binding in narcolepsy.

Pharmacologic studies showed that narcoleptic canines are sensitive to α-1b blockade and α-2 stimulation (as well as DA D2/D3 stimulation) and exhibit cataplexy.[7] They are also sensitive to cholinergic M2/3 stimulation and have cataplexy, and upregulation of muscarinic receptors in the pons was reported.[7]

Three independent studies reported altered catecholamine contents in the brains of narcoleptic dogs.[43,47] The studies found an increase in DA and NE in many brain structures, especially DA in the amygdala and NE in the pontis reticularis oralis.[43,47] These changes are not caused by a reduction in the turnover of these monoamines, because the turnover of these monoamines is high or not altered.[48] Considering that the drugs that enhance dopaminergic neurotransmission

(such as amphetaminelike stimulants and modafinil for EDS) and NE neurotransmission (such as noradrenaline uptake blockers for cataplexy) are needed to treat the symptoms in these animals,[7] increases in DA and NE contents may be compensatory, either mediated by Hcrtr 1 or by other neurotransmitter systems, but these findings are inconsistent with the CSF findings.

Most of these abnormalities are likely secondary to the deficiency in hypocretin neurotransmission, but alterations in these systems may actively mediate some of the sleep-related symptoms of narcolepsy.

The most recent neurochemical studies in canine narcolepsy specifically pointed out the involvement of histamine in narcolepsy. Histamine content in the brain was measured in genetically narcoleptic (n = 9) and control Dobermans (n = 9). For reference, contents of DA, NE, and 5-HT and their metabolites were also measured.[48] The histamine content in the cortex and thalamus (the areas important in the control of wakefulness via histaminergic input) was significantly lower in narcoleptic Dobermans compared with controls. The brain tissue was collected during the daytime, and separate sleep studies showed that sleep amounts of narcoleptic dogs during the daytime do not significantly differ (but are more fragmented) from those in control dogs,[49] suggesting that these changes are not simply secondary to the change in sleep amount in these animals.

Considering that hypocretins strongly excite TMN histaminergic neurons in vitro through Hcrtr2 stimulation,[50,51] the decrease in histaminergic content found in narcoleptic dogs may be caused by the lack of excitatory input of hypocretin on TMN histaminergic neurons. Uncompensated low histamine levels in narcolepsy may suggest that the hypocretin system may be the major excitatory input to histaminergic neurons (through Hcrtr2).

Histamine in the brains was also measured in 3 sporadic (ligand-deficient) narcoleptic dogs, and the histamine content in these animals was also as low as in the Hcrtr2-mutated narcoleptic Dobermans,[48] thus suggesting that a decrease in histamine neurotransmission may also exist in ligand-deficient human narcolepsy.

Idiopathic Hypersomnia

CSF analyses in idiopathic hypersomnia have shown normal cell counts, cytology, and protein content. Montplaisir and colleagues[42] found a decrease in dopamine and indoleacetic acid in both patients with idiopathic hypersomnia and with narcolepsy. Faull and colleagues[52] found similar mean concentrations of monoamine metabolites in subjects with narcolepsy or idiopathic hypersomnia and with controls, but, using a principal component analysis, they also found a dysregulation of the DA system in narcolepsy and of the NE system in idiopathic hypersomnia. These metabolic data may support the hypothesis of a primary deficient arousal system in patients with idiopathic hypersomnia.

HISTAMINE AND HYPERSOMNIA
Hypocretin/Histamine Interactions were Emphasized After the Discovery of the Involvement of the Hypocretin System in Narcolepsy

Research evidence suggests that central histaminergic neurotransmission is involved in the control of vigilance (see Ref.[53] for review). It is widely known that histaminergic H1 blockers such as promethazine or diphenhydramine produce sedation, sleep, and temporal disruptions of attention and cognition, and these effects are less prominent with the second generation of H1 blockers with low central penetration. The first-generation H1 blockers, such as diphenhydramine, as well as doxylamine, are available as over-the-counter hypnotics.

Histamine neurons are located exclusively in the TMN of the posterior hypothalamus, from where they project to almost all brain regions, including areas important for vigilance control, such as the hypothalamus, basal forebrain, thalamus, cortex, and brainstem structures (see Ref.[54] for review).

After discovering the involvement of the hypocretin system in narcolepsy, several researchers studied how these deficits in neurotransmission induce narcolepsy. One of the keys to solving this question is revealing the functional differences between Hcrtr 1 and Hcrtr 2, because it is evident that Hcrtr 2-mediated function plays more critical roles (more than Hcrtr 1–mediated function) in generating narcoleptic symptoms in animals.[14,22] In situ hybridization experiments in rats show that Hcrtr 1 and Hcrtr 2 mRNA have marked differential distribution.[4] Hcrtr 1 is enriched in the ventromedial hypothalamic nucleus, tenia tecta, the hippocampal formation, dorsal raphe, and LC. In contrast, Hcrtr 2 is enriched in the paraventricular nucleus, cerebral cortex, nucleus accumbens, ventral tegmental area, substantia nigra, and histaminergic TMN.[4]

The TMN exclusively expresses Hcrtr 2,[4] and a series of electrophysiologic studies consistently showed that hypocretin potently excites TMN histaminergic neurons through Hcrtr 2.[50,51] Furthermore, it has recently been shown that the wake-promoting effects of hypocretins were abolished in histamine H1 receptor knockout mice, suggesting that the wake-promoting effects of hypocretin depend on histaminergic neurotransmission.[55]

Two groups have previously reported fluctuations of extracellular levels of histamine in the brains of animals using in vivo microdialysis techniques. Mochizuki and colleagues[56] reported that histamine levels in the hypothalamus of rats show a clear diurnal variation: high during the active period and low during the resting period. Strecker and colleagues[57] also showed that histamine levels in the preoptic anterior hypothalamus in cats were also high during sleep deprivation and became lower during recovery sleep. These patterns of fluctuation in histamine levels are similar to those of extracellular hypocretin levels in the LHT and thalamus in rats.[32]

We also observed that the CSF histamine levels exhibit clear diurnal fluctuations in rats: the mean of the CSF histamine levels during the dark period was significantly higher than that during the light period.[58] After 6 hours of sleep deprivation from ZT0, CSF histamine levels increased significantly compared with controls whose sleep was not deprived. We also found that thioperamide (an H3 antagonist, 5 mg/kg, intraperitoneal) significantly increased CSF histamine levels with little effect on locomotor activation. Because H3 autoreceptor antagonists are known to enhance terminal histamine releases from histaminergic neurons, the activity of neuronal histamine is likely to be reflected in the CSF histamine levels.

Human Narcolepsy and Idiopathic Hypersomnia are also Associated with Decreased Histaminergic Neurotransmission

Because the results of our animal experiment suggest that CSF histamine levels at least partially reflect the central histamine neurotransmission and vigilance state changes, we evaluated histaminergic neurotransmission in human narcolepsy using CSF. We conducted 2 clinical studies for evaluating the CSF histamine in narcolepsy. The first study included narcolepsy with low CSF hypocretin-1 ($\leq$110 pg/mL, n = 34, 100% with cataplexy), narcolepsy without low CSF hypocretin-1 (n = 24, 75% with cataplexy), and normal controls (n = 23).[5] Narcoleptic subjects with and without hypocretin deficiency were included to determine whether histamine neurotransmission depends on the hypocretin-deficient status of

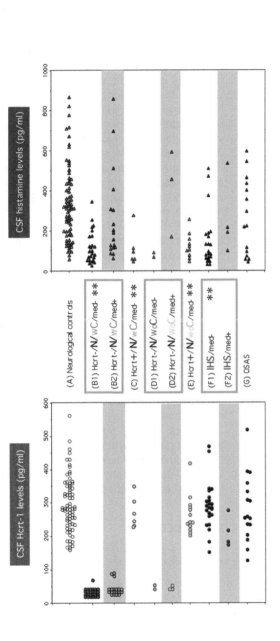

Fig. 5. CSF hyocretin-1 (Hcrt-1) and histamine values for each individual with sleep disorders. CSF Hcrt-1 (*left panel*) and histamine (*right panel*) values for each individual are plotted. The patient groups are indicated as group A to group G from the top. The results of the subjects with CNS stimulants (*shadowed*) and without CNS stimulants are presented separately in the figure. None of the patients with idiopathic hypersomnia (IHS) and obstructive sleep apnea (OSAS) showed hypocretin deficiency (Hcrt-). We found significant reductions in CSF histamine levels in hypocretin deficient (B, 176 ± 25.8 pg/mL) and nondeficient (Hcrt+) narcolepsy with cataplexy (N/C) (C, 97.8 ± 38.4 pg/mL), hypocretin nondeficient narcolepsy without cataplexy (N/woC) (E, 113.6 ± 16.4 pg/mL) and idiopathic hypersomnia (F, 161.0 ± 29.3 pg/mL), whereas those in hypocretin-deficient narcolepsy without cataplexy (D, 273.6 ± 105 pg/mL) and OSAS (G, 259.3 ± 46.6 pg/mL) were not statistically different from those in the control range (A, 333.8 ± 22.0 pg/mL). The low CSF histamine levels were observed in nonmedicated patients, and significant reductions in histamine levels were observed only in nonmedicated patients with hypocretin-deficient narcolepsy with cataplexy (B1, 112.1 ± 16.3 pg/mL) and idiopathic hypersomnia (F1, 143.3 ± 28.8 pg/mL). The levels in the medicated subjects are in the normal range (B2, 256.6 ± 51.7 pg/mL and F2, 259.5 ± 94.9 pg/mL). Nonmedicated subjects had a tendency for low CSF histamine levels in hypocretin-deficient narcolepsy without cataplexy (D1, 77.5 ± 11.5 pg/mL). (*Data from* Kanbayashi T, Kodama T, Kondo H, et al. CSF histamine contents in narcolepsy, idiopathic hypersomnia and obstructive sleep apnea syndrome. Sleep 2009;32(2):181–7.)

each subject. A significant reduction of CSF histamine levels was found in the cases with low CSF hypocretin-1, and levels were intermediate in other narcolepsy cases: mean CSF histamine levels were 133.2 (±20.1) pg/mL in narcoleptic subjects with low CSF hypocretin-1, 233.3 (±46.5) pg/mL in patients with normal CSF hypocretin-1, and 300.5 (±49.7) pg/mL in controls. Our results suggest impaired histaminergic neurotransmission in human narcolepsy, but that this does not dependent on the hypocretin-deficient status.

We therefore also examined CSF histamine levels in narcolepsy and other sleep disorders in a Japanese population. This second clinical study included 67 subjects with narcolepsy, 26 subjects with idiopathic hypersomnia, 16 subjects with obstructive sleep apnea syndrome (OSAS), and 73 neurologic controls.[6]

We found significant reductions in CSF histamine levels in hypocretin-deficient narcolepsy with cataplexy (mean ± standard error of the mean; 176.0 ± 25.8 pg/mL), hypocretin nondeficient narcolepsy with cataplexy (97.8 ± 38.4 pg/mL), hypocretin nondeficient narcolepsy without cataplexy (113.6 ± 16.4 pg/mL), and idiopathic hypersomnia (161.0 ± 29.3 pg/mL), whereas the levels in OSAS (259.3 ± 46.6 pg/mL) did not statistically differ from those in the controls (333.8 ± 22.0 pg/mL) (**Fig. 5**). Low CSF histamine levels were mostly observed in nonmedicated patients, and significant reductions in histamine levels were evident in nonmedicated patients with hypocretin-deficient narcolepsy with cataplexy (112.1 ± 16.3 pg/mL) and idiopathic hypersomnia (143.3 ± 28.8 pg/mL), whereas the levels in the medicated patients were in the normal range. Similar degrees of reduction, as seen in hypocretin-deficient narcolepsy with cataplexy, were also observed in hypocretin nondeficient narcolepsy and in idiopathic hypersomnia, whereas those in OSAS (non–central nervous system hypersomnia) were not altered. These results confirmed the result of the first study, but suggest that an impaired histaminergic system may be involved in mediating sleepiness in a broader category of patients with EDS than those with hypocretin-deficient narcolepsy. The decrease in histamine in these subjects was more specifically observed in nonmedicated subjects, suggesting CSF histamine is a biomarker reflecting the degree of hypersomnia of central origin. It is not known whether decreased histamine could either passively reflect or partially mediate daytime sleepiness in these disorders. Further studies are essential, because central histamine compounds, such as H3 antagonists, may be developed as a new class of wake-promoting compounds for EDS with various causes.

SUMMARY

This article describes the current understanding of neurochemistry and possible biomarkers for EDS with various causes.

The recent progress in understanding the pathophysiology of EDS stems particularly from the discovery of hypocretin ligand deficiency in human narcolepsy. The hypocretin deficiency can be clinically detected by CSF hypocretin-1 measures; low CSF hypocretin-1 levels are seen in more than 90% of patients with narcolepsy-cataplexy. Because the specificity of the CSF finding is also high (no hypocretin deficiency was seen in patients with idiopathic hypersomnia), low CSF hypocretin-1 levels have been included in ICSD-2 as a positive diagnosis for narcolepsy-cataplexy.

Although prevalence of primary hypersomnia such as narcolepsy and idiopathic hypersomnia is not high, that of symptomatic EDS is considerably high, and the pathophysiology of symptomatic EDS likely overlaps with that of primary hypersomnia, including recently identifying MS/NMO cases with bilateral symmetric hypothalamic damage.

The pathophysiology of hypocretin nondeficient narcolepsy is debated. The pathophysiology of idiopathic hypersomnia is also largely unknown, but hypocretin deficiency is not likely to be involved in this condition. Decreased histaminergic neurotransmission is observed in narcolepsy and idiopathic hypersomnia, regardless of hypocretin-deficient status. The functional significance of this finding (whether it mediates sleepiness or passively reflects sleepiness) further needs to be evaluated.

Although much progress was made regarding the pathophysiology and neurochemistry of EDS, this new knowledge has not yet been incorporated into the development of new treatments, and further research is needed.

REFERENCES

1. ICSD-2, editor. ICSD-2-International classification of sleep disorders, diagnostic and coding manual. 2nd edition. Westchester (IL): American Academy of Sleep Medicine; 2005.
2. Verma A, Anand V, Verma NP. Sleep disorders in chronic traumatic brain injury. J Clin Sleep Med 2007;3(4):357–62.
3. Nishino S, Kanbayashi T. Symptomatic narcolepsy, cataplexy and hypersomnia, and their implications in the hypothalamic hypocretin/orexin system. Sleep Med Rev 2005;9(4):269–310.
4. Marcus JN, Aschkenasi CJ, Lee CE, et al. Differential expression of orexin receptors 1 and 2 in the rat brain. J Comp Neurol 2001;435(1):6–25.

5. Nishino S, Sakurai E, Nevsimalova S, et al. Decreased CSF histamine in narcolepsy with and without low CSF hypocretin-1 in comparison to healthy controls. Sleep 2009;32(2):175–80.

6. Kanbayashi T, Kodama T, Kondo H, et al. CSF histamine contents in narcolepsy, idiopathic hypersomnia and obstructive sleep apnea syndrome. Sleep 2009; 32(2):181–7.

7. Nishino S, Mignot E. Pharmacological aspects of human and canine narcolepsy. Prog Neurobiol 1997;52(1):27–78.

8. Nishino S, Taheri S, Black J, et al. The neurobiology of sleep in relation to mental illness. In: Charney DS, Nestler EJ, editors. Neurobiology of mental illness. New York: Oxford University Press; 2004. p. 1160–79.

9. Saper CB, Scammell TE, Lu J. Hypothalamic regulation of sleep and circadian rhythms. Nature 2005; 437(7063):1257–63.

10. Aldrich MS, Chervin RD, Malow BA. Value of the multiple sleep latency test (MSLT) for the diagnosis of narcolepsy. Sleep 1997;20(8):620–9.

11. Sakurai T, Amemiya A, Ishii M, et al. Orexins and orexin receptors: a family of hypothalamic neuropeptides and G protein-coupled receptors that regulate feeding behavior. Cell 1998;92:573–85.

12. De Lecea L, Kilduff TS, Peyron C, et al. The hypocretins: hypothalamus-specific peptides with neuroexcitatory activity. Proc Natl Acad Sci U S A 1998;95:322–7.

13. Peyron C, Tighe DK, van den Pol AN, et al. Neurons containing hypocretin (orexin) project to multiple neuronal systems. J Neurosci 1998;18(23):9996–10015.

14. Lin L, Faraco J, Li R, et al. The sleep disorder canine narcolepsy is caused by a mutation in the hypocretin (orexin) receptor 2 gene. Cell 1999;98(3):365–76.

15. Chemelli RM, Willie JT, Sinton CM, et al. Narcolepsy in orexin knockout mice: molecular genetics of sleep regulation. Cell 1999;98:437–51.

16. Nishino S, Ripley B, Overeem S, et al. Hypocretin (orexin) deficiency in human narcolepsy. Lancet 2000;355(9197):39–40.

17. Peyron C, Faraco J, Rogers W, et al. A mutation in a case of early onset narcolepsy and a generalized absence of hypocretin peptides in human narcoleptic brains. Nat Med 2000;6(9):991–7.

18. Mignot E, Lammers GJ, Ripley B, et al. The role of cerebrospinal fluid hypocretin measurement in the diagnosis of narcolepsy and other hypersomnias. Arch Neurol 2002;59(10):1553–62.

19. Crocker A, Espana RA, Papadopoulou M, et al. Concomitant loss of dynorphin, NARP, and orexin in narcolepsy. Neurology 2005;65(8):1184–8.

20. Honda M, Eriksson KS, Zhang S, et al. IGFBP3 co-localizes with and regulates hypocretin (orexin). PLoS One 2009;4(1):e4254.

21. Yoshida Y, Okun M, Mignot E, et al. CSF dynorphine A(1-8) levels are not altered in hypocretin-deficient human narcolepsy. Sleep 2002;25(Abstract Suppl): A472.2002.

22. Ripley B, Fujiki N, Okura M, et al. Hypocretin levels in sporadic and familial cases of canine narcolepsy. Neurobiol Dis 2001;8(3):525–34.

23. Thannickal TC, Nienhuis R, Siegel JM. Localized loss of hypocretin (orexin) cells in narcolepsy without cataplexy. Sleep 2009;32(8):993–8.

24. Roth B. Narkolepsie und hypersomnie. Berlin: VEB Verlag Volk und Gesundheit; 1962.

25. Bassetti C, Aldrich MS. Idiopathic hypersomnia. A series of 42 patients. Brain 1997;120(Pt 8):1423–35.

26. Bassetti C, Gugger M, Bischof M, et al. The narcoleptic borderland: a multimodal diagnostic approach including cerebrospinal fluid levels of hypocretin-1 (orexin A). Sleep Med 2003;4(1):7–12.

27. Sakurai T. Roles of orexins in regulation of feeding and wakefulness. Neuroreport 2002;13(8):987–95.

28. Willie JT, Chemelli RM, Sinton CM, et al. To eat or to sleep? Orexin in the regulation of feeding and wakefulness. Annu Rev Neurosci 2001;24:429–58.

29. Fujiki N, Yoshida Y, Ripley B, et al. Changes in CSF hypocretin-1 (orexin A) levels in rats across 24 hours and in response to food deprivation. Neuroreport 2001;12(5):993–7.

30. Lee MG, Hassani OK, Jones BE. Discharge of identified orexin/hypocretin neurons across the sleep-waking cycle. J Neurosci 2005;25(28):6716–20.

31. Aston-Jones G, Chen S, Zhu Y, et al. A neural circuit for circadian regulation of arousal. Nat Neurosci 2001;4(7):732–8.

32. Yoshida Y, Fujiki N, Nakajima T, et al. Fluctuation of extracellular hypocretin-1 (orexin A) levels in the rat in relation to the light-dark cycle and sleep-wake activities. Eur J Neurosci 2001;14(7):1075–81.

33. Saper CB, Chou TC, Scammell TE. The sleep switch: hypothalamic control of sleep and wakefulness. Trends Neurosci 2001;24(12):726–31.

34. Nishino S, Kanbayashi T, Fujiki N, et al. CSF hypocretin levels in Guillain-Barre syndrome and other inflammatory neuropathies. Neurology 2003;61(6):823–5.

35. Overeem S, Dalmau J, Bataller L, et al. Hypocretin-1 CSF levels in anti-Ma2 associated encephalitis. Neurology 2004;62(1):138–40.

36. Kanbayashi T, Shimohata T, Nakashima I, et al. Symptomatic narcolepsy in MS and NMO patients; new neurochemical and immunological implications. Arch Neurol 2009;66:1563–6.

37. Poirier G, Montplaisir J, Dumont M, et al. Clinical and sleep laboratory study of narcoleptic symptoms in multiple sclerosis. Neurology 1987;37(4):693–5.

38. Ripley B, Overeem S, Fujiki N, et al. CSF hypocretin/orexin levels in narcolepsy and other neurological conditions. Neurology 2001;57(12):2253–8.

39. Amiry-Moghaddam M, Ottersen OP. The molecular basis of water transport in the brain. Nat Rev Neurosci 2003;4(12):991–1001.

40. Pittock SJ, Weinshenker BG, Lucchinetti CF, et al. Neuromyelitis optica brain lesions localized at sites of high aquaporin 4 expression. Arch Neurol 2006; 63(7):964–8.

41. Lennon VA, Kryzer TJ, Pittock SJ, et al. IgG marker of optic-spinal multiple sclerosis binds to the aquaporin-4 water channel. J Exp Med 2005; 202(4):473–7.

42. Montplaisir J, de Champlain J, Young SN, et al. Narcolepsy and idiopathic hypersomnia: biogenic amines and related compounds in CSF. Neurology 1982;32(11):1299–302.

43. Faull KF, Zeller-DeAmicis LC, Radde L, et al. Biogenic amine concentrations in the brains of normal and narcoleptic canines: current status. Sleep 1986;9(1):107–10.

44. Aldrich MS, Hollingsworth Z, Penney JB. Dopamine-receptor autoradiography of human narcoleptic brain. Neurology 1992;42:410–5.

45. Hublin C, Launes J, Nikkinen P, et al. Dopamine D2-receptors in human narcolepsy: a SPECT study with 123I-IBZM. Acta Neurol Scand 1994;90(3): 186–9.

46. Rinne J, Hublin C, Partinen M, et al. PET study of human narcolepsy: no increase in striatal dopamine D2-receptors. Neurology 1995;45:1735–8.

47. Mefford IN, Baker TL, Boehme R, et al. Narcolepsy: biogenic amine deficits in an animal model. Science 1983;220:629–32.

48. Nishino S, Fujiki N, Ripley B, et al. Decreased brain histamine contents in hypocretin/orexin receptor-2 mutated narcoleptic dogs. Neurosci Lett 2001; 313(3):125–8.

49. Nishino S, Riehl J, Hong J, et al. Is narcolepsy REM sleep disorder? Analysis of sleep abnormalities in narcoleptic Dobermans. Neurosci Res 2000;38(4): 437–46.

50. Eriksson KS, Sergeeva O, Brown RE, et al. Orexin/hypocretin excites the histaminergic neurons of the tuberomammillary nucleus. J Neurosci 2001;21(23): 9273–9.

51. Yamanaka A, Tsujino N, Funahashi H, et al. Orexins activate histaminergic neurons via the orexin 2 receptor. Biochem Biophys Res Commun 2002; 290(4):1237–45.

52. Faull KF, Guilleminault C, Berger PS, et al. Cerebrospinal fluid monoamine metabolites in narcolepsy and hypersomnia. Ann Neurol 1983;13(3):258–63.

53. Lin JS. Brain structures and mechanisms involved in the control of cortical activation and wakefulness, with emphasis on the posterior hypothalamus and histaminergic neurons. Sleep Med Rev 2000;4(5): 471–503.

54. Haas H, Panula P. The role of histamine and the tuberomamillary nucleus in the nervous system. Nat Rev Neurosci 2003;4(2):121–30.

55. Huang ZL, Qu WM, Li WD, et al. Arousal effect of orexin A depends on activation of the histaminergic system. Proc Natl Acad Sci U S A 2001;98(17): 9965–70.

56. Mochizuki T, Yamatodani A, Okakura K, et al. Circadian rhythm of histamine release from the hypothalamus of freely moving rats. Physiol Behav 1992; 51(2):391–4.

57. Strecker RE, Nalwalk J, Dauphin LJ, et al. Extracellular histamine levels in the feline preoptic/anterior hypothalamic area during natural sleep-wakefulness and prolonged wakefulness: an in vivo microdialysis study. Neuroscience 2002; 113(3):663–70.

58. Soya S, Song YH, Kodama T, et al. CSF histamine levels in rats reflect the central histamine neurotransmission. Neurosci Lett 2008;430: 224–9.

Primary and Secondary Neurogenic Hypersomnias

Claudio L. Bassetti, MD[a,b,*]

KEYWORDS

- Neurogenic • Hypersomnia • Excessive daytime sleepiness • Naps • MSLT • MWT • Actigraphy
- Narcolepsy • Idiopathic hypersomnia • Stroke • Parkinson • Traumatic brain injury • Therapy

KEY POINTS

- The clinical presentation of neurogenic hypersomnias is pleomorphic and includes excessive daytime sleepiness, hypersomnia and involuntary naps.
- Pathophysiologically neurogenic hypersommnias can be due to decreased sleep length or depth, insufficient wakefulness, circadian disturbances, or a combination of these factors.
- Secondary forms (e.g. after stroke, in Parkinsonian syndromes, after traumatic brain injury) are more common than primary neurogenic hypersomnias (e.g. narcolepsy). Treatment with stimulants is well established only for primary neurogenic hypersomnias.

INTRODUCTION
Clinical Spectrum and Differential Diagnosis

The term hypersomnia is used to cover a broad range of clinical manifestations of reduced wakefulness (**Box 1**).

The most frequent manifestations are an excessive daytime sleepiness (EDS; increased sleep propensity) and an increased sleep need/behavior over 24 hours (hypersomnia sensu strictu). Other forms of decreased wakefulness include increased voluntary and involuntary napping (sleep attacks), automatic behaviors, and sudden lapses of vigilance (blackouts).

A patient with hypersomnia of neurologic origin (eg, poststroke hypersomnia) may present with one or several of these symptoms, which may overlap.

The clinical differential diagnosis of hypersomnia includes fatigue (lack of energy, increased fatigability, increased sleep desire without an increase in sleep propensity), apathy/abulia (lack of initiative), depression, athymhormia (lack of autoactivation), clinophilia (increased desire to lay down), and reduced levels of vigilance (somnolence/sopor) preceding coma.

Clinical Significance

Hypersomnia is linked with decreased well-being and level of functioning, as well as an increased risk of accidents. cognitive (eg, attention, memory deficits) and psychiatric disturbances (eg, irritability, depression/euphoria) are frequently observed. Despite the absence of systematic data, clinical experience suggests a decreased quality of life in patients with neurologic hypersomnia.

Epidemiology and Classification

Primary neurogenic hypersomnias are relatively rare (<10% of patients seen in a sleep clinic), are not due to a specific underlying disorder, and include narcolepsy, behaviorally induced sleep insufficiency syndrome, idiopathic hypersomnia, and Kleine-Levin syndrome/periodic hypersomnias.

Secondary neurogenic hypersomnias are more frequent and are due to an underlying neurologic disorder such as stroke, traumatic brain injury, or Parkinsonism. In some neurologic disorders hypersomnia can be found in up to 25% to 50% of patients (see later discussion).

[a] Department of Neurology, University Hospital (Inselspital), Freiburgstrasse 1, 3010 Bern, Switzerland; [b] Neurocenter of Southern Switzerland, Via Tesserete 46, 6903 Lugano, Switzerland
* Department of Neurology, University Hospital (Inselspital), Freiburgstrasse 1, 3010 Bern, Switzerland.
E-mail address: claudio.bassetti@insel.ch

Sleep Med Clin 7 (2012) 249–261
doi:10.1016/j.jsmc.2012.03.016
1556-407X/12/$ – see front matter © 2012 Published by Elsevier Inc.

Box 1
Clinical approach to neurogenic hypersomnias

Spectrum of manifestations

  Excessive daytime sleepiness

  Hypersomnia sensu strictu

  Increased voluntary napping

  Involuntary napping (sleep attacks)

  Sudden lapses of vigilance (blackouts)

Clinical differential diagnosis

  Fatigue

  Apathy/abulia

  Depression

  Athymhormia (lack of autoactivation)

  Clinophilia (increased desire to lay down)

  Somnolence/sopor[a]/coma

Etiologic differential diagnosis

  Primary

    Decreased sleep length

    Decreased sleep depth

    Insufficient wake drive

    Disturbed timing of the sleep-wake cycle

    Combinations of the above

  Secondary (due to associated conditions/disorders causing hypersomnia)

    Sleep-disordered breathing

    Insomnia

    Excessive motor activity in sleep

    Depression

    Drugs

[a] The term "stupor" (from the Latin for "frozen") was introduced in medicine to describe a condition characterized by loss/reduction of speech and movement (akinetic mutism) usually, but not invariably, of psychiatric origin. Conversely, the term "sopor" (from the Latin term for "deep sleep") was/is reserved for a condition characterized by a decreased state of vigilance and arousability.

Pathophysiology

Neurophysiologically, hypersomnia in patients with neurologic disorders may be due to (1) a decreased sleep length, (2) a decreased sleep depth/continuity, (3) an insufficient wake drive, (4) an incorrect timing of the sleep-wake cycle, or (5) a combination of more than 1 of these factors.

Neurochemically, hypersomnia may be due to a reduced transmission in wakefulness-maintaining neurons (eg, noradrenaline, acetylcholine, dopamine, histamine) and/or increased/disinhibited transmission of sleep-inducing neurons (eg, γ-aminobutyric acid). In a few disorders changes in hypocretinergic transmission (eg, narcolepsy, severe head trauma, advanced Parkinson disease) and the prostaglandin-cytokine systems have also been found.

Assessment and Diagnostic Pitfalls

The assessment of hypersomnia includes subjective and objective measurements.

Subjectively, estimation of sleep propensity (Epworth Sleepiness Scale), sleep needs (sleep/24 hours), and fatigue (eg, Fatigue Severity Scale[1]) are typically used. Objectively, the most common sleep-wake tests include assessments of sleep propensity (multiple sleep latency test [MSLT]) and of the ability to stay awake (maintenance of wakefulness test), and a wrist actigraphy.

The correlation between results of subjective and objective sleep-wake tests is generally not very good in the general population, and this correlation is even worse in patients with neurologic disorders (in which brain areas responsible for sleep-wake and electroencephalographic (EEG) generation may be affected in association).[2]

According to the specific diagnostic hypothesis, additional ancillary tests such as brain magnetic resonance imaging, cerebrospinal fluid, and genetic analyses may be also needed.

PRIMARY NEUROGENIC HYPERSOMNIAS
Narcolepsy

Epidemiology
The frequency of narcolepsy has been estimated to be 1 in 2000.[3–5] The disease typically starts in the second or third decade of life. In 10% to 20% of cases narcolepsy begins in childhood or late adulthood, and in most cases it is sporadic and idiopathic. In 10% of cases a positive family history or an underlying brain disease are found.

Clinical features
The main and often first symptom of narcolepsy is an overwhelming ("irresistible") EDS with involuntary naps and sleep attacks. Naps are typically short and refreshing.

Cataplexy occurs in 70% to 90% of cases with episodes of sudden, bilateral, short-lasting (usually <1–2 minutes) partial loss of muscle tone (jaw sagging, knee buckling) triggered by sudden (often positive, eg, laughing, surprise) emotions, with preserved consciousness (**Fig. 1**).

Sleep paralysis and hallucinations are observed in about 50% of cases.

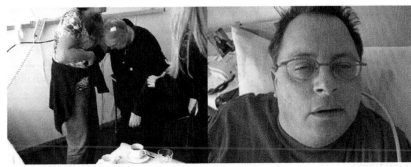

Fig. 1. Narcolepsy-cataplexy. Cataplectic attacks with a fall in a 77-year-old woman (*left*) and with loss of facial muscle control in a 42 year-old man (*right*).

Nighttime sleep is typically disturbed, with sleep-maintenance insomnia, sleep-disordered breathing, and excessive motor activity. Patients typically have no difficulties awakening.

Psychiatric and psychosocial problems are not infrequent, and may be related to the basic brain dysfunction and not only to the reactive mechanism to a chronic disorder. Remissions are unusual.

Pathophysiology/etiology
Idiopathic narcolepsy represents a hypocretin-deficient syndrome accompanied by a sleep-wake instability with dissociation/intermingling of states of being. The hypocretin deficiency is due to a neuronal loss of unknown origin. The latter arises from a genetic predisposition (HLA DQB1*0602+ in 95% of cases) and environmental factors or triggers (infections, trauma, stress). Specific (anti-Tribbles) autoantibodies may be involved, being found in a minority of cases in the acute phase. Secondary narcolepsy is rare and can be observed in association with head trauma, hypothalamus-brainstem lesions, and paraneoplastic encephalitis. Narcolepsy-like syndromes have been described in the course of Norrie, Coffin-Lowry, Prader-Willi, and Moebius syndromes.

Diagnosis
History of cataplexy, if unequivocal, is pathognomonic for narcolepsy. Polysomnography with sleep-onset rapid eye movement episodes (SOR-EMPs), MSLT with short sleep latency (<5–8 minutes), and 2 or more SOREMPs support the diagnosis of narcolepsy. Decreased/abolished cerebrospinal fluid hypocretin (orexin) levels are found in 95% of cases of narcolepsy with cataplexy, and can be found in familial narcolepsy, narcolepsy without cataplexy, and secondary narcolepsy. HLA positivity for DQB1*0602 is found in 95% of patients with narcolepsy with cataplexy, but also in 15% to 30% of normal controls.

Differential diagnosis
Other causes of EDS (behaviorally induced insufficient sleep syndrome, idiopathic hypersomnia) must be considered in patients without or with equivocal (rare, mild, or atypical) cataplexy (cataplexy-like episodes).

The differential diagnosis of cataplexy-like episodes is broad and includes "weak with laughter" in normal subjects, psychogenic falls/spells, astatic seizures, and vascular drop attacks.

Treatment
Modafinil is the drug of first choice for narcoleptic EDS. Methylphenidate, sodium oxybate, venlafaxine, and fluctine can also be used (**Table 1**).

Sodium oxybate is the drug of first choice for cataplexy. Amitriptyline, venlafaxine, and fluctine can also be used. These drugs typically also improve sleep paralysis and hallucinations.

Behaviorally Induced Insufficient Sleep Syndrome

Epidemiology
In the author's experience, at least 10% of EDS cases in a specialized sleep clinic are due to a behaviorally induced insufficient sleep syndrome (BIISS).[6–8] This condition appears to be more frequent in adolescents and young adults.

Clinical features
The clinical presentation is highly variable and includes EDS, accidents, involuntary napping, unclear blackouts or absences, and cognitive complaints. EDS typically improves during weekends and vacations.

The course is fluctuating, and remissions are not uncommon.

Pathophysiology/etiology
Insufficient and/or irregular sleep times are the cause of BIISS. Occasionally a psychiatric comorbidity is present. A genetic predisposition (HLA DQB1*0602) may play a role.

Table 1
Treatment of the most important neurogenic hypersomnias

	Modafinil	Methylphenidate	Others
Narcolepsy	+++	++	Venlafaxine, fluoxetine sodium oxybate
Behaviorally induced insufficient sleep syndrome	+	+	Sleep extension
Idiopathic hypersomnia	+	+	Melatonin, stimulating antidepressants
Kleine-Levin syndrome	+	+	Lithium, valproic acid (prevention)
Hypersomnia after stroke	+	+	Dopaminergic drugs
Hypersomnia and parkinsonism	+/++	+	Withdrawal from dopamine agonists, activating antidepressants
Hypersomnia after traumatic brain injury	+++	+	

+++, excellent evidence (randomized trials); ++, fair evidence (case series); +, poor evidence (case reports).

Diagnosis

This diagnosis may be difficult in the absence of a typical or reliable history. In the author's experience, actigraphy with irregular/insufficient sleep times is necessary, and sometimes crucial, to make the diagnosis (**Fig. 2**).

Polysomnography presents short non–rapid eye movement (NREM)/REM sleep latency, high sleep efficiency, and increased amounts of slow-wave sleep. The MSLT may present with narcolepsy-like features with short sleep latency (<5 minutes) and SOREMPs, which disappear after sleep extension.

Differential diagnosis

Idiopathic hypersomnia, narcolepsy without cataplexy, psychiatric EDS/hypersomnia are included in the differential.

Treatment

Sleep extension can be rapidly effective. Subjective EDS improves more rapidly than objective EDS (eg, MSLT results). Patients, however, not infrequently have difficulties in changing their sleep-wake schedule and in improving their sleep insufficiency (**Fig. 3**).

Idiopathic Hypersomnia

Epidemiology

This condition is about 10 times less frequent than narcolepsy (1/20,000 in the general population).[9,10] In most cases the disease starts in adolescence. About 50% of patients report a positive family history.

Clinical features

Idiopathic hypersomnia presents with a nonoverwhelming EDS with long and nonrefreshing naps.

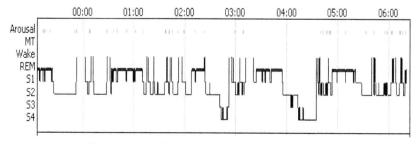

Fig. 2. Narcolepsy-cataplexy. Sleep-onset REM episode in a 42-year-old hypocretin-deficient patient with narcolepsy-cataplexy. REM sleep is denoted by the purple horizontal bars in the hypnogram below. The x-axis shows hours of sleep recordings (11 PM to 6 AM) plotted against sleep staging: arousals, movement time (MT), wake, rapid eye movement (REM), stages S1 (N1 sleep stage), S2 (N2 sleep stage), S3, and S4 (sleep wave sleep, or N3 sleep stage).

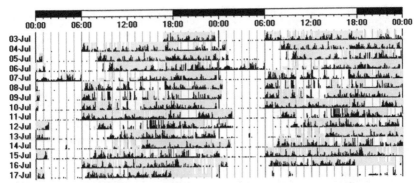

Fig. 3. Behaviorally induced insufficient sleep syndrome (BIISS). Actigraphy demonstrates irregular/insufficient sleep times in a 22-year-old patient with EDS, sleep paralysis, and sleep-onset REM episodes (but normal cerebrospinal fluid hypocretin-1 levels and dramatic improvement after sleep extension) secondary to BIISS. Black trace, intensity of activity/time interval; yellow highlight, light exposure.

Nighttime sleep is deep and undisturbed (the existence of a variant with normal sleep time is suggested by the current diagnostic criteria of the American Academy of Sleep Medicine, but remains controversial). Difficulties awakening ("sleep drunkenness") and daytime automatic behaviors with "nonsense acts" are typical hallmarks of the condition. Patients may report headache and psychiatric symptoms. Remissions are not infrequent.

Pathophysiology/etiology
The etiology and pathophysiology of idiopathic hypersomnia are unknown. A circadian disorder, an insufficient wake drive, and a deficient dopaminergic transmission have been proposed. Because of the high familiarity, genetic factors probably play a role in idiopathic hypersomnia.

Diagnosis
Idiopathic hypersomnia is a diagnosis of exclusion. A typical history, a normal polysomnography (occasionally with increased slow-wave sleep), an MSLT with short or borderline sleep latency (5–10 minutes) but without SOREMPs, and the absence of other potential causes of EDS (see later discussion) are necessary for the diagnosis. Increased times "asleep" on actigraphy can support the diagnosis.

Differential diagnosis
Behaviorally induced insufficient sleep syndrome, psychiatric disorders with clinophilia/pseudohypersomnia, narcolepsy without cataplexy, and hypersomnia due to drugs/medical disorders can mimic idiopathic hypersomnia and should be considered.

Treatment
Modafinil and methlyphenidate are most frequently used but are often ineffective. Sleep extension worsens EDS in these patients (see **Table 1**). Stimulating antidepressants and melatonin have been reported to be effective in single case reports.

Kleine-Levin Syndrome/Recurrent Hypersomnias

Epidemiology
The Kleine-Levin syndrome (KLS) is at least 20 times less common than narcolepsy.[11,12] In most cases it starts in adolescence. It is more common in males and can be familial, and is more common in the Jewish population.

Clinical features
KLS presents with recurrent episodes/attacks (duration: a few days to weeks, frequency: 1–10 times per year) of EDS/hypersomnia with megahyperphagia and behavioral abnormalities. In women the condition maybe associated with the menstrual cycle. Remissions are frequent.

Etiology/pathophysiology
A thalamic-hypothalamic dysfunction is suggested and is supported by neuroimaging observations (**Fig. 4**).

Diagnosis
History is diagnostic. Sleep-wake tests with increased sleep time, and reduced sleep latency and efficiency are conversely nonspecific.

Differential diagnosis
Psychiatric (bipolar, seasonal, somatoform) disorders, hypothalamic lesions (including tumors),

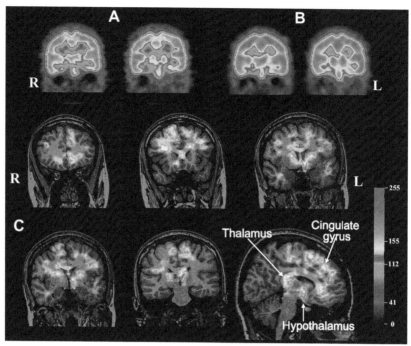

Fig. 4. Neuroimaging in KLS demonstrating episodic hypoperfusion. Brain areas depicting episodic hypofunction, demarcated by single photon emission computer tomography (SPECT) hypoperfusion. (*A*) Brain SPECT during to symptomatic phase demonstrating hypoperfusion in the bilateral frontal and temporal lobes and deincephalic structures (thalami and hypothalamus). (*B*) Brain SPECT during the convalescent phase depicting recovery in the hypofunction shown in *A*, with the exception of the right mesial temporal period. (*C*) Subtraction of brain SPECT images between *A* and *B*, revealing dramatic hypoperfusion in the diencephalic structures (bilateral thalami, left hypothalamus), basal ganglia, bilateral medial and dorsolateral frontal regions, and left temporal areas during the period of active KLS disease state. L, left side; R, right side. (*From* Hong SB, Joo EY, Tae WS, et al. Episodic diencephalic hypoperfusion in Kleine-Levin syndrome. Sleep 2006;29:1091–3; with permission.)

and encephalitis can present with a KLS-like syndrome.

Treatment
Lithium and antiepileptics may reduce the duration and frequency of the attacks.

SECONDARY NEUROGENIC HYPERSOMNIAS
Hypersomnia After Stroke

Epidemiology
Hypersomnia is present in 20% to 30% of patients after stroke. It is observed most commonly in bilateral thalamic and mesencephalic, or large, multifocal, or bilateral cortical lesions (**Fig. 5**).[1,2,13–16] Less commonly, hypersomnia is seen with small subcortical or cortical lesions (**Fig. 6**).

Clinical features
The clinical presentation of poststroke hypersomnia is pleomorphic and includes EDS, increased sleep needs (see **Fig. 5**), sleep-wake inversion, and fatigue. A few patients may rapidly change/fluctuate from hypersomnia to insomnia. EDS is

rarely very severe, whereas hypersomnia can be very profound (with sleep needs/behavior exceeding 16–20 hours per day).

An overlap of hypersomnia with apathy, athymhormia, and depression can be observed. Hypersomnia is often associated with cognitive, behavioral, and emotional disturbances.

Hypersomnia often improves within a few months after stroke.

Pathophysiology/etiology
A decreased wake drive, an increased sleep pressure (rarely), or a combination of both (eg, in patients with bithalamic lesions) have been postulated.

Other, nonneurogenic causes of hypersomnia must be considered in this population (see differential diagnosis).

Diagnosis
A high degree of clinical attention is necessary to suspect the presence of hypersomnia after stroke. This disturbance may in fact be overshadowed by other stroke manifestations/complications or may

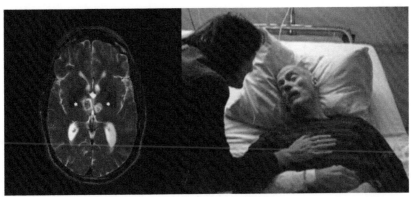

Fig. 5. Poststroke hypersomnia. A 65-year-old patient with bithalamic ischemic stroke (yellow marks in the *left panel*) and severe, initially almost nonarousable hypersomnia (*right panel*).

become evident only after discharge from hospital and a return to normal life.

In the author's experience, history and actigraphy (**Fig. 7**) can be diagnostic. As pointed out earlier (see introduction), a dissociation between clinical symptoms and sleep-wake findings is not infrequent in stroke patients with hypersomnia.

Differential diagnosis

Nonneurogenic causes of hypersomnias (such as sleep-disordered breathing, drugs, depression, sleep fragmentation/insomnia due to pain or infections) must first be ruled out.

Treatment

Modafinil, methylphenidate, and dopamine agonists have been reported to help in single patients (see **Table 1**).

Hypersomnia and Parkinsonism

Epidemiology

Hypersomnia is frequent in parkinsonian disorders.[2,17–24] Its frequency ranges in different studies

between 25% and 50% of patients. Male patients with more advanced disease, cognitive and psychiatric disturbances, hallucinations, and multiple medications are more often affected.

Clinical features

The clinical presentation of hypersomnia in parkinsonian patients is highly variable and includes EDS, sleep attacks (in 1%–30% of patients, with/without awareness), accidents, increased sleep needs, fatigue, and a fluctuating vigilance. In a minority of patients EDS can be very severe or narcolepsy-like. Cataplexy-like episodes and sleep paralysis, however, appear not to be more frequent than in the general population. Hypersomnia usually worsens in the course of parkinsonism.

Pathophysiology/etiology

An insufficient wake drive attributable to neurodegeneration of ascending aminergic-cholinergic pathways is supposed to be the cause of primary hypersomnia in parkinsonian patients.

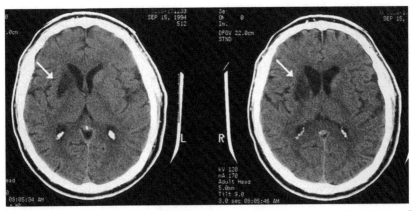

Fig. 6. Poststroke hypersomnia in a 61-year-old patient with caudate stroke (*arrow*) and severe (but transient) hypersomnia.

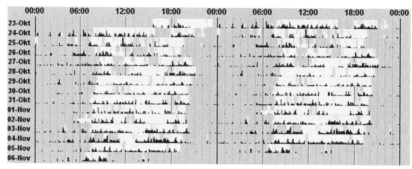

Fig. 7. Poststroke hypersomnia. Actigraphy of the patient shown in **Fig. 5** recorded in the acute phase of stroke. This test documents a reduced overall motor activity (yellow bars between 6 AM and 6 PM) and a dramatically increased time "asleep" (>12–13 hours per day). Black trace, intensity of activity/time interval; yellow highlight, light exposure.

A reduction of hypocretin cells/transmission may contribute to hypersomnia in patients with advanced forms of Parkinson disease.

Other, nonneurogenic (secondary) causes of hypersomnia must be considered in this population (see differential diagnosis).

Diagnosis

Assessment of hypersomnia is mandatory in all patients with parkinsonism because of the high frequency of this symptom (see above) and its possible exacerbation with dopaminergic and other drugs.

Sleep-wake questionnaires, polysomnography, and MSLT are typically used (**Figs. 8** and **9**). On MSLT the mean sleep latency is not infrequently less than 5 minutes; SOREMPs, conversely, are infrequent.

Differential diagnosis

Nonneurogenic causes of hypersomnia such as sleep-disordered breathing, depression, sleep deprivation (occasionally in the course of a dopamine overuse), insomnia (eg, due to urinary problems or pain), and drugs (dopamine agonists, sedative antidepressants) must be considered in all parkinsonian patients with hypersomnia.

Treatment

Change of medication (eg, dopamine agonists) and modafinil (as shown in some but not all systematic studies thus far performed) can improve hypersomnia (see **Table 1**). Cholinesterase inhibitors, activating antidepressants, and sodium oxybate may be of help in single cases.

Hypersomnia After Traumatic Brain Injury

Epidemiology

Hypersomnia is observed in up to 30% of patients after traumatic brain injury (TBI). Hypothalamic,[14,25–28] frontobasal, and thalamo-diencephalic traumatic lesions are more often complicated by hypersomnia (**Fig. 10**).

Clinical features

The clinical presentation of hypersomnia after TBI includes fatigue, EDS, and increased sleep needs. Few cases of posttraumatic narcolepsy have been reported (typically, however, without cataplexy and without hypocretin deficiency).

Hypersomnia usually improves within months after TBI. Fatigue may persist and even worsen after the acute-subacute phase.

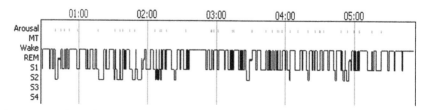

Fig. 8. Multisystem atrophy. Polysomnography of a 70-year-old patient with multisystem atrophy, insomnia/sleep fragmentation, and EDS. The x-axis shows hours of sleep recordings (11 PM to 6 AM) plotted against sleep staging: arousals, movement time (MT), wake, rapid eye movement (REM), stages S1 (N1 sleep stage), S2 (N2 sleep stage), S3, and S4 (sleep wave sleep, or N3 sleep stage).

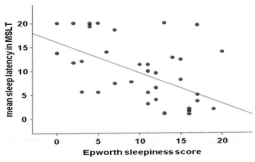

Fig. 9. Parkinsonism. Correlation between mean sleep latency on multiple sleep latency test (MSLT) and Epworth Sleepiness Scale score (ESS) in 37 parkinsonian patients ($r = 0.6$, $P<.001$) (for more details see Ref.[24]). The graph shows a correlation between objective measures of daytime sleepiness using the mean sleep latency on MSLT, and subjective assessment using the ESS. It demonstrates that the sleepier the patient is objectively, the worse is the subjective sleepiness as measured by sleep propensity.

Pathophysiology/etiology
Hypothalamic acceleration-deceleration injury and widespread white matter injury are involved. The role of initial hypocretin deficiency and mild hypocretin cell loss remains unclear. In some patients a disturbed circadian rhythm may play a role.

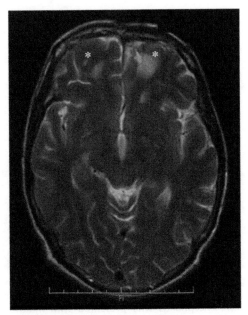

Fig. 10. Traumatic brain injury (TBI). Brain magnetic resonance (MR) image of a 62-year-old patient with severe EDS and hypersomnia after TBI with bilateral frontobasal lesions (*yellow marks*).

Other, nonneurogenic (secondary) causes of hypersomnia must be considered in this population (see differential diagnosis).

Diagnosis
History, questionnaires, actigraphy, polysomnography, MSLT, and brain magnetic resonance (MR) imaging are useful in the workup of posttraumatic hypersomnia.

Differential diagnosis
Nonneurogenic causes of hypersomnias (eg, sleep-disordered breathing, drugs, depression, sleep fragmentation/insomnia due to pain or infections) must be specifically searched for.

Treatment
Modafinil was shown recently in a double-blind controlled trial to improve EDS after TBI (see **Table 1**).

Hypersomnia and Epilepsy

Epidemiology
In most studies hypersomnia appears to affect 10% to 30% of patients with epilepsy.[29–31] The risk of driving in the presence of hypersomnia is increased in this patient population.

Clinical features
EDS and increased sleep needs are the best known and most commonly studied characteristics. The presence of severe EDS in male epileptic patients is frequently associated with sleep-disordered breathing. Sleep deprivation, but also EDS, can worsen seizure control.

Pathophysiology/etiology
Severity and cause of epilepsy, presence of nocturnal seizures, and number and type of antiepileptic drugs (eg, levetiracetam), but also concomitant disorders (sleep-disordered breathing, restless legs syndrome [RLS], depression) may cause (alone or in combination) hypersomnia in epileptic patients.

Diagnosis
History, questionnaires, polysomnography with multiple EEG channels, MSLT, and blood levels of antiepileptic drugs are usually used to identify the cause of hypersomnia in this clinical setting.

Differential diagnosis
The diagnostic challenge consists in differentiating between epilepsy-related and epilepsy-unrelated causes of hypersomnia.

Treatment
Treatment is directed against the underlying cause.

Hypersomnia and Restless Legs Syndrome

Epidemiology
Hypersomnia is found in at least 20% to 30% of patients with RLS.[2,32–34] Hypersomnia may be linked to younger age (whereas insomnia is more common in elderly RLS patients).

Clinical features
In RLS patients hypersomnia manifests with EDS and fatigue, and less commonly with prolonged sleep needs. It rarely manifests with sleep attacks or short sleep latencies on MSLT (<5 minutes).

Pathophysiology/etiology
An insufficient dopaminergic transmission has been postulated to explain primary hypersomnia in RLS. Concomitant sleep disorders (eg, sleep-disordered breathing) are not uncommonly involved (secondary hypersomnia). Rarely, hypersomnia may be due to dopaminergic medication and or its abrupt withdrawal.

Diagnosis
History, questionnaires, polysomnography, and MSLT are usually necessary for the diagnostic workup of hypersomnia in RLS patients.

Differential diagnosis
Hypersomnia should be differentiated in RLS patients from depression, which is not infrequent in this population.

Treatment
Hypersomnia usually improves (and rarely worsens, see above) with dopaminergic medication.

Hypersomnia and Infectious/Autoimmune Disorders of the Nervous System

Epidemiology
The frequency of hypersomnia in infectious and autoimmune disorders of the central nervous system is poorly studied and not well known,[2,16,35–40] with the exception of fatigue in multiple sclerosis, which was recently found using the Fatigue Severity Scale score to be present in 45% of 188 consecutive patients, and to be correlated with degree of physical disability and presence of depression.

Clinical features
Fatigue is frequently present in multiple sclerosis (see above). Severe, narcolepsy-like EDS is seen with infectious (eg, Morbus Behcet) and autoimmune processes (eg, multiple sclerosis, neuromyelitis optica, paraneoplastic encephalitis, **Figs. 11–13**) involving the hypothalamus and other subcortical structures. Hypersomnia sensu strictu (occasionally in form of an encephalitis lethargica–like syndrome) can be a feature of cerebral

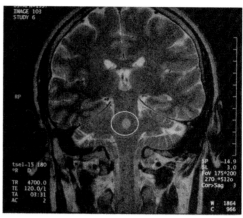

Fig. 11. Acute demyelinating encephalomyelitis. Brain MR image of a 62-year-old patient with narcolepsy-like syndrome caused by a single, acute demyelinating lesion in the pontine tegmentum (*red circle*) ("carrefour narcoleptique") (for details see Ref.[45])

trypanosomiasis (sleeping sickness), viral-postviral (eg, infections with influenza, Epstein-Barr virus, and human immunodeficiency virus), postbacterial (eg, after streptococcal infection), and autoimmune disorders.

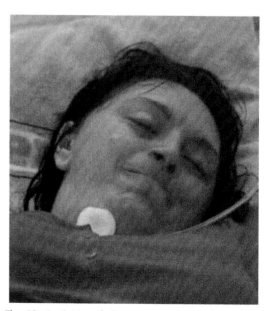

Fig. 12. Anti–*N*-methyl-D-aspartate (NMDA) encephalitis. A 39-year-old patient with paraneoplastic, anti-NMDA encephalitis who presented with multifocal seizure-like involuntary movements (including face grimacing), psychotic changes, and complex sleep-wake changes including hypersomnia and REM sleep-behavior disorder.

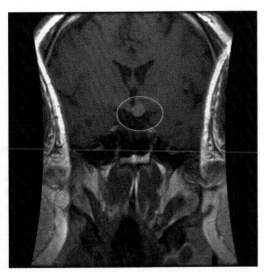

Fig. 13. Hypothalamic histiocytosis X. Brain MR image of a 50-year-old patient with severe EDS, hyperphagia, and hypothalamic histiocytosis (*red circle*).

Pathophysiology/etiology
Number and topography of brain lesions (eg, hypothalamic site) as well as neuroinflammatory factors (eg, changes in cytokine or hypocretin levels) may be involved. Genetic factors may account for different effects on vigilance of similar underlying lesions/disorders.

Diagnosis
History, questionnaires, actigraphy, polysomnography, MSLT, brain MR imaging, and cerebrospinal fluid analysis may be needed to clarify the origin of hypersomnia in this clinical setting.

Differential diagnosis
Nonneurogenic factors related to sleep-disordered breathing, depression, sleep fragmentation, insomnia, and drugs should always be considered.

Treatment
Amantidine, selegiline, methylphenidate, and modafinil have been shown to improve fatigue and EDS in patients with multiple sclerosis. Treatment of the underlying cause may lead to improvement and resolution of hypersomnia.

Hypersomnia and Neuromuscular Disorders

Epidemiology
The frequency of hypersomnia in neuromuscular disorders is poorly studied and is not known.[41–44]

Clinical features
Fatigue, apathy, and EDS are the most common presentations. Severe, narcolepsy-like EDS (eg,

in association with myotonic dystrophy) and increased sleep needs are occasionally seen.

Pathophysiology/etiology
Central neurogenic factors (including a deficient hypocretin transmission in myotonic dystrophy) as well as sleep-disordered breathing (including central apneas, mixed/obstructive apneas, and alveolar hypoventilation) resulting from muscular weakness have been suggested as possible causes of hypersomnia in neuromuscular disorders.

Diagnosis
History, questionnaires, polysomnography (with Pco_2 coregistration), MSLT, and respiratory functions are needed to clarify the origin of hypersomnia in this clinical setting.

Differential diagnosis
Nonneurogenic hypersomnias attributable to sleep-disordered breathing, depression, sleep fragmentation, insomnia, and medications should always be considered.

Treatment
Stimulants (eg, modafinil) as well as noninvasive ventilation have been shown to improve EDS and fatigue in single patients and small series of patients with neuromuscular disorders.

REFERENCES

1. Bassetti CL, Valko P. Poststroke hypersomnia. Sleep Med Clin 2006;1:139–55.
2. Valko PP, Bassetti CL, Bloch K, et al. Validation of the Fatigue Severity Scale in a Swiss cohort. Sleep 2008;31:1601–7.
3. Sturzenegger C, Bassetti C. The clinical spectrum of narcolepsy with cataplexy: a reappraisal. J Sleep Res 2004;13:395–406.
4. Dauvilliers Y, Arnulf I, Mignot E. Narcolepsy with cataplexy. Lancet 2007;369:499–511.
5. Billiard M, Bassetti C, Dauvilliers Y, et al. EFNS guidelines on management of narcolepsy. Eur J Neurol 2006;13:1049–65.
6. Roehrs T, Zorick F, Sicklesteel J, et al. Excessive daytime sleepiness associated with insufficient sleep. Sleep 1983;6:319–25.
7. Mignot E, Lin L, Finn L, et al. Correlates of sleep-onset REM periods during the Multiple Sleep Latency Test in community adults. Brain 2006;129:1609–23.
8. Marti I, Valko PO, Khatami RB, et al. Multiple sleep latency measures in narcolepsy and behaviourally insufficient sleep syndrome. Sleep Med 2009;10:1146–50.
9. Bassetti C, Aldrich M. Idiopathic hypersomnia. A study of 42 patients. Brain 1997;120:1423–35.

10. Anderson KN, Pilsworth S, Sharples LD, et al. Idiopathic hypersomnia: a study of 77 cases. Sleep 2007;30:1274–81.

11. Arnulf I, Zeitzer JM, File J, et al. Kleine-Levin syndrome: a systematic review of 186 cases in the literature. Brain 2005;128:2763–76.

12. Billiard M, Jaussent I, Dauvilliers Y, et al. Recurrent hypersomnia: a review of 339 cases. Sleep Med Rev 2011;15(4):247–57.

13. Bassetti C, Mathis J, Gugger M, et al. Hypersomnia following thalamic stroke. Ann Neurol 1996;39: 471–80.

14. Autret A, Lucas B, Mondon K, et al. Sleep and brain lesions: a critical review of the literature and additional new cases. Neurophysiol Clin 2001;31: 356–75.

15. Hermann DM, Siccoli M, Brugger P, et al. Evolution of neurological, neuropsychological and sleep-wake disturbances after paramedian thalamic stroke. Stroke 2008;39:62–8.

16. Brioschi A, Gramigna S, Werth E, et al. Effect of modafinil on subjective fatigue in multiple sclerosis and stroke patients. Eur Neurol 2010;62:243–9.

17. Arnulf I. Excessive daytime sleepiness in Parkinsonism. Sleep Med Rev 2005;9:185–200.

18. Baumann C, Ferini-Strambi L, Waldvogel D, et al. Parkinsonism with excessive daytime sleepiness A narcolepsy-like disorder? J Neurol 2005;252: 139–45.

19. Ondo WG, Foyle R, Atassi F, et al. Modafinil for daytime somnolence in Parkinson's disease: double blind, placebo controlled parallel trial. J Neurol Neurosurg Psychiatry 2005;76:1636–9.

20. Fronczeck R, Overeem S, Lee SY, et al. Hypocretin (orexin) loss in Parkinson's disease. Brain 2007; 130:1577–85.

21. Ondo WG, Perkins T, Swick T, et al. Sodium oxybate for excessive daytime sleepiness in Parkinson's disease. Arch Neurol 2008;65:1337–40.

22. Lou JS, Dimitrova DM, Park BS, et al. Using modafinil to treat fatigue in Parkinson disease: a double-blind, placebo controlled pilot study. Clin Neuropharmacol 2009;32:305–10.

23. Compta Y, Santamaria J, Ratti L, et al. Cerebrospinal hypocretin, daytime sleepiness and sleep architecture in Parkinson's disease dementia. Brain 2009; 132:3308–17.

24. Poryazova R, Benninger D, Waldvogel D, et al. Excessive daytime sleepiness in Parkinson's disease: characteristics and determinants. Eur Neurol 2010;63:129–35.

25. Baumann CR, Werth E, Stocker R, et al. Sleep-wake disturbances 6 months after traumatic brain injury. Brain 2007;130:1873–83.

26. Baumann CR, Bassetti CL, Valko PP, et al. Loss of hypocretin (orexin) neurons with traumatic brain injury. Ann Neurol 2009;66:555–9.

27. Kempf J, Werth E, Kaiser PR, et al. Sleep-wake disturbances 3 years after traumatic brain injury. J Neurol Neurosurg Psychiatry 2010;81:1402–4.

28. Kaiser PR, Valko PO, Werth E, et al. Modafinil ameliorates excessive daytime sleepiness after traumatic brain injury. Neurology 2010;75:1780–5.

29. Malow BE, Bowes RJ, Lin X. Predictors of sleepiness in epilepsy patients. Sleep 1997;20:1105–10.

30. Khatami R, Siegel AM, Bassetti CL. Hypersomnia in an epilepsy patient treated with levetiracetam. Epilepsia 2005;46:588–9.

31. Khatami R, Zutter D, Siegel A, et al. Sleep-wake habits and disorders in a series of 100 adult epilepsy patients- A prospective study. Seizure 2006;15:299–306.

32. Bassetti C, Clavadetscher S, Gugger M, et al. Pergolide-associated "sleep attacks" attacks in a patient with restless legs syndrome. Sleep Med 2002;3: 275–7.

33. Kallweit U, Siccoli M, Poryazova R, et al. Excessive daytime sleepiness in idiopathic restless legs syndrome: characteristics and evolution under dopaminergic treatment. Eur Neurol 2009; 62:176–9.

34. Kallweit U, Khatami R, Pizza F, et al. Dopaminergic treatment in restless legs syndrome: effects on vigilance. Clin Neuropharmacol 2010;33:276–8.

35. Baumann CR, Bassetti CL, Hersberger M, et al. Excessive daytime sleepiness in Behcet's disease with diencephalic lesions and hypocretin dysfunction. Eur Neurol 2010;63:190.

36. Dale RC, Chruch AJ, Surtes RA, et al. Encephalitis lethargica: 20 new cases and evidence of basal ganglia autoimmunity. Brain 2004;127:21–33.

37. Carlander B, Vincent T, Le Flich A, et al. Hypocretinergic dysfunction in neuromyelitis optica with coma-like episodes. J Neurol Neurosurg Psychiatry 2008;79:333–4.

38. Stankoff B, Waubant E, Confavreux C, et al. Modafinil for fatigue in MS: a randomized placebo-controlled double-blind study. Neurology 2005;64: 1139–43.

39. Nishino S, Kanbayashi T. Symptomatic narcolepsy, cataplexy and hypersomnia and their implications in the hypothalamic hypocretin/orexin system. Sleep Med Rev 2005;9:269–310.

40. Overeem S, Dalmau J, Bataller L, et al. Hypocretin-1 CSF levels in anti-Ma2 associated encephalitis. Neurology 2004;62:138–40.

41. Labanowski M, Schmidt-Nowara W, Guilleminault C. Sleep and neuromuscular disease: frequency of sleep disordered breathing in a neuromuscular disease clinic population. Neurology 1996;47: 1173–80.

42. Laberge L, Begin P, Montplaisir J, et al. Sleep complaints in patients with myotonic dystrophy. J Sleep Res 2004;13:95–100.

43. Damian MS, Gerlach A, Schmidt F, et al. Modafinil for excessive daytime sleepiness in myotonic dystrophy. Neurology 2001;56:794–6.

44. Poryazova R, Schnepf B, Boesiger P, et al. Magnetic resonance spectroscopy in a patient with Kleine-Levin syndrome. J Neurol 2007;254: 1445–6.

45. Mathis J, Hess CW, Bassetti C. Isolated medioteg-mental lesion causing narcolepsy and rapid eye movement sleep behaviour disorder: a case evidencing a common pathway in narcolepsy and rapid eye movement sleep behaviour disorder. J Neurol Neurosurg Psychiatry 2007;78(4): 427–9.

Narcolepsy

Sebastiaan Overeem, MD, PhD[a,b,*],
Paul Reading, FRCP, PhD[c], Claudio L. Bassetti, MD[d,e]

KEYWORDS

• Narcolepsy • Cataplexy • Hypocretin • Orexin • Excessive daytime sleepiness • Hypersomnia

KEY POINTS

- The typical phenotype of narcolepsy extends beyond excessive daytime sleepiness and cataplexy with numerous other sleep-related symptoms such as sleep maintenance insomnia.
- A range of non-sleep-related symptoms may dominate the clinical picture in some narcoleptics and require specific attention. Examples include mood or anxiety disorders and obesity.
- The expression of cataplexy often changes with age such that children typically exhibit brief generalized episodes with more prominent facial involvement and abnormal posturing compared to adults.
- Most now regard full-blown narcolepsy as a hypocretin (orexin) deficiency syndrome. However, the distinction between narcolepsy with and without cataplexy needs further clarification as the role of hypocretin is not established in all forms of narcolepsy.

Narcolepsy is widely regarded as the prototypical hypersomnia of central origin and has been the focus of both scientific and clinical attention for a considerable time.[1–3] In the last decade, enormous progress has been made in our understanding of the pathophysiology of narcolepsy, providing additional valuable insights into mechanisms regulating normal sleep and wakefulness.[4] This review focuses particularly on the clinical aspects and diagnostic approach toward patients with narcolepsy, emphasizing the severe impact the disease has on all aspects of daily life.[5,6] Current views on the pathophysiology of narcolepsy are also discussed while highlighting remaining crucial gaps in our knowledge.

In 1877, Westphal[7] reported the first unequivocal case of a disease subsequently called narcolepsy ("seized by somnolence") by Gelineau[8] 3 years later. Based on several index cases, Westphal and Gelineau described the combination of severe daytime sleepiness and attacks of muscle weakness triggered by emotions, later termed cataplexy.[8] Gelineau proposed that narcolepsy could either be a primary disorder or be triggered by other pathologic conditions, the most common example at the time being neurosyphilis. His early theories provoked a long debate centered on whether narcolepsy was indeed a specific disease entity and, if so, whether cataplexy was truly essential for the diagnosis. This debate continues and essentially remains unresolved.

It is now established that full-blown idiopathic narcolepsy with cataplexy is almost invariably associated with impaired hypothalamic hypocretin (orexin) signaling, fueling the notion that narcolepsy

Financial support: Sebastiaan Overeem is supported by a VIDI grant from the Netherlands Organization for Scientific Research (grant number 016.116.371).
Financial disclosures/conflicts of interest: The authors have nothing to disclose.
[a] Department of Neurology, Donders Institute for Brain, Cognition, and Behaviour, Radboud University Nijmegen Medical Centre, Reinier Postlaan 4, PO Box 9101, 6500 HB Nijmegen, The Netherlands; [b] Sleep Medicine Centre 'Kempenhaeghe', Sterkselseweg 65, 5590 AB Heeze, The Netherlands; [c] Department of Neurology, The James Cook University Hospital, Marton Road, Middlesbrough TS4 3BW, UK; [d] Department of Neurology, University Hospital (Inselspital), Freiburgstrasse 1, Bern 3010, Switzerland; [e] Neurocenter of Southern Switzerland, Via Tesserete 46, 6903 Lugano, Switzerland
* Corresponding author. Department of Neurology, Radboud University Nijmegen Medical Centre, PO Box 9101, 6500 HB Nijmegen, The Netherlands.
E-mail address: s.overeem@neuro.umcn.nl

Sleep Med Clin 7 (2012) 263–281
doi:10.1016/j.jsmc.2012.03.013

might be better defined as a syndrome of hypocretin deficiency. This simple approach is challenged, however, by the concept of familiar/secondary narcolepsy and narcolepsy without cataplexy, which are much less tightly linked to hypocretin deficiency. In addition, the narcoleptic syndrome forms a wider spectrum than previously appreciated both in terms of severity and the nature of symptoms.[9]

Early attempts to refine the clinical diagnosis were made by Yoss and Daly[10] who added the phenomena of hallucinations and sleep paralysis to obtain the classical tetrad of narcolepsy. However, only a minority of patients with narcolepsy routinely reports the full tetrad, and it is increasingly recognized that the typical phenotype of narcolepsy is actually much broader. In particular, most patients with narcolepsy have nocturnal sleep that is both dysregulated and fragmented, often in the presence of a variety of parasomnias. Furthermore, a range of nonsleep problems are recognized, reflecting metabolic, emotional, and cognitive dysfunctions. Common examples include obesity and mood and eating disorders.[11–13]

EPIDEMIOLOGY

In Western countries, narcolepsy has an estimated prevalence of 20 to 60 per 100,000 inhabitants.[14–16] Globally, however, there may be significant differences, with the highest reported prevalence in Japan and the lowest in Israel.[17,18] These disparities have not been causally explained and may also result from variations in diagnostic criteria or study design. Little information is available on the incidence of narcolepsy, but it has been estimated around 1.4 per 100,000 person-years.[19] It should be emphasized that narcolepsy often goes unrecognized and it is not uncommon for patients to wait more than 10 years between symptom onset and final diagnosis.[20]

Men and women are affected equally, with an average age of 24 years. A bimodal distribution in the age at onset has been described with a first peak occurring at adolescence (14.7 years) and a second at 35 years of age as shown in **Fig. 1**.[21] Recent studies highlight the fact that narcolepsy in young children may present somewhat differently, especially in regard to cataplexy, potentially leading to errors in gauging the age of onset.[22] Reassuringly, increasing awareness of narcolepsy is almost certainly improving its recognition in younger populations.

Narcoleptic symptoms typically develop in a gradual fashion with excessive daytime sleepiness (EDS) as the presenting problem and cataplexy appearing in the following few years.[23] Only a minority of patients develops the full-blown picture of narcolepsy, with around 10% to 15% displaying the classical tetrad.[3] Once symptoms have fully developed, there tends to be only minor fluctuations in severity, although cataplexy may lessen slightly with age.

PATHOPHYSIOLOGY
Animal Models

Research into the pathophysiology of narcolepsy was greatly stimulated in the early 1970s when

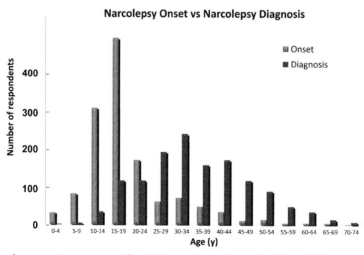

Fig. 1. Age of narcolepsy onset versus age of actual narcolepsy diagnosis. Although better recognition of narcolepsy in children may lower the number, previous studies demonstrate a delay in diagnosing narcolepsy. While the majority (70%–80%) of narcolepsy symptoms occur before age 25, the average peak age of onset is in the late teens. Unfortunately, the average delay in diagnosis is approximately 10 years. (*From* Dauvilliers Y, Montplaisir J, Molinari N, et al. Age at onset of narcolepsy in two large populations of patients in France and Quebec. Neurology 2001;57(11):2029–33; with permission.)

a canine model was discovered.[24] In several breeds, it was soon shown that narcolepsy was transmitted as a monogenetic, autosomal recessive trait.[25] In 1999, the hunt for the responsible canine gene was completed when mutations coding for a hypothalamic neuropeptide (hypocretin or orexin) receptor were identified.[26] In the same year, it was shown that preprohypocretin knockout mice, effectively unable to produce hypocretin, have fragmented nighttime sleep, sudden transitions form wakefulness into rapid eye movement (REM) sleep, and peculiar episodes of sudden behavioral arrest, reminiscent of cataplexy.[27] These findings in animal models were the basis for the final conclusion that defects in hypocretin neurotransmission are responsible for human idiopathic and sporadic narcolepsy.

The canine narcolepsy model has also been invaluable in characterizing the neuropharmacology of narcolepsy. This characterization has allowed testing of a broad range of drugs for their effect on sleepiness and cataplexy, in particular.[28] More recent rodent models of narcolepsy models are becoming increasingly influential.[29–32] Besides peptide knockouts, mice lacking hypocretin receptors 1, 2, or both are available. Moreover, using advanced genetic techniques, it is possible to destroy hypocretin neurons after birth in mice, yielding perhaps the model most closely resembling human narcolepsy.[33]

In several research areas, it is crucial to obtain a precise behavioral characterization of the symptoms produced in the various animal models. Cataplexy attacks witnessed in the canine model closely mimic the human condition, presumably reflecting the emotional range expressed by dogs. Understandably, in rodent models, cataplexy is less defined and more difficult to differentiate from simple REM sleep onset periods (SOREMPs). However, useful attempts have been undertaken in coming to a consensus when defining cataplexy in the various animal models (**Table 1**).[34]

Table 1
Cataplexy across species

	Human	Dog	Mouse
Behavioral features	Abrupt loss of postural muscle tone	Abrupt loss of postural muscle tone	Abrupt loss of postural muscle tone
Level of consciousness	Awake (memory of episodes intact)	Probably awake (visual tracking intact)	Uncertain but possibly awake at onset (response to visual stimuli intact)
Triggers	Strong, generally positive emotions (eg, laughter, joking, playing) immediately before cataplexy	Probably positive emotions (eg, playing, eating palatable food) immediately before cataplexy	Active behaviors with likely emotional content (eg, running, climbing, vigorous grooming, social interaction)
Duration	Brief (seconds to a few minutes)	Brief (seconds to a few minutes)	Brief (seconds to a few minutes)
EEG	Wake pattern and sometimes features of REM sleep	Wake pattern in cortex with theta activity in hippocampus	Theta activity similar to REM sleep
EMG	Atonia, sometimes with intermittent lapses in tone at onset	Atonia, sometimes with intermittent lapses in tone at onset	Atonia, sometimes with intermittent lapses in tone at onset
Response to therapy	Suppressed by monoamine reuptake blockers (eg, antidepressants) and sodium oxybate	Suppressed by monoamine reuptake blockers	Suppressed by clomipramine

Cataplexy has many similarities in people, dogs, and mice with narcolepsy, including abrupt postural atonia and improvement with clomipramine. During cataplexy in people and dogs, some investigators report an EEG pattern similar to wake, whereas others describe characteristics of REM sleep despite preservation of consciousness.

Abbreviations: EEG, electroencephalogram; EMG, electromyogram.

From Scammell TE, Willie JT, Guilleminault C, et al. A consensus definition of cataplexy in mouse models of narcolepsy. Sleep 2009;32:113; with permission.

Narcolepsy as a Hypocretin-Deficiency Syndrome

Following initial skepticism, it is now firmly established that human narcolepsy also reflects dysfunction of the hypocretin system. Almost 95% of patients with narcolepsy and clear-cut cataplexy have very low levels of hypocretin-1 in cerebrospinal fluid (CSF).[35-39] This deficiency is highly specific to narcolepsy and has not been found in healthy controls or other sleep disorders.[40,41] Low hypocretin levels have also been described in some cases of secondary narcolepsy caused by hypothalamic damage from different causes, a small number of cases with a severe form of Guillain-Barré syndrome (in Asiatic but not European patients), and in head trauma.[41-46] Pathologic studies in postmortem brain tissue from patients with narcolepsy have shown a clear loss of preprohypocretin messenger RNA, hypocretin peptides in the hypothalamus, and in hypocretin neuron projection areas.[47-49] Because 2 independent markers of hypocretin neurons (prodynorphin and neuronal activity-regulated pentraxin) were also depleted, it is most likely that the hypocretin deficiency in patients with narcolepsy is caused by a destruction of hypocretin-producing neurons.[50,51] If so, this process would be highly selective because melanin-concentrating hormone-producing neurons, which are intermingled with hypocretin neurons in the hypothalamus, were shown to be unaffected.[47]

The Cause of the Hypocretin Deficiency

Understandably, a major goal of current research is to identify the ultimate cause of the hypocretin deficiency in narcolepsy. One intense area of interest centers on the genetic aspects of the disorder. Although true familial narcolepsy is rare, most patients with sporadic narcolepsy are thought to carry a genetic susceptibility.[52,53] Of note, the risk of narcolepsy in a first-degree relative of a patient with narcolepsy is 2%, which is 10 to 40 times higher than the prevalence observed in the general population. Twin studies, although limited, indicated that more than 75% of monozygotic pairs are discordant for narcolepsy, suggesting a major contribution of environmental factors.[54-57] The first genetic factor in narcolepsy was identified in the early 1980s when it was shown that all Japanese patients with narcolepsy were human leukocyte antigen (HLA) DR2 positive.[58] Subsequent work in Caucasians confirmed this strong association. Molecular HLA typing revealed that HLA DRB1*1501, DQA1*0102, and DQB1*0602 alleles were present in more than 95% of the patients, compared to 25% in controls.[59,60] This established the tightest HLA association ever found in a disease. However, the HLA association in narcolepsy has proven to be complex. A recent genome-wide association study (GWAS) found that the HLA DRB1*1301-DQB1*0603 haplotype was almost never present in patients, suggesting a protective effect of this haplotype.[61] Another recent GWAS yielded a highly interesting association between narcolepsy and polymorphisms in the T cell receptor alpha subtype gene.[62] Only one patient has been found so far with a mutation in a gene directly related to hypocretin, in this case the preprohypocretin locus. This mutation was detected in a very atypical HLA DQB1*0602 negative narcolepsy case with a very young age at onset and a strikingly severe phenotype.[47] Other genetic predisposition factors are likely to play a role in narcolepsy, although their contribution to disease expression is not known. Associations with the tumor necrosis factor (TNF) alpha 2, as well as TNF receptor 2 genes, have been variably identified as important factors.[63,64] A recent finding that implicates an immunologic mechanism confirms an association with the purinergic receptor gene P2Y11, which has immune-modulatory effects.[65]

Narcolepsy and Autoimmunity

The strong HLA association in narcolepsy quickly led to the hypothesis that autoimmunity was a likely etiologic mechanism, potentially explaining the astonishing selectivity of neuronal destruction in the hypothalamus.[66,67] It has been hypothesized that the T cell receptor alpha subtype polymorphism could contribute to the presumed autoimmunity toward hypocretin neurons by influencing specific recombination of T cell receptor variable joining segments capable of interacting with HLA DQB1*0602.[62,67]

Repeated efforts were directed toward finding a marker of humoral autoimmunity in narcolepsy with particular emphasis on the proposed presence of circulating antibodies against various elements of the hypocretin system.[66,68] Although one study found an increased CSF immunoglobulin G (IgG) fraction cross-reacting with rat hypothalamic extract, most studies have been negative in this respect.[68-72] Recently, increased titers of antibodies against Tribbles homologue 2, expressed in hypocretin neurons, have been found in a small percentage of patients studied close to disease onset.[73-75] In addition, increased IgG titers of antistreptolysin O have also been found in recent onset cases.[76,77]

However, definitive proof for autoimmunity remains elusive. In contrast to established autoimmune disorders, narcolepsy is only rarely associated with other manifestations of autoimmunity.[67]

Furthermore, treatments with immune-modulating drugs have largely been negative, except for a possible reduction of symptoms in a few cases after repeated high doses of intravenous immunoglobulins (IvIG).[78–80] However, this positive result has not been easy to replicate.[81–83] In addition, the effects of IvIG are complex and may also produce a large placebo effect for symptoms, such as cataplexy.[81]

In 2010, a significant increase in new cases of narcolepsy in young children was reported in Finland and Sweden, which seemed to have a temporal association with vaccination against pandemic H1N1 influenza.[84–86] A comparable increase in incidence has not been reported in other countries to date, and case-control studies are currently underway to confirm or refute a possible causal association. Of interest, a large retrospective analysis of narcolepsy onset in China suggested a possible 3-fold increase following the 2009 H1N1 pandemic.[87] In that study, a relation with vaccination was unlikely because only 5% of the population were actually vaccinated.

Overall, therefore, an autoimmune-mediated destruction of hypocretin neurons as the primary cause of narcolepsy is a tantalizing possibility but remains to be confirmed.

From Hypocretin-Deficiency to Clinical Symptoms

Several models have been developed to link the defects in hypocretin neurotransmission to the clinical symptoms of narcolepsy. Hypocretin neurons exert a major excitatory influence on both monoaminergic and cholinergic systems involved in the regulation of vigilance states.[88,89] Hypocretin deficiency may, therefore, explain abnormalities in these classical sleep-regulating neurotransmitter systems reported in narcolepsy.[28] An influential perspective on the effects of hypocretin deficiency comes from the description of the so-called sleep switch.[90] In this model, the normal mutual inhibitory connections between key sleep and wake regulating brain structures result in an inherently unstable flip-flop system. In this system, intermediate states of wake and sleep are avoided and any change in state occurs quickly.[90] The hypocretin system is ideally situated to act as a stabilizing factor, keeping the sleep switch fixed in the wake position. In the absence of hypocretin, the switch reverts to an unstable system with frequent changes between vigilance states, a prominent feature of hypocretin-deficient mice.[91,92] This system also perfectly fits with the phenotype of human narcolepsy, a key component of which is an inability to sustain either wakefulness or sleep for appropriate periods of time.[93]

For cataplexy, the theoretical framework is less clear. Based on the fact that strong emotions, such as laughter, can induce subclinical signs of motor inhibition even in healthy subjects,[94–96] it may be necessary to have a brain system that suppresses this tendency for paralysis.[97] Recent studies measuring the activity of hypocretin neurons in freely moving rats may support this view.[98] Hypocretin neurons were relatively silent during most of the day but were activated most when the animals were confronted with emotional stimuli, such as types of food not encountered previously. It was hypothesized that the hypocretin system is necessary to prevent the normal onset of motor inhibition seen in emotionally charged situations.[98] Another explanation is based on the REM-sleep dissociation theory of cataplexy, portraying it as the physiologic atonia that occurs during REM sleep intruding into the wakeful state.[99] Deficits in the hypocretin system are thought to result in dysregulation and disinhibition of REM sleep in this model, leading to cataplexy and other REM sleep–related phenomena. Regardless of the effector system, there is increasing evidence that the hypocretin system is integrated in a circuit involving the amygdala and, more generally, emotional processing, which could partly explain the triggering of cataplexy.[100,101]

CLINICAL FEATURES
General Aspects

The classical tetrad of narcolepsy described more than 50 years ago is still often quoted despite only applying to a minority of patients.[3,10] Many have argued that fragmented or poor quality nocturnal sleep is so common and troublesome in patients with narcolepsy that it warrants inclusion as a core symptom, creating a pentad.[9,102] The clinical phenotype of narcolepsy is even broader and includes persistently impaired vigilance together with automatic behaviors that occur in presumed microsleeps. Obesity, pain syndromes, and mood and anxiety disorders are common.

Excessive Daytime Sleepiness

EDS is the primary, most recognized symptom of narcolepsy and usually the most debilitating. It may take various forms, with reports of continuous somnolence at one end of the spectrum and intermittent sudden or irresistible sleep attacks at the other. Some experience a combination of these 2 patterns. As in healthy individuals, the tendency to fall asleep is more pronounced during monotonous, nonstimulating activities. Indeed, a proportion of patients are able to fight the need to sleep simply by engaging in physical activity, for example. Typically, sleep episodes in narcolepsy are short, often lasting less than 20 minutes. In many patients, such short naps are refreshing or restorative, which is a feature that can help with the differential diagnosis.[3,103] Although sleep episodes may recur throughout the day, the total amount of sleep is normal or only minimally increased over a 24-hour period because of nocturnal sleep fragmentation.[93] Different patterns of sleepiness, such as prolonged daytime naps or continuous sleepiness with superimposed naps, are also described and should not necessarily suggest an alternative diagnosis.

EDS can be an incapacitating symptom but is not always recognized as such. Especially in the young, napping at inopportune times is often dismissed as laziness or as a simple consequence of over doing it. This view is, in part, because many commentators consider themselves experts, having experienced mild daytime sleepiness as a result of bad or reduced nocturnal sleep.

Cataplexy

The presence of cataplexy is of paramount diagnostic importance because it is virtually pathognomonic for narcolepsy. Because there are no practical or objective measures of cataplexy, its presence needs to be established based on the clinical interview alone. In the current *International Classification of Sleep Disorders* (ICSD-2), cataplexy is descriptively defined as "sudden and transient episodes of loss of muscle tone triggered by emotions."[104] In addition, "episodes must be triggered by strong emotions - most reliably laughing or joking- and must be generally bilateral and brief (less than two minutes)."[104] In practice, this definition is often difficult to apply for various reasons. The cataplexy phenotype differs widely between patients, ranging from rare instances of partial attacks triggered by laughter to frequent complete attacks of collapse brought about by a variety of emotions.[3,105–107] A further complication is that feelings of muscle weakness potentially causing knee buckling when laughing out loud are regularly reported in healthy individuals in many cultures.[3,95]

Cataplexy results from a temporary loss of voluntary muscle tone causing flaccid paresis or paralysis. It can affect virtually all skeletal muscles, although some muscle groups are preferentially involved.[3,105–107] Neck weakness is a common complaint, producing head drop, whereas facial weakness may lead to sagging of the jaw and dysarthria. Knee buckling is also frequently reported in full-blown attacks. Respiratory muscles are not involved, although patients sometimes describe shortness of breath when symptomatic.

In most attacks, cataplexy is bilateral, although patients sometimes report one side of the body to be more affected. Cataplectic attacks are often partial, preferentially involving the muscle groups described previously. Partial attacks can be subtle and sometimes only recognized by experienced observers, such as the patient's partner. Attacks start abruptly and usually build up over several seconds, especially in attacks producing complete peripheral weakness and collapse.[3,107] Although the central characteristic of cataplexy is atonia, positive motor phenomena are often observed, with muscle twitching or small jerks, particularly of the face, potentially leading to diagnostic confusion.[3,107]

The key involvement of emotion or its anticipation as a trigger for cataplexy is a defining feature.[3,107] In **Table 2**, a list of most frequently reported cataplexy triggers is shown, ordered in the frequency of likely occurrence. Although the whole gamut of emotions can potentially lead to cataplexy, those associated with mirth are usually the most potent. Laughing out loud, telling a joke, or making a witty remark are typical examples, with some reporting the anticipation of laughter, typically as a punch line approaches, to be the most effective precipitant.[3,107] Collapse induced by surprise on unexpectedly meeting a friend is also a commonly reported scenario. Although rare, spontaneous cataplectic attacks are also possible in the absence of a clear identifiable trigger. Cataplexy has been linked also with orgasm (orgasmolepsia).

The frequency of cataplexy is variable, ranging from less than one attack per month to more than 20 attacks per day. However, in an individual patient, the attack frequency remains relatively stable.[108] Because a certain intimacy is often required for attacks to occur in company, cataplexy is rarely observed or elicited during medical consultation. Many patients develop an awareness that a cataplectic attack is about to happen, reporting warning signs, such as strange feelings in the head or sensations of warmth or nervousness. Indeed, many patients develop tricks to try and prevent cataplectic attacks from evolving.[107]

Cataplexy is generally short lived, lasting a matter of seconds, with most attacks lasting less than 2 minutes. However, if a particular trigger continues, consecutive attacks may merge together to form what seems to be one long episode. Sudden withdrawal of anticataplectic medication, especially antidepressants, can also result in so-called status cataplecticus in which long-lasting attacks happen virtually continuously, rendering patients severely disabled.[109]

Table 2
Cataplexy triggers

Trigger	Percentage of Patients[a]
Laughing excitedly	61.7
Making a sharp-minded remark	53.8
Telling a joke	48.1
Before reaching the punch line of a joke	47.2
Being tickled	42.1
Hearing a joke	39.6
Being angry	36.2
Unexpectedly meeting someone well known	34.9
Being startled	29.9
Tickling someone	25.0
Laughing	21.9
Chuckling	16.2
Experiencing an orgasm	15.9
Being the center of attention	14.3
Expectedly meeting someone well known	13.6
Unexpectedly meeting an acquaintance	12.5
Feeling stressed	10.6
Feeling ashamed	8.9
Hearing an unexpected sound	6.8
Spontaneously	6.8
In the waiting room at the doctor	4.8
Hearing an expected sound	4.8
While eating	3.9
In pain	1.0

[a] Percentage of patients reporting that a trigger could often or always trigger their cataplexy.
Data from Overeem S, van Nues SJ, van der Zande WL, et al. The clinical features of cataplexy: a questionnaire study in narcolepsy patients with and without hypocretin-1 deficiency. Sleep Med 2011;12:12–8.

Cataplexy in Children

In recent years, increasing attention has been given to the clinical presentation of narcolepsy in childhood. Several studies, especially by Plazzi and colleagues in Bologna, have now shown that cataplexy in children can seem phenotypically different to typical episodes seen in adulthood.[22,110–112] In addition to typical attacks triggered by positive emotions, children can also present with more generalized hypotonia. Weakness particularly involves the face, eyelids, and mouth (**Fig. 2**).[22] Together with tongue protrusion, this characteristic pattern has been termed a cataplectic facies.[110] In addition, children with cataplexy may also display positive motor phenomena, ranging from perioral dyskinetic or dystonic movements to frank stereotypies. Although follow-up data are limited, it seems this phenotype gradually evolves over subsequent months and years to the typical adult form.[22]

Hallucinations

About one-third of the patients with narcolepsy have frequent hypnagogic hallucinations, which are defined as vivid dreamlike experiences occurring at the transition between wake and sleep. If present at the point of waking from sleep, the term hypnopompic hallucinations is used. Typically, hypnagogic hallucinations have a multimodal or holistic character, often combining visual, auditory, and tactile phenomena.[3,113] Not infrequently, visual elements of the sleeping environment are incorporated into the hallucination producing bizarre and often disturbing experiences. In some patients, hallucinations are so intense that they may be misdiagnosed as psychotic symptoms.[114] However, the multimodal nature of the hallucination and retained insight into its dreamlike quality are usually sufficient to avoid a misdiagnosis of conditions, such as schizophrenia.[113]

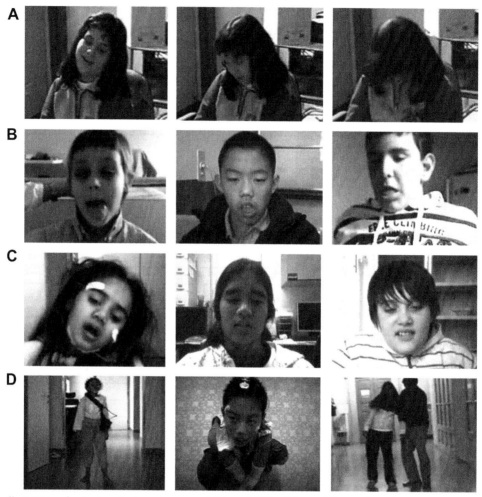

Fig. 2. Illustration of cataplexy features in young children. (*A*) Head drop while watching funny cartoons. (*B*) Ptosis and tongue protrusion in 3 patients. (*C*) Facial hypotonia in 3 patients. (*D*) Persisting generalized hypotonia in 3 patients with a wide based gate, forced squatting position and unsteady gate respectively. (*From* Plazzi G, Pizza F, Palaia V, et al. Complex movement disorders at disease onset in childhood narcolepsy with cataplexy. Brain 2011;134:3484; with permission.)

Sleep Paralysis

Sleep paralysis describes the disturbing temporary inability to move voluntary muscles at sleep-wake transitions.[3] The phenomenon usually occurs at the point of waking, although patients with narcolepsy also experience episodes as they drift to sleep. Despite being awake and conscious of the sleeping environment, it is impossible for patients to move their limbs or even open their eyes. The experience may last for several minutes and it can be extremely distressing, especially when occurring for the first time. An inability to take a voluntary deep breath often gives the disturbing sensation of chest constriction. Concomitant visual or tactile hypnagogic or hypnopompic hallucinations may occur, adding to the unpleasant nature

of the experience. Stress, sleep deprivation, or an uncomfortable sleep position may increase the frequency of episodes. Sensory stimulation, typically being touched by a bed partner, usually terminates an episode, although some patients report such attempts cause further distress.

Disturbed Nocturnal Sleep

Although sleep onset is rarely a problem, an inability to maintain continuous sleep is extremely common and often a major concern for patients with narcolepsy and their partners.[2,3,9,102] Numerous arousals from sleep may be reported, some of which are prolonged and severely disruptive. Polysomnography typically shows destructuring of the normal sleep architecture with an increased frequency of shifts between sleep states and frequent awakenings (**Fig. 3**).[115,116] In some patients, disturbing dream or hallucinatory experiences are largely responsible for the sleep fragmentation, whereas, in others, it simply seems to reflect an inability simply to stay in a state of sleep. Attempts to improve the quality of overnight sleep may help to alleviate daytime sleepiness to some extent. However, a direct relationship between the severity of nocturnal sleep disruption and daytime sleepiness has not been established.[117]

An increased frequency of numerous other sleep disorders has been described in narcolepsy, including sleep talking, periodic limb movement disorder, sleep-disordered breathing, and REM sleep behavior disorder (RBD).[3,102,118,119] However, with the possible exception of sleep apnea, the clinical relevance of any potential comorbid sleep disturbance is often unclear. On overnight testing, patients with narcolepsy are frequently observed to move abnormally during REM sleep, although any resulting dream enactment is rarely aggressive or troublesome in contrast to idiopathic RBD. The striking male preponderance usually seen in RBD is not seen in narcolepsy, and the age of onset is typically young, highlighting further differences. However, in common with other forms of RBD, the phenomenon can be exacerbated or even induced by concomitant treatment with antidepressant drugs.[119]

Decreased Vigilance, Automatic Behavior, and Memory Complaints

Narcolepsy is typically characterized by excessive sleepiness and the intrusion of unwanted naps during the day. However, it is important to appreciate that even when appearing alert, patients with narcolepsy often display significant problems with decreased vigilance that interferes with cognition and performance. Assessments of maintained attention or vigilance are sensitive markers of sleep-wake disturbance compared with the multiple sleep latency test (MSLT), for example, and may probe different aspects.[120] It has been advocated that tests of vigilance should be incorporated in the diagnostic workup of narcolepsy, especially given the likely impact that impaired attention may have on daily activities.[120] Reduced vigilance or the presence of so-called microsleeps may explain the frequent occurrence of automatic behaviors reported in narcolepsy. Typical examples of semipurposeful but inappropriate automatic behaviors are placing unusual objects in a refrigerator or writing nonsense prose down a page. A further likely consequence of reduced vigilance is impaired memory and an inability to focus adequately. Indeed, most patients with narcolepsy complain of a poor short-term memory, although formal deficits are minimal on objective testing.[121]

Obesity

From as early as the 1930s, it has been reported that patients with narcolepsy tend to be overweight.[122] This finding has usually been attributed to the inactivity associated with EDS and has, therefore, received little attention. However, epidemiologic studies have now clearly shown that obesity is likely to be a primary symptom of narcolepsy. Obesity (defined as a body mass index [BMI] $\geq$30 kg/m^2) occurs more than twice as often in patients with narcolepsy compared with control groups.[11,123,124] Nearly 40% of patients with narcolepsy have a waist circumference large enough to warrant intervention to prevent possible long-term complications.[11] Weight gain can be a major issue for many patients and an important issue to address even though effective management is often difficult.

The precise cause of excessive weight gain in narcolepsy remains unknown. On direct enquiry, although many patients report a tendency to binge eat (see later discussion), the limited data on actual caloric intake do not support overeating

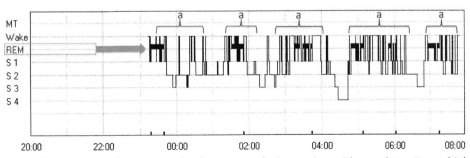

Fig. 3. Typical hypnogram based on nocturnal polysomnography in a patient with narcolepsy. Note a highly fragmented sleep pattern with numerous awakenings (a) and frequent shifts between sleep states. In addition a sleep-onset REM period is present (*red arrow*). MT, movement time; REM, rapid eye movement sleep; S1, N1 sleep stage, S2, N2 sleep stage; S3, S4, N3 sleep stage (slow wave sleep).

as a primary cause. In a study using cross-checked dietary histories, it was shown that patients with narcolepsy actually tended to consume fewer calories over a 24-hour period compared with controls.[125] Inactivity secondary to EDS is also unlikely to account for significant obesity because patients suffering from idiopathic hypersomnia with equivalent levels of EDS have been shown to have a lower BMI than patients with narcolepsy.[11] It has, therefore, been speculated that the hypocretin deficiency in narcolepsy may directly affect metabolism and possibly lower basal metabolic rates. However, studies on this topic have yielded conflicting results with no systematic decreases in objective metabolic parameters. Initial interesting data suggesting abnormalities in the neuropeptide systems regulating satiety and body weight have also been difficult to replicate.[126–130]

Mood Disorders

For a considerable time, there have been suggestions of increased levels of depression in narcolepsy. More recently, the relationship has been addressed in various ways: either as a secondary outcome in quality-of-life studies, generally using self-report depression-severity scales, or with more formal psychiatric diagnostic instruments. Self-reporting with the Beck Depression Inventory, for example, has invariably implied a high prevalence of depression.[131,132] However, self-report scales may be particularly unreliable in the patients with narcolepsy because of the potential overlap of many symptoms that may characterize both conditions. Disordered nocturnal sleep, reduced powers of attention, changes in body weight, and general fatigue are clearly common examples. Using more formal psychiatric evaluations, Vourdas and colleagues[133] did not find an overrepresentation of major depression in narcolepsy. In a recent study using a structured psychiatric interview, no higher prevalence of major depression in narcolepsy compared with a population control group was found.[12] However, there were suggestions that many reported symptoms, such as pathologic guilt and anhedonia, could not be easily attributed to narcolepsy. As with many long-term conditions, paying attention to mood status is of paramount importance. Indeed, the presence of depressive symptoms has been shown to be an important independent predictor of health-related quality of life in narcolepsy.[6] Recent neuroimaging studies have demonstrated an altered emotional processing in narcolepsy suggesting the possibility that

psychiatric disturbances may be at least in part nonreactive/related to the disease per se.[101,134]

Anxiety

Anxiety symptoms have received less attention compared with depression in narcolepsy. However, in a recent study, the authors found a strikingly high level of anxiety disorders, such as panic attacks or social phobias, which affected 20% of patients. Indeed, more than one-third fulfilled criteria for a formal anxiety disorder.[12] It remains unclear whether anxiety symptoms are related to the disease itself or are secondary phenomena. The latter explanation is perhaps favored by the loss of control reported by many patients with narcolepsy. Particular examples include experiencing unpredictable cataplexy in public environments or anxiety triggered by daytime recollection of hallucinatory experiences. The latter might fuel specific phobias, such as a fear of insects.[12]

Other Psychiatric Symptoms

Although it is important to clearly differentiate EDS from fatigue when assessing patients with a suspected hypersomnia, there are indications that fatigue is not an uncommon additional complaint in narcolepsy.[135,136] In one study, more than 60% of patients with narcolepsy and cataplexy reported severe fatigue separable from actual EDS.[135] Although often overlooked, fatigue may warrant more attention because it was independently associated with functional impairment and a lowered quality of life.

When specifically questioned, patients with narcolepsy often report changes in their appetite or eating habits. For example, many patients tend to eat during prolonged nocturnal arousals or report episodes of carbohydrate craving. More formal studies have confirmed that eating disorders may be overrepresented in narcolepsy, with a form of binge eating disorder as a frequent association.[13,137] Sexual dysfunction is also common, including erectile problems and loss of libido. Occasionally, severe EDS or even cataplexy may interfere with sexual activity.[138] It is important to address the possibility of drug side effects as contributors to such problems, especially if antidepressants are prescribed.

Psychosocial Consequences

Narcolepsy has a striking negative effect on quality of life and affects virtually every domain.[5,6,131,139–143] Psychosocial problems are frequent, incapacitating, and occur across all cultures. To the surprise of some, the impact of narcolepsy is often more severe than that of other chronic diseases, such as epilepsy.[144] Many patients have educational and occupational problems, even when taking optimum drug treatment. In particular, narcolepsy has deleterious effects on work performance, promotion, earning capacity, and interpersonal relations, including marriage and sexual function. There is an increased risk of job loss, accidents, and additional insurance payments. Stringent driving regulations in many countries may also impair job prospects. Children and adolescents with narcolepsy report embarrassment, academic decline, and loss of self-esteem, often accentuated by a long delay before diagnosis. The psychosocial impact of narcolepsy is not limited to the adverse effects of EDS because significant cataplexy can also be extremely debilitating. Many such patients become severely reclusive to avoid stimuli that provoke attacks.

DIAGNOSTIC TOOLS
Clinical Approach

In every patient, the whole gamut of potential symptoms needs to be assessed, especially because many may not be spontaneously reported or even suspected as a likely consequence of narcolepsy. In **Table 3**, a suggested outline is

Table 3 Important topics to cover in the clinical interview	
General	Age at onset and initial presenting symptom; Are there any possible triggers around onset (eg, infection, vaccination, trauma)?
Sleepiness	What is the pattern of excessive sleepiness: continuous somnolence or sleep attacks? What is the frequency and duration of both involuntary and planned sleep episodes? Are sleep episodes refreshing? Can sleep be resisted? Are there dreams or similar phenomena during short naps? What circumstances worsen or improve sleepiness?
Cataplexy	What is the description of a typical attack, including pattern of weakness? Are attacks mostly partial or complete? What is the frequency and duration of episodes? Ensure there is no loss of consciousness. Enquire about spectrum of triggers. Have there been physical injuries?
Nocturnal sleep	Habitual sleep duration and sleep-wake schedule; subjective sleep latency, number and duration of awakenings; symptoms of possible other sleep disorders (such as sleep-disordered breathing, restless legs syndrome). Assess sleep hygiene
Hypnagogic hallucinations	Duration, frequency, and content; associated symptoms of fear and anxiety
Sleep paralysis	Duration and frequency; Co-occurrence with hypnagogic hallucinations?
Weight change	Current weight and height to calculate body mass index; Is there any change around onset of narcolepsy symptoms? current stability of weight; Is there any influence of medication on weight?
Eating habits	Abnormal appetite (eg, binge eating, eating at night); influence of meals and their type (eg, high carbohydrate load) on (postprandial) sleepiness
Mood/anxiety	Are there mood disturbances? Is there a history of depression, anxiety, panic attacks, or phobias?
Automatic behavior	Establish any examples of automatic behaviors and their circumstances and frequency
Other symptoms	Are there memory complaints? If appropriate, ask about sexual problems. Specifically assess fatigue (separate from actual sleepiness)
Psychosocial aspects	Have the symptoms (sleepiness or cataplexy) influenced social interactions at school or work? Ask about driving
Family history	Are their any relatives with narcolepsy, daytime sleepiness, or other sleep disorders?

given of topics to cover in the clinical interview. The precise pattern of sleepiness and features of naps, such as length and restorative value, are important differential diagnostic clues. The diagnostic classification of narcolepsy (see later discussion) is highly dependent on the presence of cataplexy, which is established solely from history taking. Besides the presence of specific symptoms, the impact of sleep-related symptoms on daily living should be probed. The relative burden that a specific symptom poses on patients will also direct the course and aims of subsequent treatment. In most patients, the clinical symptoms remain stable over years. However, the actual expression of symptoms and the associated functional disability depends greatly on a patient's circumstances. It is, therefore, strongly advised to keep patients under long-term follow-up even if symptom control seems stable.

Nocturnal Polysomnography

Polysomnography is most often performed to exclude other nocturnal sleep disorders as a possible cause of EDS, such as sleep-disordered breathing. However, it also provides a useful indication of associated sleep disturbances frequently observed in narcolepsy, including RBD. A SOREMP during nighttime recording can be observed in up to 50% of cases, although this finding is not part of the diagnostic criteria.[104] Frequent arousals, often from deep sleep, are commonly observed, and the distribution of deep non-REM sleep may seem abnormal, with episodes occurring late in the night. Ideally, polysomnography should always be performed before an MSLT to establish the preceding total nocturnal sleep time.[145]

Multiple Sleep Latency Test

The MSLT remains a cornerstone in the diagnosis of narcolepsy, despite its many shortcomings. In most protocols, patients are given 5 nap opportunities at 2 hourly intervals through the morning and early afternoon after a routine nocturnal sleep. Each nap opportunity is terminated after 20 minutes whether sleep is achieved or not. Across naps, the mean latency to sleep onset (stage 1) in narcolepsy is usually around 2 to 3 minutes. However, given the considerable variability between patients and even within patients when repeated tests are performed, a criterion of 8 minutes has been adopted to indicate the presence of significant EDS.[104] If EDS is established, the occurrence of REM sleep on at least 2 naps within 15 minutes of recording (sudden-onset REM or SOREM periods) is used as a diagnostic

indicator for narcolepsy.[104] Although these diagnostic criteria are widely accepted, clinical experience and formal studies have indicated that both their sensitivity and specificity are suboptimal.[146–148] False negative and false positive results are common, in part reflecting the difficulty in standardizing the test. For example, some patients with proven hypocretin-1 deficiency fail to fulfill the MSLT criteria for narcolepsy. In addition, the presence of typical cataplexy is a better predictor for hypocretin-1 deficiency than seemingly more objective MSLT results.

CSF Hypocretin-1 Measurements

Following the earliest reports of hypocretin deficiency in human narcolepsy by Nishino and colleagues,[35] it was anticipated that hypocretin-1 measurements would grow into an important new diagnostic tool. Indeed, an extended study in more than 40 patients with narcolepsy confirmed that more than 90% of patients with classical narcolepsy (ie, with cataplexy and HLA DQB1*0602) had undetectable hypocretin-1 levels.[36] This finding has been replicated in numerous studies across different populations.[37,38,41,149–153] Increasing data on hypocretin-1 levels in the narcolepsy borderland, such as atypical cases of narcolepsy (no cataplexy, familial cases, HLA DQB1*0602 negative), and other sleep disorders (eg, idiopathic hypersomnia) are available to help clarify the role of hypocretin measurements in the diagnosis of narcolepsy.[40] The sensitivity and specificity of low hypocretin-1 levels in a randomly selected subset of patients with cataplexy are high (87% and 99% respectively), resulting in both a positive and a negative predictive value of about 90% to 95%.[40,153] In patients without cataplexy, the specificity of low hypocretin values is still high but sensitivity is much lower (about 15%), with most people having normal levels.

Hypocretin-1 levels can be measured in CSF, using a commercially available radioimmunoassay. Standards for the application of the assay have been published.[154] The interassay variability of the test is high, prompting recommendations to include a reference sample in each assay to obtain comparable results. Using the Stanford reference sample, a hypocretin-1 concentration less than 110 pg/mL is considered to be diagnostic.[40] Alternatively, normal values can be established locally using healthy subjects or patients with disorders known not to affect hypocretin levels.

Currently, there are several clinical situations in which hypocretin measurements are particularly useful. Sometimes the MSLT is difficult to interpret, for example, in patients using sleep-modulating medications or with concomitant sleep disorders, such as sleep apnea. Likewise, interpretation of the MSLT can be problematic in young children because of a lack of normative data and practical issues with the test in this group. Hypocretin measurements are also valuable when cataplexy is doubtful or atypical. Finally, for research purposes, hypocretin measurements make it possible to define homogenous patient groups.

Other Diagnostic Tools

More than 90% of patients with typical sporadic narcolepsy with cataplexy are positive for the HLA subtype DQB1*0602 compared with around 25% in control groups.[59] The low specificity of this finding means HLA typing is rarely a useful clinical tool for diagnosis. Furthermore, in clinically difficult cases (no cataplexy, very young onset, a positive family history), HLA positivity is considerably less common. HLA typing remains an important research tool, however, helping to define homogenous patient groups and providing insights into pathophysiology.

Actigraphy can be used to obtain an estimate of the habitual sleep-wake patterns of patients over long periods. In the absence of clear-cut cataplexy, actigraphy can be useful in assessing the possibility of behaviorally induced insufficient sleep as a cause of EDS.[155,156] Questionnaires, such as the Epworth Sleepiness Scale, and the Swiss Narcolepsy Scale[3] can also be applied to measure subjective sleepiness. These scales do not help with the differential diagnosis but provide a useful indication of the severity of the perceived sleepiness and may sometimes be helpful in monitoring treatment effects. Vigilance tests, such as the Sustained Attention to Response Task, have been shown to be abnormal in patients with narcolepsy.[120] Future studies are required to study the specificity and usefulness of the test. However, a measure that has practical implications and is capable of assessing functional status has intuitive appeal.

DIAGNOSTIC CLASSIFICATION

The current ICSD-2 classification of narcolepsy makes an explicit distinction between narcolepsy with and without cataplexy.[104] The diagnostic criteria are listed in **Box 1**. In the presence of otherwise unexplained EDS and clear-cut

---

Box 1
ICSD-2 narcolepsy criteria

Narcolepsy with cataplexy

1. The patient has a complaint of excessive daytime sleepiness occurring almost daily for at least 3 months.

2. A definite history of cataplexy, defined as sudden and transient episodes of loss of muscle tone triggered by emotions, is presen.

3. The diagnosis of narcolepsy with cataplexy *should, whenever possible,* be confirmed by nocturnal polysomnography followed by an MSLT. The mean sleep latency on MSLT is less than or equal to 8 minutes and 2 or more SOREMPs are observed following sufficient nocturnal sleep (minimum 6 hours) during the night before the test. Alternatively, hypocretin-1 levels in the CSF are less than or equal to 110 pg/mL or one-third of the mean normal control values.

4. The hypersomnia is not better explained by another sleep disorder, medical or neurologic disorder, mental disorder, medication use, or substance use disorder.

Narcolepsy without cataplexy

1. The patient has a complaint of excessive daytime sleepiness occurring almost daily for at least 3 months.

2. Typical cataplexy is not present, although doubtful or atypical cataplexylike episodes may be reported.

3. The diagnosis of narcolepsy without cataplexy *must* be confirmed by nocturnal polysomnography followed by an MSLT. In narcolepsy without cataplexy, the mean sleep latency on MSLT is less than or equal to 8 minutes and 2 or more SOREMPs are observed following sufficient nocturnal sleep (minimum 6 hours) during the night before the test.

4. The hypersomnia is not better explained by another sleep disorder, medical or neurologic disorder, mental disorder, medication use, or substance use disorder.

From American Academy of Sleep Medicine. The International Classification of Sleep Disorders: diagnostic and coding manual. 2nd edition. Chicago: AASM; 2005; with permission.

cataplexy, a diagnosis of narcolepsy with cataplexy can be made based solely on patients' history. However, a confident determination of cataplexy can be difficult, especially when there are only partial or atypical attacks. Even if a confident clinical diagnosis is made, confirmatory objective investigations are usually recommended because of the implications of a positive diagnosis (both socially and therapeutically). Using the ICSD-2 criteria, diagnosis can be made either when an MSLT demonstrates sleep latency less than 8 minutes together with at least 2 SOREMPs or if CSF hypocretin-1 levels are less than 110 pg/mL.

In the absence of clear cataplexy, it can be difficult to establish a diagnosis of narcolepsy, either clinically or with tests, and it is mandatory to exclude other causes of EDS, such as sleep-disordered breathing. In young patients, chronic sleep curtailment may frequently masquerade as possible narcolepsy without cataplexy. The standard MSLT criteria or hypocretin-1 deficiency are mandatory to make the diagnosis but their application and reliability in this situation are debated. There may well be an overlap between narcolepsy without cataplexy and idiopathic hypersomnia. Alternatively, whether narcolepsy without cataplexy is truly part of a continuum with narcolepsy and cataplexy, sharing a common pathophysiology, remains uncertain.[3,157] In particular, it is unclear whether levels of CSF hypocretin should have a more important role in diagnosis, especially in the context of narcolepsy without cataplexy.[3,153]

Given the possible difficulties in assessing the presence of cataplexy and the suboptimal reliability of objective testing, one approach is to recommend a grading system with increasing levels of diagnostic probability. Such a system was proposed by Silber and colleagues[158] just before hypocretin measurements were integrated into clinical practice. Given the current state of knowledge, levels could range from definite narcolepsy with proven hypocretin-1 deficiency, to probable narcolepsy with clear cataplexy and an abnormal MSLT, to possible narcolepsy based solely on the presence of clinical symptoms. A comparable grading system could also be applied to individual symptoms, such as cataplexy. Classification could then be based on the number of key features that are present, such as muscle atonia, specifically defined emotional triggers, short duration, preserved consciousness, and quick recovery.[107] Even though these types of classification systems may be too complex to apply in everyday practice, they could prove highly valuable in research studies.

SUMMARY AND FUTURE PERSPECTIVES

In the last 2 decades, giant leaps have been made in our understanding of the pathophysiology of narcolepsy alongside increasing appreciation of the wide spectrum and disabling array of symptoms patients are confronted with. However much remains to be learned. In the following years further insights into the precise causal mechanisms leading to hypocretin deficiency are expected, with the ultimate aim of preventing the disease. Increased knowledge of the pathophysiology of narcolepsy may also lead to significant therapeutic advances. In the meantime, clinical efforts to delineate the spectrum of narcolepsy are important. For example, more knowledge is needed to confidently diagnose narcolepsy without cataplexy and understand its pathophysiology. New approaches toward the clinical classification of narcolepsy are likely to benefit patients by allowing a more precise diagnosis. In turn, clinical advances will aid research efforts, particularly in genetic association studies in which diagnostic accuracy is of paramount importance. Describing the particular features of childhood narcolepsy will be important for early recognition, potentially leading to future disease-modifying therapies. Finally, narcolepsy is likely to remain an extremely influential model to probe our understanding of normal sleep-wake regulation and the role of sleep regulation systems in other diseases.

REFERENCES

1. Mignot E. A hundred years of narcolepsy research. Arch Ital Biol 2001;139:207–20.
2. Dauvilliers Y, Arnulf I, Mignot E. Narcolepsy with cataplexy. Lancet 2007;369:499–511.
3. Sturzenegger C, Bassetti C. The clinical spectrum of narcolepsy with cataplexy: a reappraisal. J Sleep Res 2004;13:395–406.
4. Nishino S. Hypothalamus, hypocretins/orexin, and vigilance control. Handb Clin Neurol 2011;99:765–82.
5. Dodel R, Peter H, Spottke A, et al. Health-related quality of life in patients with narcolepsy. Sleep Med 2007;8:733–41.
6. Vignatelli L, Plazzi G, Peschechera F, et al. A 5-year prospective cohort study on health-related quality of life in patients with narcolepsy. Sleep Med 2011;12:19–23.
7. Westphal C. Eigenthümliche mit Einschlafen verbundene Anfälle. Arch Psychiatr Nervenkr 1877;7:631–5.
8. Gélineau JB. De la narcolepsie. Gaz Hôp (Paris) 1880;53:626–8.
9. Overeem S, Mignot E, van Dijk JG, et al. Narcolepsy: clinical features, new pathophysiologic

insights, and future perspectives. J Clin Neurophysiol 2001;18:78–105.

10. Yoss RE, Daly DD. Criteria for the diagnosis of the narcoleptic syndrome. Proc Staff Meet Mayo Clin 1957;32:320–8.

11. Kok SW, Overeem S, Visscher TL, et al. Hypocretin deficiency in narcoleptic humans is associated with abdominal obesity. Obes Res 2003;11: 1147–54.

12. Fortuyn HA, Lappenschaar MA, Furer JW, et al. Anxiety and mood disorders in narcolepsy: a case-control study. Gen Hosp Psychiatry 2010; 32:49–56.

13. Fortuyn HA, Swinkels S, Buitelaar J, et al. High prevalence of eating disorders in narcolepsy with cataplexy: a case-control study. Sleep 2008;31: 335–41.

14. Longstreth WT Jr, Koepsell TD, Ton TG, et al. The epidemiology of narcolepsy. Sleep 2007;30:13–26.

15. Ohayon MM, Priest RG, Zulley J, et al. Prevalence of narcolepsy symptomatology and diagnosis in the European general population. Neurology 2002;58:1826–33.

16. Hublin C, Kaprio J, Partinen M, et al. The prevalence of narcolepsy: an epidemiological study of the Finnish twin cohort. Ann Neurol 1994; 35:709–16.

17. Lavie P, Peled R. Narcolepsy is a rare disease in Israel. Sleep 1987;10:608–9.

18. Honda Y. Census of narcolepsy, cataplexy and sleep life among teenagers in Fujisawa city. Sleep Res 1979;8:191.

19. Silber MH, Krahn LE, Olson EJ, et al. The epidemiology of narcolepsy in Olmsted County, Minnesota: a population-based study. Sleep 2002; 25:197–202.

20. Morrish E, King MA, Smith IE, et al. Factors associated with a delay in the diagnosis of narcolepsy. Sleep Med 2004;5:37–41.

21. Dauvilliers Y, Montplaisir J, Molinari N, et al. Age at onset of narcolepsy in two large populations of patients in France and Quebec. Neurology 2001; 57:2029–33.

22. Plazzi G, Pizza F, Palaia V, et al. Complex movement disorders at disease onset in childhood narcolepsy with cataplexy. Brain 2011;134:3480–92.

23. Ohayon MM, Ferini-Strambi L, Plazzi G, et al. How age influences the expression of narcolepsy. J Psychosom Res 2005;59:399–405.

24. Mitler MM, Boysen BG, Campbell L, et al. Narcolepsy-cataplexy in a female dog. Exp Neurol 1974;45:332–40.

25. Foutz AS, Mitler MM, Cavalli-Sforza LL, et al. Genetic factors in canine narcolepsy. Sleep 1979; 1:413–21.

26. Lin L, Faraco J, Li R, et al. The sleep disorder canine narcolepsy is caused by a mutation in the hypocretin (orexin) receptor 2 gene. Cell 1999;98: 365–76.

27. Chemelli RM, Willie JT, Sinton CM, et al. Narcolepsy in orexin knockout mice: molecular genetics of sleep regulation. Cell 1999;98:437–51.

28. Nishino S, Mignot E. Pharmacological aspects of human and canine narcolepsy. Prog Neurobiol 1997;52:27–78.

29. De La Herran-Arita AK, Zomosa-Signoret VC, Millan-Aldaco DA, et al. Aspects of the narcolepsy-cataplexy syndrome in O/E3-null mutant mice. Neuroscience 2011;183:134–43.

30. Gerashchenko D, Kohls MD, Greco M, et al. Hypocretin-2-saporin lesions of the lateral hypothalamus produce narcoleptic-like sleep behavior in the rat. J Neurosci 2001;21:7273–83.

31. Mieda M, Hasegawa E, Kisanuki YY, et al. Differential roles of orexin receptor-1 and -2 in the regulation of non-REM and REM sleep. J Neurosci 2011;31:6518–26.

32. Willie JT, Chemelli RM, Sinton CM, et al. Distinct narcolepsy syndromes in orexin receptor-2 and orexin null mice: molecular genetic dissection of non-REM and REM sleep regulatory processes. Neuron 2003;38:715–30.

33. Hara J, Beuckmann CT, Nambu T, et al. Genetic ablation of orexin neurons in mice results in narcolepsy, hypophagia, and obesity. Neuron 2001;30:345–54.

34. Scammell TE, Willie JT, Guilleminault C, et al. A consensus definition of cataplexy in mouse models of narcolepsy. Sleep 2009;32:111–6.

35. Nishino S, Ripley B, Overeem S, et al. Hypocretin (orexin) deficiency in human narcolepsy. Lancet 2000;355:39–40.

36. Nishino S, Ripley B, Overeem S, et al. Low cerebrospinal fluid hypocretin (orexin) and altered energy homeostasis in human narcolepsy. Ann Neurol 2001;50:381–8.

37. Bassetti C, Gugger M, Bischof M, et al. The narcoleptic borderland: a multimodal diagnostic approach including cerebrospinal fluid levels of hypocretin-1 (orexin A). Sleep Med 2003;4:7–12.

38. Kanbayashi T, Inoue Y, Chiba S, et al. CSF hypocretin-1 (orexin-A) concentrations in narcolepsy with and without cataplexy and idiopathic hypersomnia. J Sleep Res 2002;11:91–3.

39. Krahn LE, Pankratz VS, Oliver L, et al. Hypocretin (orexin) levels in cerebrospinal fluid of patients with narcolepsy: relationship to cataplexy and HLA DQB1*0602 status. Sleep 2002;25:733–6.

40. Mignot E, Lammers GJ, Ripley B, et al. The role of cerebrospinal fluid hypocretin measurement in the diagnosis of narcolepsy and other hypersomnias. Arch Neurol 2002;59:1553–62.

41. Ripley B, Overeem S, Fujiki N, et al. CSF hypocretin/orexin levels in narcolepsy and other neurological conditions. Neurology 2001;57:2253–8.

42. Nishino S, Kanbayashi T. Symptomatic narcolepsy, cataplexy and hypersomnia, and their implications in the hypothalamic hypocretin/orexin system. Sleep Med Rev 2005;9:269–310.

43. Baumann CR, Stocker R, Imhof HG, et al. Hypocretin-1 (orexin A) deficiency in acute traumatic brain injury. Neurology 2005;65:147–9.

44. Kanbayashi T, Ishiguro H, Aizawa R, et al. Hypocretin-1 (orexin-A) concentrations in cerebrospinal fluid are low in patients with Guillain-Barre syndrome. Psychiatry Clin Neurosci 2002;56:273–4.

45. Nishino S, Kanbayashi T, Fujiki N, et al. CSF hypocretin levels in Guillain-Barre syndrome and other inflammatory neuropathies. Neurology 2003;61:823–5.

46. Overeem S, Dalmau J, Bataller L, et al. Hypocretin-1 CSF levels in anti-Ma2 associated encephalitis. Neurology 2004;62:138–40.

47. Peyron C, Faraco J, Rogers W, et al. A mutation in a case of early onset narcolepsy and a generalized absence of hypocretin peptides in human narcoleptic brains. Nat Med 2000;6:991–7.

48. Thannickal TC, Moore RY, Nienhuis R, et al. Reduced number of hypocretin neurons in human narcolepsy. Neuron 2000;27:469–74.

49. Thannickal TC, Siegel JM, Nienhuis R, et al. Pattern of hypocretin (orexin) soma and axon loss, and gliosis, in human narcolepsy. Brain Pathol 2003; 13:340–51.

50. Blouin AM, Thannickal TC, Worley PF, et al. Narp immunostaining of human hypocretin (orexin) neurons: loss in narcolepsy. Neurology 2005;65:1189–92.

51. Crocker A, Espana RA, Papadopoulou M, et al. Concomitant loss of dynorphin, NARP, and orexin in narcolepsy. Neurology 2005;65:1184–8.

52. Chabas D, Taheri S, Renier C, et al. The genetics of narcolepsy. Annu Rev Genomics Hum Genet 2003; 4:459–83.

53. Mignot E. Genetic and familial aspects of narcolepsy. Neurology 1998;50:S16–22.

54. Dauvilliers Y, Maret S, Bassetti C, et al. A monozygotic twin pair discordant for narcolepsy and CSF hypocretin-1. Neurology 2004;62:2137–8.

55. Honda M, Honda Y, Uchida S, et al. Monozygotic twins incompletely concordant for narcolepsy. Biol Psychiatry 2001;49:943–7.

56. Khatami R, Maret S, Werth E, et al. Monozygotic twins concordant for narcolepsy-cataplexy without any detectable abnormality in the hypocretin (orexin) pathway. Lancet 2004;363:1199–200.

57. Partinen M, Hublin C, Kaprio J, et al. Twin studies in narcolepsy. Sleep 1994;17:S13–6.

58. Juji T, Satake M, Honda Y, et al. HLA antigens in Japanese patients with narcolepsy. All the patients were DR2 positive. Tissue Antigens 1984;24:316–9.

59. Mignot E, Hayduk R, Black J, et al. HLA DQB1*0602 is associated with cataplexy in 509 narcoleptic patients. Sleep 1997;20:1012–20.

60. Mignot E, Kimura A, Lattermann A, et al. Extensive HLA class II studies in 58 non-DRB1*15 (DR2) narcoleptic patients with cataplexy. Tissue Antigens 1997;49:329–41.

61. Hor H, Kutalik Z, Dauvilliers Y, et al. Genome-wide association study identifies new HLA class II haplotypes strongly protective against narcolepsy. Nat Genet 2010;42:786–9.

62. Hallmayer J, Faraco J, Lin L, et al. Narcolepsy is strongly associated with the T-cell receptor alpha locus. Nat Genet 2009;41:708–11.

63. Hohjoh H, Nakayama T, Ohashi J, et al. Significant association of a single nucleotide polymorphism in the tumor necrosis factor-alpha (TNF-alpha) gene promoter with human narcolepsy. Tissue Antigens 1999;54:138–45.

64. Hohjoh H, Terada N, Kawashima M, et al. Significant association of the tumor necrosis factor receptor 2 (TNFR2) gene with human narcolepsy. Tissue Antigens 2000;56:446–8.

65. Kornum BR, Kawashima M, Faraco J, et al. Common variants in P2RY11 are associated with narcolepsy. Nat Genet 2011;43:66–71.

66. Overeem S, Black JL 3rd, Lammers GJ. Narcolepsy: immunological aspects. Sleep Med Rev 2008;12:95–107.

67. Fontana A, Gast H, Reith W, et al. Narcolepsy: autoimmunity, effector T cell activation due to infection, or T cell independent, major histocompatibility complex class II induced neuronal loss? Brain 2010;133:1300–11.

68. Scammell TE. The frustrating and mostly fruitless search for an autoimmune cause of narcolepsy. Sleep 2006;29:601–2.

69. Overeem S, Verschuuren JJ, Fronczek R, et al. Immunohistochemical screening for autoantibodies against lateral hypothalamic neurons in human narcolepsy. J Neuroimmunol 2006;174:187–91.

70. Black JL 3rd, Krahn LE, Pankratz VS, et al. Search for neuron-specific and nonneuron-specific antibodies in narcoleptic patients with and without HLA DQB1*0602. Sleep 2002;25:719–23.

71. Black JL 3rd, Silber MH, Krahn LE, et al. Studies of humoral immunity to preprohypocretin in human leukocyte antigen DQB1*0602-positive narcoleptic subjects with cataplexy. Biol Psychiatry 2005;58:504–9.

72. Black JL 3rd, Avula RK, Walker DL, et al. HLA DQB1*0602 positive narcoleptic subjects with cataplexy have CSF IgG reactive to rat hypothalamic protein extract. Sleep 2005;28:1191–2.

73. Cvetkovic-Lopes V, Bayer L, Dorsaz S, et al. Elevated Tribbles homolog 2-specific antibody levels in narcolepsy patients. J Clin Invest 2010;120:713–9.

74. Kawashima M, Lin L, Tanaka S, et al. Anti-Tribbles homolog 2 (TRIB2) autoantibodies in narcolepsy are associated with recent onset of cataplexy. Sleep 2010;33:869–74.

75. Toyoda H, Tanaka S, Miyagawa T, et al. Anti-Tribbles homolog 2 autoantibodies in Japanese patients with narcolepsy. Sleep 2010;33:875–8.

76. Aran A, Lin L, Nevsimalova S, et al. Elevated anti-streptococcal antibodies in patients with recent narcolepsy onset. Sleep 2009;32:979–83.

77. Longstreth WT Jr, Ton TG, Koepsell TD. Narcolepsy and streptococcal infections. Sleep 2009;32: 1548.

78. Dauvilliers Y. Follow-up of four narcolepsy patients treated with intravenous immunoglobulins. Ann Neurol 2006;60:153.

79. Dauvilliers Y, Carlander B, Rivier F, et al. Successful management of cataplexy with intravenous immunoglobulins at narcolepsy onset. Ann Neurol 2004;56:905–8.

80. Lecendreux M, Maret S, Bassetti C, et al. Clinical efficacy of high-dose intravenous immunoglobulins near the onset of narcolepsy in a 10-year-old boy. J Sleep Res 2003;12:347–8.

81. Fronczek R, Verschuuren J, Lammers GJ. Response to intravenous immunoglobulins and placebo in a patient with narcolepsy with cataplexy. J Neurol 2007;254:1607–8.

82. Plazzi G, Poli F, Franceschini C, et al. Intravenous high-dose immunoglobulin treatment in recent onset childhood narcolepsy with cataplexy. J Neurol 2008;255:1549–54.

83. Valko PO, Khatami R, Baumann CR, et al. No persistent effect of intravenous immunoglobulins in patients with narcolepsy with cataplexy. J Neurol 2008;255:1900–3.

84. Bardage C, Persson I, Ortqvist A, et al. Neurological and autoimmune disorders after vaccination against pandemic influenza A (H1N1) with a monovalent adjuvanted vaccine: population based cohort study in Stockholm, Sweden. BMJ 2011; 343:d5956.

85. Dauvilliers Y, Montplaisir J, Cochen V, et al. Post-H1N1 narcolepsy-cataplexy. Sleep 2010;33: 1428–30.

86. Zarocostas J. WHO backs further probes into possible link between H1N1 vaccine and narcolepsy in children. BMJ 2011;342:d909.

87. Han F, Lin L, Warby SC, et al. Narcolepsy onset is seasonal and increased following the 2009 H1N1 pandemic in China. Ann Neurol 2011;70: 410–7.

88. Bayer L, Eggermann E, Serafin M, et al. Orexins (hypocretins) directly excite tuberomammillary neurons. Eur J Neurosci 2001;14:1571–5.

89. Peyron C, Tighe DK, van den Pol AN, et al. Neurons containing hypocretin (orexin) project to multiple neuronal systems. J Neurosci 1998;18:9996–10015.

90. Saper CB, Chou TC, Scammell TE. The sleep switch: hypothalamic control of sleep and wakefulness. Trends Neurosci 2001;24:726–31.

91. Diniz Behn CG, Klerman EB, Mochizuki T, et al. Abnormal sleep/wake dynamics in orexin knockout mice. Sleep 2010;33:297–306.

92. Mochizuki T, Crocker A, McCormack S, et al. Behavioral state instability in orexin knock-out mice. J Neurosci 2004;24:6291–300.

93. Broughton R, Dunham W, Newman J, et al. Ambulatory 24 hour sleep-wake monitoring in narcolepsy-cataplexy compared to matched controls. Electroencephalogr Clin Neurophysiol 1988; 70:473–81.

94. Lammers GJ, Overeem S, Tijssen MA, et al. Effects of startle and laughter in cataplectic subjects: a neurophysiological study between attacks. Clin Neurophysiol 2000;111:1276–81.

95. Overeem S, Lammers GJ, van Dijk JG. Weak with laughter. Lancet 1999;354:838.

96. Overeem S, Reijntjes R, Huyser W, et al. Corticospinal excitability during laughter: implications for cataplexy and the comparison with REM sleep atonia. J Sleep Res 2004;13:257–64.

97. Overeem S, Lammers GJ, van Dijk JG. Cataplexy: 'tonic immobility' rather than 'REM-sleep atonia'? Sleep Med 2002;3:471–7.

98. Mileykovskiy BY, Kiyashchenko LI, Siegel JM. Behavioral correlates of activity in identified hypocretin/orexin neurons. Neuron 2005;46:787–98.

99. Hishikawa Y, Shimizu T. Physiology of REM sleep, cataplexy, and sleep paralysis. Adv Neurol 1995; 67:245–71.

100. Poryazova R, Schnepf B, Werth E, et al. Evidence for metabolic hypothalamo-amygdala dysfunction in narcolepsy. Sleep 2009;32:607–13.

101. Schwartz S, Ponz A, Poryazova R, et al. Abnormal activity in hypothalamus and amygdala during humour processing in human narcolepsy with cataplexy. Brain 2008;131:514–22.

102. Plazzi G, Serra L, Ferri R. Nocturnal aspects of narcolepsy with cataplexy. Sleep Med Rev 2008; 12:109–28.

103. Mullington J, Broughton R. Scheduled naps in the management of daytime sleepiness in narcolepsy-cataplexy. Sleep 1993;16:444–56.

104. American Academy of Sleep Medicine. The International Classification of Sleep Disorders: diagnostic and coding manual. 2nd edition. Chicago: AASM; 2005.

105. Anic-Labat S, Guilleminault C, Kraemer HC, et al. Validation of a cataplexy questionnaire in 983 sleep-disorders patients. Sleep 1999;22:77–87.

106. Guilleminault C, Gelb M. Clinical aspects and features of cataplexy. Adv Neurol 1995;67:65–77.

107. Overeem S, van Nues SJ, van der Zande WL, et al. The clinical features of cataplexy: a questionnaire study in narcolepsy patients with and without hypocretin-1 deficiency. Sleep Med 2011;12: 12–8.

108. Gelb M, Guilleminault C, Kraemer H, et al. Stability of cataplexy over several months–information for the design of therapeutic trials. Sleep 1994;17: 265–73.

109. Poryazova R, Siccoli M, Werth E, et al. Unusually prolonged rebound cataplexy after withdrawal of fluoxetine. Neurology 2005;65:967–8.

110. Serra L, Montagna P, Mignot E, et al. Cataplexy features in childhood narcolepsy. Mov Disord 2008;23:858–65.

111. Dhondt K, Verhelst H, Pevernagie D, et al. Childhood narcolepsy with partial facial cataplexy: a diagnostic dilemma. Sleep Med 2009;10: 797–8.

112. Peraita-Adrados R, Garcia-Penas JJ, Ruiz-Falco L, et al. Clinical, polysomnographic and laboratory characteristics of narcolepsy-cataplexy in a sample of children and adolescents. Sleep Med 2011;12: 24–7.

113. Fortuyn HA, Lappenschaar GA, Nienhuis FJ, et al. Psychotic symptoms in narcolepsy: phenomenology and a comparison with schizophrenia. Gen Hosp Psychiatry 2009;31:146–54.

114. Douglass AB, Hays P, Pazderka F, et al. Florid refractory schizophrenias that turn out to be treatable variants of HLA-associated narcolepsy. J Nerv Ment Dis 1991;179:12–7 [discussion: 8].

115. Montplaisir J, Billiard M, Takahashi S, et al. Twenty-four-hour recording in REM-narcoleptics with special reference to nocturnal sleep disruption. Biol Psychiatry 1978;13:73–89.

116. Montplaisir J, Godbout R. Nocturnal sleep of narcoleptic patients: revisited. Sleep 1986;9:159–61.

117. Broughton R, Dunham W, Weisskopf M, et al. Night sleep does not predict day sleep in narcolepsy. Electroencephalogr Clin Neurophysiol 1994;91: 67–70.

118. Nightingale S, Orgill JC, Ebrahim IO, et al. The association between narcolepsy and REM behavior disorder (RBD). Sleep Med 2005;6:253–8.

119. Schenck CH, Mahowald MW. Motor dyscontrol in narcolepsy: rapid-eye-movement (REM) sleep without atonia and REM sleep behavior disorder. Ann Neurol 1992;32:3–10.

120. Fronczek R, Middelkoop HA, van Dijk JG, et al. Focusing on vigilance instead of sleepiness in the assessment of narcolepsy: high sensitivity of the Sustained Attention to Response Task (SART). Sleep 2006;29:187–91.

121. Aguirre M, Broughton R, Stuss D. Does memory impairment exist in narcolepsy-cataplexy? J Clin Exp Neuropsychol 1985;7:14–24.

122. Daniels LE. Narcolepsy. Medicine 1934;13:1–122.

123. Dahmen N, Bierbrauer J, Kasten M. Increased prevalence of obesity in narcoleptic patients and relatives. Eur Arch Psychiatry Clin Neurosci 2001; 251:85–9.

124. Schuld A, Hebebrand J, Geller F, et al. Increased body-mass index in patients with narcolepsy. Lancet 2000;355:1274–5.

125. Lammers GJ, Pijl H, Iestra J, et al. Spontaneous food choice in narcolepsy. Sleep 1996;19:75–6.

126. Arnulf I, Lin L, Zhang J, et al. CSF versus serum leptin in narcolepsy: is there an effect of hypocretin deficiency? Sleep 2006;29:1017–24.

127. Dahmen N, Engel A, Helfrich J, et al. Peripheral leptin levels in narcoleptic patients. Diabetes Technol Ther 2007;9:348–53.

128. Kok SW, Meinders AE, Overeem S, et al. Reduction of plasma leptin levels and loss of its circadian rhythmicity in hypocretin (orexin)-deficient narcoleptic humans. J Clin Endocrinol Metab 2002;87:805–9.

129. Overeem S, Kok SW, Lammers GJ, et al. Somatotropic axis in hypocretin-deficient narcoleptic humans: altered circadian distribution of GH-secretory events. Am J Physiol Endocrinol Metab 2003;284:E641–7.

130. Schuld A, Blum WF, Uhr M, et al. Reduced leptin levels in human narcolepsy. Neuroendocrinology 2000;72:195–8.

131. Dauvilliers Y, Paquereau J, Bastuji H, et al. Psychological health in central hypersomnias: the French Harmony study. J Neurol Neurosurg Psychiatry 2009;80:636–41.

132. Kales A, Soldatos CR, Bixler EO, et al. Narcolepsy-cataplexy. II. Psychosocial consequences and associated psychopathology. Arch Neurol 1982;39:169–71.

133. Vourdas A, Shneerson JM, Gregory CA, et al. Narcolepsy and psychopathology: is there an association? Sleep Med 2002;3:353–60.

134. Ponz A, Khatami R, Poryazova R, et al. Reduced amygdala activity during aversive conditioning in human narcolepsy. Ann Neurol 2010;67:394–8.

135. Droogleever Fortuyn HA, Fronczek R, Smitshoek M, et al. Severe fatigue in narcolepsy with cataplexy. J Sleep Res 2012;21(2):163–9.

136. Valko PO, Bassetti CL, Bloch KE, et al. Validation of the fatigue severity scale in a Swiss cohort. Sleep 2008;31:1601–7.

137. Chabas D, Foulon C, Gonzalez J, et al. Eating disorder and metabolism in narcoleptic patients. Sleep 2007;30:1267–73.

138. Poryazova R, Khatami R, Werth E, et al. Weak with sex: sexual intercourse as a trigger for cataplexy. J Sex Med 2009;6:2271–7.

139. Broughton WA, Broughton RJ. Psychosocial impact of narcolepsy. Sleep 1994;17:S45–9.

140. Campbell AJ, Signal TL, O'Keeffe KM, et al. Narcolepsy in New Zealand: pathway to diagnosis and effect on quality of life. N Z Med J 2011;124: 51–61.

141. David A, Constantino F, Santos JM, et al. Health-related quality of life in Portuguese patients with narcolepsy. Sleep Med 2012;13(3):273–7.

142. Ervik S, Abdelnoor M, Heier MS, et al. Health-related quality of life in narcolepsy. Acta Neurol Scand 2006;114:198–204.

143. Vignatelli L, D'Alessandro R, Mosconi P, et al. Health-related quality of life in Italian patients with narcolepsy: the SF-36 health survey. Sleep Med 2004;5:467–75.

144. Broughton RJ, Guberman A, Roberts J. Comparison of the psychosocial effects of epilepsy and narcolepsy/cataplexy: a controlled study. Epilepsia 1984;25:423–33.

145. Littner MR, Kushida C, Wise M, et al. Practice parameters for clinical use of the multiple sleep latency test and the maintenance of wakefulness test. Sleep 2005;28:113–21.

146. Lammers GJ, van Dijk JG. The multiple sleep latency test: a paradoxical test? Clin Neurol Neurosurg 1992;94(Suppl):S108–10.

147. Aldrich MS, Chervin RD, Malow BA. Value of the multiple sleep latency test (MSLT) for the diagnosis of narcolepsy. Sleep 1997;20:620–9.

148. Bishop C, Rosenthal L, Helmus T, et al. The frequency of multiple sleep onset REM periods among subjects with no excessive daytime sleepiness. Sleep 1996;19:727–30.

149. Arii J, Kanbayashi T, Tanabe Y, et al. CSF hypocretin-1 (orexin-A) levels in childhood narcolepsy and neurologic disorders. Neurology 2004; 63:2440–2.

150. Heier MS, Jansson TS, Gautvik KM. Cerebrospinal fluid hypocretin 1 deficiency, overweight, and metabolic dysregulation in patients with narcolepsy. J Clin Sleep Med 2011;7:653–8.

151. Kubota H, Kanbayashi T, Tanabe Y, et al. Decreased cerebrospinal fluid hypocretin-1 levels near the onset of narcolepsy in 2 prepubertal children. Sleep 2003;26:555–7.

152. Tsukamoto H, Ishikawa T, Fujii Y, et al. Undetectable levels of CSF hypocretin-1 (orexin-A) in two prepubertal boys with narcolepsy. Neuropediatrics 2002;33:51–2.

153. Baumann CR, Bassetti CL. Hypocretins (orexins) and sleep-wake disorders. Lancet Neurol 2005;4: 673–82.

154. Lin L, Bassetti C, Lammers GJ, et al. Guidelines for the appropriate use of CSF measurements to diagnose narcolepsy. In: Bassetti C, Billiard M, Mignot E, editors. Narcolepsy and Hypersomnia. New York: Informa Health Care; 2007. p. 663–71.

155. Marti I, Valko PO, Khatami R, et al. Multiple sleep latency measures in narcolepsy and behaviourally induced insufficient sleep syndrome. Sleep Med 2009;10:1146–50.

156. Sadeh A. The role and validity of actigraphy in sleep medicine: an update. Sleep Med Rev 2011; 15:259–67.

157. Aldrich MS. The clinical spectrum of narcolepsy and idiopathic hypersomnia. Neurology 1996;46: 393–401.

158. Silber MH, Krahn LE, Olson EJ. Diagnosing narcolepsy: validity and reliability of new diagnostic criteria. Sleep Med 2002;3:109–13.

Idiopathic Hypersomnia

Tony J. Masri, MD[a], Carmella G. Gonzales, MD[b],
Clete A. Kushida, MD, PhD[c],*

KEYWORDS

- Idiopathic hypersomnia • Idiopathic hypersomnia with long sleep
- Idiopathic hypersomnia with short sleep • Hypersomnolence • Epidemiology • Pathophysiology
- Treatment

KEY POINTS

- Idiopathic hypersomnia is a rare sleep disorder characterized by excessive daytime sleepiness without the rapid eye movement sleep disturbances seen in narcolepsy. Our understanding of this condition is limited. Therefore, the diagnosis and treatment of idiopathic hypersomnia can be challenging.
- Idiopathic hypersomnia is a diagnosis of exclusion. The differential diagnosis should include narcolepsy, sleep related breathing disorders, restless leg syndrome, behaviorally induced insufficient sleep syndrome, chronic sleep insufficiency, long sleepers, chronic fatigue syndrome, and hypersomnia induced by a psychiatric or medical condition.
- Diagnostic polysomnography (PSG) is essential to rule out other causes of excessive daytime sleepiness.
- A multiple sleep latency test (MSLT) can also be useful in the work up of idiopathic hypersomnia. Findings on MSLT typically include a mean sleep latency of less than 8 minutes and fewer than two sleep-onset REM periods (SOREMPs).
- Modafinil is considered by most clinicians as the first-line treatment for idiopathic hypersomnia. It is best to start with a low dose of 100 mg daily and slowly titrate upward to the maximum daily dose of 400 mg.

Sleep disorders comprise a myriad group of conditions. Among these disorders, the most challenging to diagnose and treat is idiopathic hypersomnia; a primary disorder of hypersomnolence that is distinguished from narcolepsy by the absence of rapid eye movement (REM) sleep disturbance. This condition is rare. Clinically, patients present with excessive daytime sleepiness (EDS), unrefreshing naps, undisturbed nocturnal sleep, and sleep drunkenness. Although the term idiopathic hypersomnia was used as early as 1892,[1] it was Bedrich Roth[2] who first described the

syndrome in the late 1950s and distinguished it clinically from narcolepsy without cataplexy after analyzing 642 patients over 30 years and identifying 174 patients with idiopathic hypersomnia. Roth was also the first to recognize 2 distinct forms of the disorder: the monosymptomatic (EDS alone) and the polysymptomatic (EDS, prolonged sleep, and sleep drunkenness) forms.

The rarity of idiopathic hypersomnia has precluded any systematic studies or randomized controlled trials on the subject, and as a result, ability to fully understand and treat this condition is greatly limited. At

a Stanford University, Stanford Sleep Medicine Clinic, 450 Broadway Street, Pavilion C, 2nd Floor, Redwood City, CA 94063, USA; b Neurology Department, Case Western Reserve University, 11100 Euclid Avenue, Cleveland, OH 44106-5040, USA; c Stanford University, Stanford Sleep Medicine Center, 450 Broadway Street, MC 5704, Pavilion C, 2nd Floor, Redwood City, CA 94063-5704, USA
* Corresponding author. Stanford University, Stanford Sleep Medicine Center, 450 Broadway Street, MC 5704, Pavilion C, 2nd Floor, Redwood City, CA 94063-5704.
E-mail address: clete@stanford.edu

Sleep Med Clin 7 (2012) 283–289
doi:10.1016/j.jsmc.2012.03.012
1556-407X/12/$ – see front matter © 2012 Published by Elsevier Inc.

present, knowledge about idiopathic hypersomnia stems from retrospective and descriptive studies. This review covers the major points regarding the clinical features and diagnosis of idiopathic hypersomnia and discusses current evidence supporting the available treatment options for this condition.

EPIDEMIOLOGY

In the absence of systematic studies, the exact prevalence of idiopathic hypersomnia is unknown. Estimates are derived from clinical experience at large sleep centers. The ratio of idiopathic hypersomnia to narcolepsy is 10.3:16.2, which places the prevalence of idiopathic hypersomnia between 2 to 8 per 100,000.[3,4] The condition is familial in up to two-thirds of cases, and instances of narcolepsy and idiopathic hypersomnia occurring in the same family have been reported.[3–5] Because of the insidious onset of the disease the exact age of onset is difficult to determine. The disease process commonly begins between the ages of 10 and 30.[6]

Predisposing Factors and Etiologic Theories

As mentioned earlier, some studies have suggested a familial component to idiopathic hypersomnia, in particular, in the form of long sleep time (**Table 1**). An autosomal dominant mode of inheritance and preponderance of women have been suggested.[7] There is currently no familial data for idiopathic hypersomnia without long sleep time.

Knowledge of the etiology and exact pathogenesis of idiopathic hypersomnia is limited, in part due to the lack of natural animal models. An early experiment published in 1970 involved lesioning of

Table 1
The 2005 International Classification of Sleep Disorders-2 criteria for the diagnosis of idiopathic hypersomnia

Criterion	IH With Long Sleep	IH Without Long Sleep
A.	The patient has a complaint of excessive daytime sleepiness occurring almost daily for at least 3 mo	The patient has a complaint of excessive daytime sleepiness occurring almost daily for at least 3 mo
B.	The patient has prolonged nocturnal sleep time (>10 h) documented by interview, actigraphy, or sleep logs. Waking up in the morning or at the end of naps is almost always laborious	The patient has normal nocturnal sleep (>6 h but <10 h), documented by interviews, actigraphy, or sleep logs
C.	Nocturnal polysomnography has excluded other causes of daytime sleepiness	Nocturnal polysomnography has excluded other causes of daytime sleepiness
D.	The polysomnogram demonstrates a short sleep latency and a major sleep period that is prolonged to >10 h in duration	Polysomnography demonstrates amajor sleep period that is normal in duration (>6 h but <10 h)
E.	If an MSLT is performed after overnight polysomnography, a mean sleep latency of <8 min is found and fewer than 2 SOREMPs are recorded. Mean sleep latency in IH with long sleep time has been shown to be 6.2 ± 3.0 min	An MSLT after overnight polysomnography demonstrates a mean sleep latency of <8 min and fewer than 2 SOREMPs. Mean sleep latency in IH has been shown to be 6.2 ± 3.0 min
F.	The hypersomnia is not better explained by another sleep disorder, medical or neurologic disorder, mental disorder, medication use, or substance use disorder	The hypersomnia is not better explained by another sleep disorder, medical or neurologic disorder, mental disorder, medication use, or substance use disorder

Abbreviations: IH, idiopathic hypersomnia; MSLT, multiple sleep latency test; SOREMPs, sleep-onset rapid eye movement periods.

Adapted from American Academy of Sleep Medicine. International Classification of Sleep Disorders. Diagnostic and coding manual. 2nd edition. Westchester (IL): American Academy of Sleep Medicine; 2005.

ascending noradrenergic pathways in the cat showed an increase in both REM and non-rapid eye movement (NREM) sleep similar to that of idiopathic hypersomnia with long sleep time.[8] This study has not been reproduced.

More recent studies have also suggested dysfunction of aminergic arousal systems as a possible mechanism behind idiopathic hypersomnia. Montplaisir and colleagues[9] found a decrease in the level of dopamine and indole-3-acetic acid in patients with idiopathic hypersomnia and narcolepsy, whereas Faull and colleagues[10–12] discovered a dysregulation of the noradrenergic and dopaminergic system in patients with idiopathic hypersomnia and narcolepsy, respectively. Another recent study has shown that cerebrospinal fluid (CSF) histamine levels were significantly lower in patients with idiopathic hypersomnia and narcolepsy than in those with obstructive sleep apnea, suggesting that low CSF histamine levels may be specific to hypersomnias of central origin.[13] Histamine has been linked to the activation of the sympathetic nervous system, arousal, and anxiety. Histamine has been observed to exhibit highest rates of firing during wakefulness and lowest rates of firing during REM sleep.[14]

Imaging studies using positron emission tomography (PET) have also shown dysfunction in dopaminergic transmission among patients with idiopathic hypersomnia.[15] However, these studies have failed to explain the pathophysiologic differences between narcolepsy and idiopathic hypersomnia, which is crucial because there is significant overlap between these 2 entities clinically. In addition, none of the neurochemical studies on the subject so far has tried to identify any differences between idiopathic hypersomnia with and without long sleep time, and none of these studies have been replicated.

Some investigators have found a significantly high level of slow-wave activity in patients with idiopathic hypersomnia, as a result of either an abnormally slow decay or a normal decay of a higher level of slow-wave sleep (SWS).[16,17] A study by Vernet and Arnulf[18] found that patients with idiopathic hypersomnia had a delayed sleep phase with SWS episodes that were more frequent at the end of the night, and to a larger degree in those with long sleep time. In addition, Nevsimalova and colleagues[19] reported increased sleep spindle activity at the beginning and at the end of sleep and a delayed initiation and decline of melatonin and cortisol secretion in idiopathic hypersomnia. These findings suggest that disturbances in circadian sleep regulation and deficient arousal systems may play a role in the pathophysiology of idiopathic hypersomnia.

Clinical Features and Diagnosis

The 2005 *International Classification of Sleep Disorders* Second Edition (ICSD-2) classifies idiopathic hypersomnia into 2 forms: with prolonged sleep time and without prolonged sleep time. Each form has 6 criteria[20] and they are listed on **Table 1**.

Idiopathic hypersomnia with prolonged sleep time, which is the polysymptomatic form of the disease, is marked by constant daytime sleepiness accompanied by long and unrefreshing naps despite an abnormally prolonged and undisturbed nocturnal sleep. Morning and nap awakenings are laborious; patients are hard to awaken and typically require vigorous stimulation (often by family members) to wake up. In some instances they may be aggressive when awakened. In addition, they may remain disoriented and confused and are unable to react to external stimuli adequately, a state called sleep drunkenness.

Idiopathic hypersomnia without long sleep time is monosymptomatic, showing isolated daytime sleepiness with normal nocturnal sleep time and absence of sleep drunkenness. Daytime naps may be more irresistible, more frequent, shorter, and more refreshing in this group similar to that seen in patients suffering from narcolepsy without cataplexy, which shows a significant overlap between idiopathic hypersomnia and narcolepsy and represents a challenge in clinically differentiating one from the other.

In both forms of idiopathic hypersomnia, patients have EDS that usually does not lead to involuntary naps. Patients, during episodes of drowsiness, may exhibit automatic behavior that leads them to act inappropriately and have reported hitting plates with utensils, driving miles away from home, putting pepper on drinks, and other similar behavior. Patients usually are unaware of these episodes unless a witness alerts them to the event. Similar to narcolepsy, sleep paralysis and hypnagogic/hypnopompic hallucinations may be present in patients with idiopathic hypersomnia. Cataplexy, however, does not occur. In one cohort of 77 patients, the most useful factor in the clinical history that distinguished idiopathic hypersomnia from narcolepsy was a nap duration greater than 60 minutes, which was 87% sensitive and specific.[6] However, this is nonspecific and shorter naps can definitely occur.

Autonomic symptoms, such as fainting episodes, orthostatic hypotension, and cold hands and feet, have also been observed. Patients may also exhibit depressive symptoms. The psychosocial handicap of patients with idiopathic hypersomnia is similar to that of patients with narcolepsy.[21]

Spontaneous remission has been reported, a phenomenon that has not been observed in patients with narcolepsy.[6]

Hypersomnolence can also be observed in certain organic disorders, and secondary causes of hypersomnia, including the α-synucleinopathies, such as Parkinson disease and multiple system atrophy; tauopathy Alzheimer disease; and lesions involving the thalamus, hypothalamus, and brainstem, must be observed in evaluating a patient with EDS. The ICSD-2 has identified differential diagnosis for idiopathic hypersomnia[18] and they are listed in **Box 1**.

As mentioned in the ICSD-2 criteria, polysomnography (PSG) is important in the workup of patients with possible idiopathic hypersomnia. The main utility of PSG is to exclude other causes of EDS. Findings on PSG include short sleep latency, long sleep time of more than 10 hours for the polysymptomatic form (6 to 10 hours for the monosymptomatic form), a high sleep efficiency, and increased amounts of slow-wave NREM sleep.[3,6,22,23] However, these findings are nonspecific and may be found in other conditions with EDS, particularly in patients with behaviorally induced insufficiency sleep syndrome (BIISS).

Another useful test in the workup of patients suspected with idiopathic hypersomnia is a multiple sleep latency test (MSLT). MSLT is done the day after PSG, which creates problems in adequately assessing patients with the polysymptomatic form. Because the patient needs to be awakened for the MSLT, the clinician is unable to document prolonged sleep time, which is one of the main components of the condition. Also, patients are usually in a state of sleep drunkenness in between naps, and it is very difficult to wake them up and keep them awake. Typical findings on MSLT include a mean sleep latency of less than 8 minutes and fewer than 2 sleep-onset REM periods (SOREMPS). These findings are also nonspecific. Some studies have shown mean sleep latencies of longer than 8 minutes in patients with idiopathic hypersomnia,[3,6,23] suggesting that this ICSD-2 criteria may not hold true for all patients.

Because of the limitations of the current PSG-MSLT procedure, some investigators have suggested an ad libitum PSG protocol as diagnostic criteria for idiopathic hypersomnia. This protocol would allow documentation of prolonged sleep time and prolonged naps (>1 hour) during the day. Despite the advantages, this protocol is very costly, adding to the economic burden of the diagnostic workup. In addition, there is no standardization regarding the level of social and physical activity during the procedure. An ad libitum PSG also does not preclude the need for an MSLT. The MSLT still has to be performed to exclude other causes of EDS.

Actigraphy, a method of monitoring human rest-activity cycles, is useful in clinical evaluation. Actigraphy can demonstrate the prolonged sleep episodes seen in idiopathic hypersomnia with long sleep time although it is difficult to differentiate actual sleep from restful wakefulness, which is also useful to rule out other causes of EDS, such as circadian rhythm disorders or BIISS. However, standardization or validation of actigraphy protocols has not been performed for idiopathic hypersomnia.

Aside from the previously mentioned methods, the rest of the workup for idiopathic hypersomnia involves identifying and excluding other causes of EDS because it is a diagnosis of exclusion. Imaging studies such as a brain MRI are typically unremarkable, hypocretin level in the CSF less than 110 ng/L is more consistent with narcolepsy, measurement of CSF hypocretin levels and HLA typing may be useful.

Treatment

Because the cause and pathogenesis of idiopathic hypersomnia are yet to be identified, available treatment is strictly symptomatic. Therapy is primarily targeted toward alleviating EDS. Therefore, pharmacologic treatment options for the EDS in idiopathic hypersomnia with and without long sleep time and narcolepsy are essentially the same. Treatment response has traditionally been thought to be less in patients with idiopathic hypersomnia, but recent research suggests otherwise.[24]

There is a paucity of research regarding therapy for idiopathic hypersomnia, and at present there

---

**Box 1
Differential diagnosis of idiopathic hypersomnia**

Narcolepsy with and without cataplexy

Chronic sleep deprivation in long sleepers

Circadian rhythm disorder (phase advance/delay)

Sleep-disordered breathing (obstructive sleep apnea , upper airway resistance syndrome)

Psychiatric disorders, especially mood disorders

Chronic fatigue syndrome

Post head trauma

Post infectious conditions

are no systematic studies on the subject. The most recent literature includes retrospective studies from major sleep centers. There has been a change in the diagnostic criteria of idiopathic hypersomnia with the advent of the ICSD-2, and as a result, the current literature on idiopathic hypersomnia involves a heterogeneous patient population that was chosen using varying inclusion criteria. Some studies did not use the current MSLT requirements, which are now mandated by the American Academy of Sleep Medicine. Hence, some of the existing data is derived from patients who technically do not meet the current criteria for idiopathic hypersomnia.

Most clinicians consider modafinil as the first-line treatment of idiopathic hypersomnia. The chief molecular target of modafanil is the dopamine transporter, although its exact mechanism of action is still unknown. Modafinil is molecularly unrelated to typical central nervous system (CNS) stimulants, such as amphetamines, and the potential for abuse is generally considered to be low. Modafinil has been found to increase hypothalamic histamine levels[25] as well as promote the release of norepinephrine and dopamine from synaptic terminals, an action similar to that of other stimulants. Modafinil has also shown some efficacy in EDS in children.[26] Patients are usually started on daily dose of 200 mg divided twice daily, with the maximum daily dose being 400 mg. In some cases, it is even better to start with a low dose of 100 mg daily and slowly titrate upward. Common side effects include headache, nausea, palpitations, anxiety, and diarrhea.

Armodafinil is a long lasting R-enantiomer of racemic modafinil. Armodafinil has a longer effective half-life close to 15 hours with a similar mean maximum plasma concentration as modafinil, which results in higher plasma concentrations toward the second half of the half-life when compared with modafinil. Hence armodafinil is especially beneficial for patients suffering from idiopathic hypersomnia with persistent EDS in the later afternoon periods. The side effect profile is similar to modafinil.

In the largest cohort study on idiopathic hypersomnia to date, Lavault and colleagues[27] treated 104 patients (59 with long sleep time and 45 without long sleep time) with modafinil alone using the Epworth Sleepiness Scale (ESS), a visual analog scale, as well as patient and clinician opinions as outcome measures. They found that modafinil caused a similar decrease in the ESS in patients with idiopathic hypersomnia and narcolepsy (-2.6 ± 5.1 vs -3 ± 5.1). Therapeutic benefits estimated by the patients (6.9 ± 2.7 vs 6.5 ± 2.5 on a visual analog scale) and clinicians were

also similar for both conditions. However, the improvement in the ESS was lower among patients with idiopathic hypersomnia also with long sleep time as compared with those without long sleep time, suggesting that this group might be more refractory to therapy.

In another cohort of patients studied by Anderson and colleagues,[6] 24 of 54 (44.4%) patients with idiopathic hypersomnia treated with modafinil had a drop of more than 4 points on their ESS, whereas 7 patients reported no efficacy. The population was more heterogeneous, comprising 61 patients with idiopathic hypersomnia treated with modafinil or amphetamines followed up for a mean of 3.8 years. The outcome measure was the ESS at every visit to the clinic. Later, similar study conducted by Ali and colleagues[24] had a cohort of 85 patients followed up over a period of 2.4 + 4.7 years, with the outcome measure being an internally developed scale using a review of the language used by patients and physicians to describe progress in follow-up visits. In this group, 18 of the 50 patients treated with modafinil reported complete symptomatic relief with 4 cohorts of patients reporting only partial relief. The study also found that even though modafinil was the most common drug initially prescribed for patients with idiopathic hypersomnia, methylphenidate was preferred as the final monotherapy agent, with 51% of cohorts remaining on the drug at the time of the last follow-up visit.

Methylphenidate is a compound structurally similar to amphetamines, and its effect is more akin to that of cocaine although methylphenidate has a longer duration of action and is less potent.[28] Methylphenidate primarily acts as a norepinephrine-dopamine reuptake inhibitor and is also thought to increase the release of both neurotransmitters although to a much lesser extent than amphetamines.[29] The side effect profile of methylphenidate is similar to that of amphetamines and represents CNS stimulation. Side effects include insomnia, anorexia, hypertension, tachycardia, palpitations, and weight loss. There is limited data on methylphenidate and idiopathic hypersomnia; most of our experience with this drug stem from patients with narcolepsy.

In a study by Ali and colleagues,[24] 25 (41%) of the 40 patients who were still on modafinil as of the last follow-up visit reported complete efficacy; 13 reported a partial response whereas 2 had a poor response. The study also noted that patients treated with methylphenidate had a higher percentage of complete or partial therapeutic responses to treatment compared with those treated with modafinil, although this difference was not found to be statistically significant.

As mentioned earlier, amphetamines also act as CNS stimulants. Their principal targets include the dopamine and monoamine receptors leading to higher concentrations of these neurotransmitters. Similar to methylphenidate, most studies and clinical experience with amphetamines come from patients with narcolepsy. Among the previously mentioned drugs, amphetamines are considered to have the highest addiction potential, thus they are used more sparingly. In the study by Ali and colleagues,[24] 7 patients were treated with dextroamphetamine, with none reporting a complete or partial response. Five patients were on methamphetamine and 3 had a complete response.

Anecdotal evidence has also been presented in favor of melatonin as a possible agent for the treatment of patients with idiopathic hypersomnia.[30] Montplaisir and Fantini[30] in 2001 reported improvement in 5 of their 10 patients who were treated with 2 mg of slow release melatonin at bedtime. There has not been any attempt currently to validate these findings. Sodium oxybate has been effectively used to treat narcolepsy but there are no systematic studies on its use in idiopathic hypersomnia.[31]

Behavioral treatment

Aside from medication, behavior modification and sleep hygiene are also part of treatment, but they are minimally effective if used alone. Counseling patients on role of good sleep hygiene and keeping a regular sleep-wake schedule is essential. Patients should avoid large meals rich in carbohydrate, which can produce significant sedating effects. In patients with idiopathic hypersomnia increasing sleep time during the weekend has not been shown to be helpful.[32] Increasing sleep time and naps have been suggested but has not shown any significant effect.[3] There is some anecdotal evidence that restricting total sleep time may be beneficial in some patients with idiopathic hypersomnia. Patients with idiopathic hypersomnia are often frustrated because of the difficulty involved in their diagnosis. Patients go undiagnosed or misdiagnosed for 10 to 15 years after the onset of their initial symptoms. Support groups such as the National Sleep Foundation and The Narcolepsy Network can be very helpful.

SUMMARY

Because idiopathic hypersomnia is such a rare disorder, large systematic randomized systematic studies that would enhance the understanding of the disease are lacking. However, recent advances in neurogenetics and basic neuroscience hold the promise of better insight into the pathophysiology of idiopathic hypersomnia. As a result, definitive diagnostic tools and more effective highly targeted therapies might be available in the near future.

REFERENCES

1. Furukawa T. Heinrich Bruno Schindler's description of narcolepsy in 1829. Neurology 1987;37:146.
2. Roth B. Narkolepsie und hypersomnie. In: Roth B, editor. Narkolepsie und hypersomnie. Berlin: VEB Verlag; 1962.
3. Bassetti C, Aldrich MS. Idiopathic hypersomnia. A series of 42 patients. Brain 1997;120(Pt 8):1423–35.
4. Billiard M, Dauvilliers Y. Idiopathic hypersomnia. Sleep Med Rev 2001;5(5):351–60.
5. Nevsimalova-Bruhova S, Roth B. Heredofamilial aspects of narcolepsy and hypersomnia. Schweiz Arch Neurol Neurochir Psychiatr 1972;110:45–54.
6. Anderson KN, Pilsworth S, Sharples LD, et al. Idiopathic hypersomnia: a study of 77 cases. Sleep 2007;30:1274–81.
7. Nevšímalová S. Differential diagnosis of narcolepsy and other hypersomnia. Vigilia-Sueno 1998; 10(Suppl):S85–6.
8. Petitjean F, Jouvet M. Hypersomnie et augmentation de l'acide 5-hydroxy-indolacétique cérébral par lésion isthmique chez le chat. C R Soc Biol 1970; 164:2288–93 [in French].
9. Montplaisir J, de Champlain J, Young SN, et al. Narcolepsy and idiopathic hypersomnia: biogenic amines and related compounds in CSF. Neurology 1982;32:1299–302.
10. Faull KF, Guilleminault C, Berger PA, et al. Cerebrospinal fluid monoamine metabolites in narcolepsy and hypersomnia. Ann Neurol 1983;13: 258–63.
11. Faull KF, Thiemann S, King RJ, et al. Monoamine interactions in narcolepsy and hypersomnia: a preliminary report. Sleep 1986;9:246–9.
12. Faull KF, Thiemann S, King RJ, et al. Monoamine interactions in narcolepsy and hypersomnia: reanalysis. Sleep 1989;12:185–6.
13. Kanbayashi T, Kodama T, Kondo H, et al. CSF histamine contents in narcolepsy, idiopathic hypersomnia and obstructive sleep apnea. Sleep 2009; 32:181–7.
14. Brown RE, Stevens DR, Haas HL. The physiology of brain histamine. Prog Neurobiol 2001;63:637–72.
15. Bassetti CL, Khatami R, Poryazova R, et al. Idiopathic hypersomnia: a dopaminergic disorder? Sleep 2009;32(Suppl 1):A248–9.
16. Sforza E, Gaudreau H, Petit D, et al. Homeostatic sleep regulation in patients with idiopathic hypersomnia. Clin Neurophysiol 2000;111:277–82.
17. Billiard M, Rondouin G, Espa F, et al. Physiopathologie de l'hypersomnie idiopathique. Rev Neurol 2001; 157(11 Pt 2):S101–6 [in French].

18. Vernet C, Arnulf I. Idiopathic hypersomnia with and without long sleep time: a controlled series of 75 patients. Sleep 2009;32(6):753–9.

19. Nevsimalova S, Blazejova K, Illnerova H, et al. A contribution to pathophysiology of idiopathic hypersomnia. Suppl Clin Neurophysiol 2000;53:366–70.

20. American Academy of Sleep Medicine. International classification of sleep disorders. Diagnostic and coding manual. 2nd edition. Westchester (IL): American Academy of Sleep Medicine; 2005.

21. Broughton R, Nevsimalova S, Roth B. The socioeconomic effects of idiopathic hypersomnia—comparison with controls and with compound narcoleptics. In: Popoviciu L, Asgian B, Badiu G, editors. Sleep 1978. Basel (Switzerland): Karger; 1980. p. 229–33.

22. Roth B, Nevsìmalovà S, Rechtschaffen A. Hypersomnia with "sleep drunkenness." Arch Gen Psychiatry 1972;26:456–62.

23. Baker TL, Guilleminault C, Nino-Murcia G, et al. Comparative polysomnographic study of narcolepsy and idiopathic central nervous system hypersomnia. Sleep 1986;9:232–42.

24. Ali M, Auger RR, Slocumb NL, et al. Idiopathic hypersomnia: clinical features and response to treatment. J Clin Sleep Med 2009;5(6):562–8.

25. Ishizuka T, Murakami M, Yamatodani A. Involvement of central histaminergic systems in modafinil-induced but not methylphenidate-induced increases in locomotor activity in rats. Eur J Pharmacol 2008; 578(2–3):209–15.

26. Ivanenko A, Tauman R, Gozal D. Modafinil in the treatment of excessive daytime sleepiness in children. Sleep Med 2003;4:579–82.

27. Lavault S, Dauvilliers Y, Drouot X, et al. Benefit and risk of modafinil in idiopathic hypersomnia vs. narcolepsy with cataplexy. Sleep Med 2011;2(6): 550–6.

28. Peter D. Why isn't methylphenidate more addictive? Neuropsychiatry Rev 2002;3(1):19.

29. Sulzer D, Sonders MS, Poulsen NW, et al. Mechanisms of neurotransmitter release by amphetamines: a review. Prog Neurobiol 2005;75(6):406–33.

30. Montplaisir J, Fantini L. Idiopathic hypersomnia: a diagnostic dilemma. Sleep Med Rev 2001;5: 361–2.

31. Wise M, Arand D, Auger R, et al. Treatment of narcolepsy and other hypersomnias of central origin. An American Academy of Sleep medicine review. Sleep 2007;30(12):1712–27.

32. Bassetti C, Pelayo R, Guilleminault C. Idiopathic hypersomnia. In: Kryger MH, Roth T, Dement WC, editors. Principle and practice of sleep medicine. 4th edition. Saint Louis (MO): Saunders; 2005. p. 791–800.

Comorbidities of Central Nervous System Hypersomnia

Alon Y. Avidan, MD, MPH

KEYWORDS

- Narcolepsy • Sleep • Comorbidities • Diabetes • Fibromyalgia • Psychosocial
- Psychiatric disorders • Migraine headaches

KEY POINTS

- Central nervous system hypersomnias are associated with and have a bidirectional impact on a variety of comorbid medical and psychiatric comorbidities.
- Narcolepsy is strongly related to obesity and eating disorders; diabetes; psychiatric disorders; fibromyalgia; neurologic disease, including migraine headaches and cognitive dysfunction, and is associated with psychosocial impairment.
- While the actual frequencies of these disorders in central nervous system hypersomnias is unclear, sleep experts need to be mindful about the spectrum of the underlying comorbidities when caring for people with hypersomnolence.

INTRODUCTION

Central nervous system (CNS) hypersomnia is a term that encompasses a variety of conditions with an underlying unified presenting symptom of excessive daytime sleepiness (EDS) and an underlying pathologic condition in the CNS. The most important type of CNS hypersomnia is narcolepsy, a chronic neurodegenerative disease characterized by severe unremitting EDS and rapid eye movement (REM) intrusion phenomena such as cataplexy, sleep paralysis, and hypnagogic and hypnopompic hallucinations.[1] The underlying pathophysiology of the disease is localizable to the hypothalamus and is attributed to a deficiency of the neuropeptide hypocretin in the hypothalamus.[2] Narcolepsy has a genetic association with certain human leukocyte antigen (HLA) alleles such as HLA-DR2 and HLA-DQB1*0602.[3] In recent years, it has been postulated that environmental factors may trigger an autoimmune process, resulting in destruction of the hypothalamic cells responsible for hypocretin production.[4] This article describes the most prevalent comorbid conditions seen in

CNS hypersomnia and discusses selected comorbid conditions in the most common CNS hypersomnias according to the International Classification of Sleep Disorders, Second Edition.

NARCOLEPSY

Narcolepsy is associated with several other comorbid medical problems, which include eating disorders; obesity; diabetes; psychiatric conditions, including schizophrenia and depression; fibromyalgia; neurologic symptoms, including migraine headaches and cognitive dysfunction; and psychosocial impairment (**Fig. 1**).

Psychosocial Comorbidities

Narcolepsy is associated with significant social impairment and reduced quality of life, affecting both children and adults. In adult patients, narcolepsy induces a negative effect on health-related quality-of-life assessments, specifically in the domains of bodily pain, social function, and general health, compared with data from the general

Disclosures: Speaker's Bureau: Purdue, Cephalon, GSK; Consultant: Merck.
Sleep Disorders Center and Department of Neurology, University of California, Los Angeles, 710 Westwood Boulevard, Room 1-169 RNRC, Los Angeles, CA 90095-6975, USA
E-mail address: avidan@mednet.ucla.edu

Sleep Med Clin 7 (2012) 291–302
doi:10.1016/j.jsmc.2012.04.001

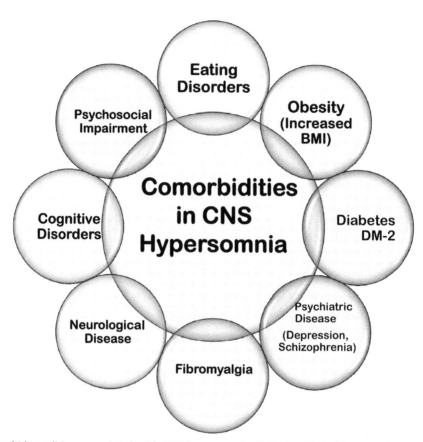

Fig. 1. Comorbid conditions associated with CNS hypersomnia. Patients affected by narcolepsy are at risk for a variety of conditions including obesity, diabetes (type 1 and type 2), psychiatric conditions including schizophrenia and depression, fibromyalgia, neurologic symptoms including migraine headaches and cognitive dysfunction, as well as psychosocial impairment. (*Modified from* Panossian LA, Avidan AY. Narcolepsy and other comorbid medical illnesses. In: Goswami M, Pandi-Perumal SR, Thorpy MJ, editors. Narcolepsy: clinical guide. New York: Humana Press; 2010. p. 105–15; with permission.)

population.[5] A study of children aged between 4 and 18 years with narcolepsy revealed significant problems in behavior, emotional state, quality of life, educational progress, and family impact when compared with healthy age- and gender-matched controls.[6] The rate of such problems was also increased among children with EDS not due to narcolepsy. Areas of problem included difficulties with peer interactions, behavioral conduct, and emotional symptoms. Children with narcolepsy as well as those with isolated EDS had significantly higher scores on the Child Depression Inventory than controls. These data suggest that the symptom of excessive sleepiness, which is present in children with narcolepsy as well as in children with idiopathic EDS, is responsible for many of the apparent psychosocial and quality-of-life issues that arise.[6] The quality of life using the 36-Item Short Form Health Survey of patients with narcolepsy had similar results and at times worse psychosocial function when compared with other neurologic

disorders including lower vitality and reduced social functioning[7] (refer to Fig. 1 in Goswani's article).

Comorbid Endocrine and Metabolic Dysregulation

Weight and appetite
For a long time, a peculiar link has been noted between narcolepsy and increased body mass index ([BMI] expressed in kilograms per meters squared). Recent data suggest an increased prevalence of high BMI and obesity in patients with narcolepsy.[8–10] One study examining 35 HLA-DR2–positive patients with narcolepsy with cataplexy revealed a significantly elevated BMI compared with population controls who never used analeptics (CNS stimulants).[10] Although the increase in BMI was noted in both genders, male patients with narcolepsy exhibited a higher mean BMI (in the 75th percentile) than female patients (BMI noted in the 61st percentile). Similar data

were seen in a group of patients with childhood-onset narcolepsy that was diagnosed before age 18 years. This cohort too had a significantly higher BMI than controls, and the historical use of analeptics did not make a significant difference in weight in these patients.[11]

A few hypotheses are proposed to describe the prevalence of higher BMI in this cohort. One proposed theory is that the effect on BMI may be due to narcolepsy-induced behavioral changes related to eating, physical activity, and reduced energy expenditure. An alternative theory is that the weight gain could be related to the underlying disease pathophysiology in those patients who are positive for the HLA-DR2 allele. This stems from the finding that although patients with narcolepsy express positivity for the HLA-DR2 haplotype, healthy nonnarcoleptic patients who are HLA-DR2 positive do not show any increased risk for elevated BMI; thus there does not seem to be a genetic linkage between the HLA-DR2 allele and obesity in and of itself.[9]

An interesting proposal to help explain the observed metabolic derangement in narcolepsy is the observation that neuroendocrine changes in narcolepsy may result in altered energy homeostasis.[2,10] Weight gain in patients with narcolepsy may be attributable to a deficiency in hypothalamic hypocretin neurons, which regulate endocrine and autonomic functions. Hypocretin, the neuropeptide that is deficient in most patients with narcolepsy, is normally thought to stimulate eating behavior as well as to regulate energy expenditure and physical activity (**Fig. 2**).[12,13] It might then be deduced that hypocretin deficiency would ultimately result in less food intake and reduced BMI; however, this is not what is observed in narcolepsy. A possible explanation may be that hypocretin deficiency reduces energy expenditure to a greater degree than it reduces food intake, resulting in net weight gain.[13]

Previous studies have also tested the possible relationship between narcolepsy and the adipose tissue–derived hormone leptin, which acts on the hypothalamus where it exerts its effect to inhibit appetite and the size of adipose cells.[14] A deficiency in leptin is predicted to reduce feedback to the CNS and result in obesity.

Leptin and hypocretin are believed to work synergistically to inhibit REM sleep.[15,16] Their loss could play a role in the increased sleep-onset REM periods that are observed on polysomnograms and multiple sleep latency tests in patients with narcolepsy. A study that assayed the levels of leptin

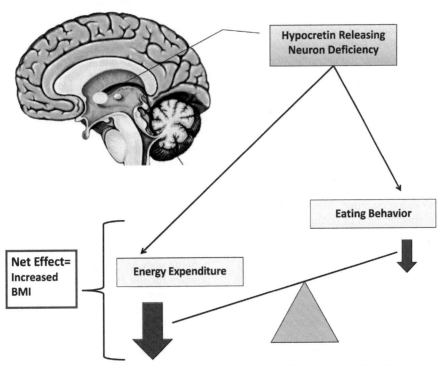

Fig. 2. Hypocretin is believed to regulate energy expenditure and physical activity. Hypocretin deficiency could induce both a decline in food intake and a reduction in BMI. However, patients with narcolepsy are observed to have a higher BMI than age-matched controls. One possible explanation for this observation is that hypocretin deficiency may lead to a worse decline of energy expenditure than reduced food intake, leading to a net weight gain.

in the serum (cerebrospinal fluid [CSF]) demonstrated a significant reduction in the level in patients with narcolepsy in comparison with the control groups.[14]

A relatively more recent study of leptin in narcolepsy has yielded contradictory results. A measurement of the CSF to serum leptin ratio as an indicator of leptin transport across the blood-brain barrier showed no significant reduction in serum leptin level in patients with narcolepsy, more than half of whom had hypocretin deficiency in comparison with normal controls.[13] The study also revealed no significant difference in CSF leptin levels or in the CSF to serum leptin ratio. Because CSF leptin levels were unchanged in patients with narcolepsy, the investigators deduced that leptin is unlikely to be involved in the weight changes seen in these patients. This finding has been corroborated by other studies showing no difference in serum leptin levels between patients with narcolepsy and controls.[17]

Increases in weight (as measured by BMI) in narcolepsy may be attributed to several behavioral factors. A study comparing food intake in patients with narcolepsy with cataplexy with that in normal controls found that those with narcolepsy consumed fewer kilojoules of food per day.[18] Although food intake in patients with narcolepsy, measured by energy consumed, may not be pathologic, several other studies found an interesting and significant association between narcolepsy and eating disorders. Patients with narcolepsy with cataplexy scored significantly higher on almost all measures on the eating disorder assessment compared with healthy controls (using a clinical assessment tool for eating disorders).[8] Patients with narcolepsy continued to demonstrate increased rates of overeating, binge eating, and cravings for food when compared with BMI-matched controls.[8] Although those with narcolepsy exhibited frequent symptoms of eating disorders (about a quarter of whom met formal criteria for an eating disorder), there was no predilection for a specific type of eating disorder. The spectrum of eating disorders present in the narcoleptic group included bulimia nervosa, anorexia nervosa, and eating disorder not otherwise specified.[8] However, as in the case of neuroendocrine metabolic indicators, conflicting data occur in this area also because other investigators have found no correlation between narcolepsy syndrome and eating disorders, including lack of observed increase in hyperphagic behavior among patients with narcolepsy.[19] A potential reason for these discrepancies may be the time in the disease course during which the symptoms of eating disorders are measured because weight gain seen in narcolepsy tends to manifest early at the time of initial diagnosis.[11,19]

Derangement of metabolic rate has been proposed and measured in narcolepsy as a possible contributor to weight gain. Because of the lack of convincing data implicating abnormal eating behavior or increased caloric intake as the cause of weight gain in narcolepsy, it has been hypothesized that attenuation of basal metabolic rate may be a cause. However, when comparing hypocretin-deficient narcoleptic subjects with healthy controls, there was no conclusive difference observed with respect to measurement of resting metabolic rate.[20]

The cause for the increased BMI observed in narcolepsy remains to be clearly defined. There are unclear associations between weight gain and positive HLA-DR2 haplotype,[9] caloric intake,[18] and resting metabolic rate.[20] More data are needed to clarify the impact that eating disorders and behavioral factors could have on weight gain in narcolepsy.[8,19] The most likely cause seems to implicate derangement of hypocretin neuroendocrinology. Although the data regarding the role of leptin have also been contradictory,[13,14] it is suggested that other yet to be identified hormonal pathways in the CNS and periphery are involved and interact with hypocretin neurons to induce weight alterations.[21]

Diabetes mellitus

Diabetes mellitus is another neuroendocrine disturbance that has an association with narcolepsy. Narcolepsy and diabetes mellitus type 1 (insulin-dependent diabetes) share a common autoimmune pathophysiology. Both involve the selective, autoimmune-mediated destruction of unique cell types (pancreatic islet cells in type 1 diabetes and hypocretin-producing hypothalamic neurons in narcolepsy).[22] Both also share a genetic association, probably mediated through specific HLA haplotypes. Although findings demonstrate that the HLA-DQB1*0602 haplotype confers susceptibility to narcolepsy with cataplexy, it is nonetheless strongly protective against type 1 diabetes.[23,24] This may lead some to suggest that patients with narcolepsy with cataplexy who are positive for the HLA-DQB1*0602 allele are likely to have much lower rates of type 1 diabetes than the general population. It may be deduced from these data that patients with narcolepsy are expected to have much lower rates of type 1 diabetes but may exhibit higher rates of type 2 diabetes because of the increased risk of insulin resistance associated with elevated BMI and obesity.[22] However, studies to determine the incidence of type 1 versus type 2 (noninsulin dependent) diabetes mellitus in narcolepsy have not yet been carried out. No clinically relevant pathologic findings in glucose metabolism were appreciated in a recent study that compared patients with narcolepsy with weight-matched controls, leading the investigators to conclude that narcolepsy is probably an unlikely a risk factor per se for impaired glucose metabolism or diabetes.[25]

Psychiatric Disorders

Patients with narcolepsy are susceptive to several comorbid psychiatric disorders, including depression and schizophrenia.[1] Depression is strongly linked as a comorbidity to the 2 most common sleep disturbances, insomnia and hypersomnia.[26,27] Major depressive disorder is a major confounder with the diagnosis of narcolepsy, particularly narcolepsy without cataplexy, because of similar presenting symptoms in the 2 conditions. Of patients with major depression, 10% to 20% have been reported to complain of EDS.[27] One extensive study attempted to investigate the presence of primary narcolepsy symptoms (sleep paralysis, hypnagogic and hypnopompic hallucinations, cataplexy, and automatic behaviors) among patients with depression but without a diagnosis of narcolepsy.[26] The finding documented a strong correlation between severe depression and sleep paralysis, hypnagogic or hypnopompic hallucinations, and automatic behaviors, even after controlling for age, sex, and BMI and concomitant use of antidepressant. In addition, both severe and milder forms of depression demonstrated a strong positive correlation with cataplexy.[26] Cataplexy has been proposed to share a common underlying pathophysiology with depression, and both conditions respond to antidepressant medications.[28] In fact, data show that in the presence of monoaminergic/cholinergic imbalance, gamma-hydroxybutyrate (GHB) may restore the imbalance, and repeated use of GHB at night may make this an effective treatment of narcolepsy and comorbid depression.[29]

A recent epidemiologic study revealed that 7.6% of the general population, 28.3% of students, and 31.9% of patients with psychiatric conditions experienced at least 1 episode of sleep paralysis in their lifetime.[30] Sleep paralysis can also occur in otherwise healthy nonnarcoleptic patients with underlying sleep disturbances, insufficient sleep, or insomnia, and it may be that the sleeping problems and insomnia in patients with depression exacerbate symptoms of sleep paralysis.[26] Nevertheless, despite the potential confounding effects of sleep insufficiency, sleep paralysis does appear to occur more frequently among patients with comorbid psychiatric disorders and in patients who use anxiolytic medication, compared with the healthy population, even after controlling for the effects of sleep problems.[31] Sleep paralysis is also strongly correlated with trauma and posttraumatic panic symptoms, with increased prevalence among patients of African American decent.[32] However, this association may be related to the disturbed sleep and insomnia that accompanies posttraumatic panic that induces sleep paralysis, rather than an independent association between sleep paralysis and a psychiatric diagnosis.[32]

Narcolepsy is frequently associated with hypnagogic and hypnopompic hallucinations and shares with the tactile and visual perceptual phenomena associated with psychosis (**Fig. 3**). The accurate diagnosis of psychotic symptoms in patients with narcolepsy may be challenging because of adverse effects of pharmacotherapy with stimulants (which may induce hallucinations) as well as primary symptoms of narcolepsy (sleep paralysis and hypnagogic and/or hypnopompic hallucinations).[33] Patients with schizophrenia are more likely to experience primarily auditory rather than visual or tactile hallucinations. Some hypnagogic hallucinations can manifest as a complex and multimodal pattern with an auditory component.[34] Patients with narcolepsy typically report multisensory "holistic" hallucinations rather than the predominantly verbal-auditory sensory pattern encountered in patients with schizophrenia.[35] A minority of patients with narcolepsy may also experience hallucinations during wakefulness, making the differentiation between narcolepsy and schizophrenia a diagnostic challenge. Indeed, patients with narcolepsy have been previously misdiagnosed as having refractory schizophrenia on the grounds of these hallucinatory experiences while awake.[34,36–38] An intriguing and a unique psychotic form of narcolepsy exists in which patients experience hallucinations while awake, as well as nocturnal hypnagogic and hypnopompic hallucinations (see **Fig. 3**). These patients with narcolepsy typically have a good insight into their illness, with preserved interpersonal interactions, appropriate effect, and no loose associations. Another key feature of the psychotic form of narcolepsy is that it does not typically respond to antipsychotic medications but rather improves with CNS stimulants such as methylphenidate or modafinil.[37] Recent data to help differentiate psychotic-like symptoms in narcolepsy from bona fide psychosis reported that delusions and formal psychotic disorders were not more frequent in patients with narcolepsy in comparison with population controls.[35]

Rarely do schizophrenia and narcolepsy coexist in the same patient.[37,39] Although some studies

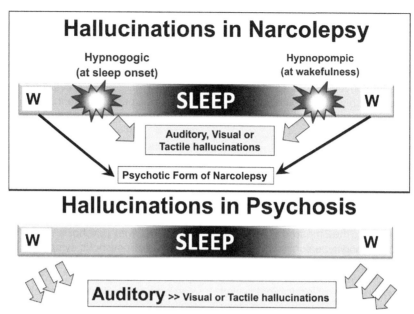

Fig. 3. Comorbid hallucinatory experiences in narcolepsy and psychosis. Both narcolepsy and psychosis are associated with hallucinations. Patients with narcolepsy may experience hypnagogic hallucinations (at sleep onset) and hypnopompic hallucinations (at wakefulness). Unlike narcolepsy, hallucinations in psychosis tend to be primarily auditory rather than visual or tactile phenomenon. W, wake.

report a higher incidence of comorbid schizophrenia among patients with narcolepsy than among the general population, the diagnosis of schizophrenia in patients with narcoleptics vary widely with reported prevalence rates ranging from 0% to 14%.[34] Some controversy exists, however, about the actual incidence of waking psychosis symptoms among patients with narcolepsy. One study found that only 8.9% of patients with narcolepsy experienced psychotic symptoms, which were temporally related to treatment with psychostimulants as patients improved after discontinuing or lowering the dose of the medication.[34] The treatments of EDS in narcolepsy, including the use of CNS stimulants, could precipitate psychotic symptoms as a result of their dopaminergic stimulatory effect.[36,39] The medication-related side effects may therefore contribute to confounding the actual data regarding the true prevalence of comorbid psychosis among patients with narcolepsy.

Headache Syndromes

Migraine headaches

Compared with the general population, patients with narcolepsy have a 2- to 4-fold increased prevalence rate of migraine headaches (either with or without aura).[40,41] However, the association of migraine headaches in patients with narcolepsy

has not been significantly linked to the severity of underlying narcolepsy symptoms, the degree of daytime sleepiness, BMI, or HLA-DR2 phenotype.[41] However, those patients with narcolepsy who do go on to develop migraine headaches tend to do so at a younger age and typically have their migraine headache onset over a decade after experiencing their initial narcolepsy symptoms.[41] The prevalence of migraine headache among patients with narcolepsy elevated even after controlling for concomitant use of psychostimulants and antidepressant medications. This finding may suggest that the migraine phenomenon is an underlying neurologic comorbidity associated with narcolepsy itself, as opposed to consequent adverse pharmacologic treatments of narcolepsy.[41] One proposed pathophysiologic mechanism is that both narcolepsy and migraine headaches arise from shared neuroanatomical regions in the brainstem, including the dorsal raphe nuclei and the locus ceruleus,[41] areas known to exhibit increased blood flow during migraine headaches, and are also involved in the origin of REM sleep control.[41] Migraine headaches may be more common among patients with narcolepsy because of the underlying primary sleep disturbances associated with narcolepsy such as poor-quality sleep and frequent nocturnal awakenings.[42] Migraines may be triggered or exacerbated by either extreme: excessive sleep or too little sleep (sleep deprivation, behaviorally induced insufficient sleep syndrome).[43]

To address the question of whether migraines and narcolepsy may have a direct genetic association, Coelho and colleagues[44] investigated the frequency of the HLA-DQB1*0602 allele in patients with migraine. As described in this issue by several other investigators, HLA subtype is present in most patients who present with narcolepsy with cataplexy, particularly in subjects with CSF hypocretin-1 levels less than 110 pg/mL.[3,45] The investigators did not find significant increase in the frequency of expression of the HLA-DQB1*0602 allele among patients with migraine with or without aura in comparison with healthy controls.[44] Although the lack of HLA antigen association may not necessarily rule out the possibility that migraines and narcolepsy may share a common association through other mechanisms, further data are needed to elucidate the association between both the disorders.

Tension headaches

A multicenter case-control study determined that the rate of nonmigrainous headaches, particularly tension-type headaches, was higher in patients with narcolepsy than in healthy controls.[46] These headache syndromes could be conceptualized as related to the underlying sleep disturbance associated with narcolepsy or may be secondary to medication use to treat narcolepsy, which was not controlled for in this study.[46]

Cluster headaches

Cluster headaches consist of episodic bouts of severe unilateral pain centered around the periorbital area, often with associated rhinorrhea and lacrimation.[47] Data showed that the onset of narcolepsy, specifically the symptoms of hypersomnia and disturbed nocturnal sleep, does not have a significant impact on cluster headache frequency or severity, suggesting a lack of pathophysiologic association between cluster headaches and narcolepsy.[47] Furthermore, the gender predilection and genetic associations are also dissimilar between both the disorders; narcolepsy has no clear gender predilection, whereas cluster headaches are much more prevalent in men than in women. Cluster headaches are generally associated with the HLA DR5 haplotype, as opposed to the HLA-DR2 linkage commonly seen in narcolepsy.[47] Although cluster headaches and narcolepsy may be conceptualized as episodic brain disorders with an underlying unified mechanism involving the hypothalamus,[48] the data thus far do not seem to be supportive of cluster headaches as a significant comorbid disorder in narcolepsy.

Fibromyalgia

Fibromyalgia is a disorder distinguished by chronic widespread pain in the presence of widespread tenderness and multiple somatic symptoms.[49,50] Approximately 2% of the population are affected by the fibromyalgia syndrome, with a higher prevalence rate in women.[50,51] Fibromyalgia is also frequently associated with fatigue and nonrestorative sleep.[50] In fact, the American College of Rheumatology has recently proposed that sleep should be a central component of the clinical assessment of patients with possible fibromyalgia.[52] Classic symptoms of fibromyalgia may be encountered in patients with long-standing narcolepsy without cataplexy as well as narcolepsy with cataplexy.[53–55] Although reports of narcolepsy with comorbid fibromyalgia are exceedingly rare, the pathophysiology of the 2 disorders may share a common underlying pathophysiologic mechanism. As described earlier, because narcolepsy is associated with headache syndromes, it is likely that the underlying pathophysiology of narcolepsy may play a role in pain sensation.[44] Hypocretin has previously been shown to interact with pain modulation and sensory input pathways[56] and has been proposed to play a role in the mediating pain syndromes such as fibromyalgia. However, this theory was not supported by a study by Taiwo and colleagues[50] who assayed the levels of hypocretin in the CSF of patients with fibromyalgia and compared it with that in healthy controls, revealing no significant difference in mean hypocretin levels between patients with fibromyalgia and healthy controls. Genetic studies on fibromyalgia found a possible association with the HLA-DR4 allele but not with the subtypes, HLA-DR2 and HLA-DQB1*0602.[57] It may therefore be conclude that thus far, the evidence of an underlying pathophysiologic association between fibromyalgia and narcolepsy is rather weak, with only rare reports of narcolepsy being associated with comorbid fibromyalgia.

Cognitive Dysfunction

Patients with narcolepsy are at risk for impairments in several cognitive domains. This association is apparent among both older and younger cohorts,[58] with tiredness and episodes of sleepiness believed to be the main reason for this impairment.[59] An epidemiologic study showed that people with narcolepsy younger than 45 years are more likely than healthy age-matched controls to experience significant impairments in attention and concentration, delayed recall, and difficulty with orientation to persons (recalling names or recognizing acquaintances).[58] However, when patients with narcolepsy older than 45 years were compared with age-matched healthy controls, the findings depicted more significant impartment across multiple domains of cognitive function. Older people with narcolepsy experience severe and worse cognitive difficulties across multiple areas, including attention and concentration, praxis, delayed recall, orientation to persons, temporal orientation, and prospective memory.[58]

Because cognitive impairment alone may contribute to EDS, the investigators subsequently controlled for confounders such as sleepiness (as measured by the Epworth Sleepiness Scale scores), age, sleep apnea, physical health, and use of psychotropic medications, confirming again that narcolepsy continued to be significantly associated with a higher risk of poor concentration, deficits in attention, and a difficulty with prospective memory.[58] Although most cognitive pathologic conditions in patients with narcolepsy seem to be secondary to EDS, some degree of cognitive decline is likely to be ascribed to the underlying disease pathophysiology and is probably independent of advanced age or the severity of sleepiness.

Data examining objective cognitive impairment in narcolepsy provide conflicting conclusions; although most patients with narcolepsy showed subjective cognitive complaints, some studies provided no evidence for specific cognitive deficits. A small study consisting of 10 untreated patients with narcolepsy demonstrated no significant difference on tests of verbal and nonverbal learning, digit span, naming, and fluency when compared with controls.[60] There was also a lack in data that demonstrated significant or dramatic difference, between patients with narcolepsy and age- and education-matched healthy controls on a spectrum of neuropsychological tests, except that those with narcolepsy experienced lapses in attention and decline of executive function when compared with controls.[61,62] Medication use also had no significant effect on memory tasks among subgroups of patients with narcolepsy.[62] These data report that patients with narcolepsy demonstrate a deficit or a decline in cognitive processing resources as opposed to a problem in a specific cognitive area.[62] A recent literature review utilized data from event-related potential (ERP) paradigms, which are useful tools in the evaluation of information processing and are markers sensitive to subtle neuropsychological changes.[63] The use of these paradigms in patients with narcolepsy confirms the presence of changes in cognitive attentive processing presumably through an association with altered functioning of the level of the prefrontal cortex.[63] ERP electromagnetic tomography showed that therapy with the wake-

promoting agent modafinil ameliorated the speed of information processing and enhanced energetic resources in prefrontal cortical areas.[63]

Human Immunodeficiency Virus Infection/ AIDS and Other Infections

In the era of life-prolonging antiretroviral (ARV) therapy, sleepiness and chronic fatigue are among the most disabling symptoms of persons with human immunodeficiency virus (HIV) infection/ AIDS, yet its management is challenging and the etiology remains elusive. There are currently an estimated 40 million patients worldwide who live with AIDS.[64] In the United States, it is estimated that more than 1 million people are living with HIV infection and approximately 56,300 people were newly infected with HIV in 2006. With an increasing proportion of AIDS survivors, it is expected that this population will face longer periods of life with potential increased comorbidities such as sleep disorders, pain, metabolic problems, and psychiatric illness, both directly caused by the virus and ARV therapy.

Sleepiness and fatigue are encountered at all stages of HIV infection and are related to several etiologic factors including the neurotropic effects of the HIV virus, ARV therapy, substance use, and psychiatric illness affecting all aspects of quality of life.[65–67] The prevalence of sleepiness among patients with HIV infection is estimated to be between 20% and 60%, and, as HIV progresses, fatigue may become even more prevalent.[68] Hypersomnolence contributes to significant morbidity and disability in HIV-infected patients.[69–72] When undiagnosed or undertreated, sleep disturbances are associated with an increased risk of depression, pain, and substance abuse, which is common among patients with HIV.[73–76] These findings underscore the need for addressing excessive sleepiness and sleep quality in developing effective care for individuals with HIV/AIDS who experience fatigue. In fact, in 1988, a specific term, AIDS-lethargy, was coined to delineate an underlying syndrome of specific apathy, tiredness, and indolence of the patients affected with HIV.[77]

During the first few months of 2010, an abrupt increased onset of narcolepsy-cataplexy diagnosed within a few months of H1N1 onset was observed leading to a proposed link between H1N1 vaccination and narcolepsy onset because of this temporal association.[78] Recently, in China, narcolepsy onset has been found to be strongly associated with both annual and seasonal patterns of upper respiratory infections, particularly H1N1 influenza. In 2010, the peak seasonal onset of narcolepsy was phase delayed by 6 months relative to winter H1N1 infections, and the correlation was independent of H1N1 vaccination in most samples.[79] Earlier streptococcal infections, which are known to trigger autoimmunity, were proposed as a significant environmental trigger for narcolepsy based on high anti–streptolysin O and anti–DNase B titers during the disease period, which improved during the convalescent phase.[80] These data depicting a strong seasonality of disease onset in children and associations with the *Streptococcus pyogenes*, and influenza A H1N1 infection as well as H1N1 vaccination, implicate processes such as molecular mimicry or bystander activation as critical for the development of narcolepsy.[81]

Kleine-Levin Syndrome

Patients with Kleine-Levin syndrome (KLS) have significant difficulties with psychiatric, physical and psychological, and eating disorders: cognitive impairment, derealization, megaphagia, hypersexuality, increased BMI, and depressed mood are frequent.[82,83] Out of 10 patients with KLS, 1 develops various genetic, inflammatory, vascular, or paraneoplastic conditions.[83] Patients may experience disturbed function of the hypothalamic-pituitary axis at adrenal and thyroid levels supportive of the hypothesis that KLS is related to an intermittent hypothalamic dysfunction.[84] Based on biomarkers such as electroencephalographic analysis and response to therapy with lithium, studies found that mood disorders are strongly correlated in KLS.[85,86] In fact, the literature on the management with lithium both as directed treatment as well as prophylactic therapy in KLS is extensive, further raising the underlying link to bipolar depression.[87–92]

SUMMARY

CNS hypersomnia, in general, and narcolepsy, in particular, are associated with a spectrum of medical and psychiatric comorbidities. Some comorbidities, such as the increased rate of obesity and overweight, have been well established in the literature. Other associations, such as between narcolepsy and schizophrenia or between narcolepsy and migraine headaches, have been inconsistent and have occasionally demonstrated contradictory findings. Although the true incidence of many of these disorders in narcolepsy is unknown or disputed, it is important to be aware of possible medical comorbidities when caring for patients with narcolepsy. Clinician vigilance in screening for these conditions can prevent delays in diagnosis and treatment of many comorbid medical illnesses.

REFERENCES

1. Benca RM. Narcolepsy and excessive daytime sleepiness: diagnostic considerations, epidemiology, and comorbidities. J Clin Psychiatry 2007; 68(Suppl 13):5–8.
2. Siegel JM. Narcolepsy: a key role for hypocretins (orexins). Cell 1999;98(4):409–12.
3. Chabas D, Taheri S, Renier C, et al. The genetics of narcolepsy. Annu Rev Genomics Hum Genet 2003; 4:459–83.
4. Dauvilliers Y, Arnulf I, Mignot E. Narcolepsy with cataplexy. Lancet 2007;369(9560):499–511.
5. Ervik S, Abdelnoor M, Heier MS, et al. Health-related quality of life in narcolepsy. Acta Neurol Scand 2006; 114(3):198–204.
6. Stores G, Montgomery P, Wiggs L. The psychosocial problems of children with narcolepsy and those with excessive daytime sleepiness of uncertain origin. Pediatrics 2006;118(4):e1116–23.
7. Beusterien KM, Rogers AE, Walsleben JA, et al. Health-related quality of life effects of modafinil for treatment of narcolepsy. Sleep 1999;22(6): 757–65.
8. Fortuyn HA, Swinkels S, Buitelaar J, et al. High prevalence of eating disorders in narcolepsy with cataplexy: a case-control study. Sleep 2008;31(3): 335–41.
9. Schuld A, Beitinger PA, Dalal M, et al. Increased body mass index (BMI) in male narcoleptic patients, but not in HLA-DR2-positive healthy male volunteers. Sleep Med 2002;3(4):335–9.
10. Schuld A, Hebebrand J, Geller F, et al. Increased body-mass index in patients with narcolepsy. Lancet 2000;355(9211):1274–5.
11. Kotagal S, Krahn LE, Slocumb N. A putative link between childhood narcolepsy and obesity. Sleep Med 2004;5(2):147–50.
12. Sakurai T. Orexins and orexin receptors: implication in feeding behavior. Regul Pept 1999;85(1):25–30.
13. Arnulf I, Lin L, Zhang J, et al. CSF versus serum leptin in narcolepsy: is there an effect of hypocretin deficiency? Sleep 2006;29(8):1017–24.
14. Schuld A, Blum WF, Uhr M, et al. Reduced leptin levels in human narcolepsy. Neuroendocrinology 2000;72(4):195–8.
15. Sinton CM, Fitch TE, Gershenfeld HK. The effects of leptin on REM sleep and slow wave delta in rats are reversed by food deprivation. J Sleep Res 1999; 8(3):197–203.
16. Piper DC, Upton N, Smith MI, et al. The novel brain neuropeptide, orexin-A, modulates the sleep-wake cycle of rats. Eur J Neurosci 2000; 12(2):726–30.
17. Dahmen N, Engel A, Helfrich J, et al. Peripheral leptin levels in narcoleptic patients. Diabetes Technol Ther 2007;9(4):348–53.

18. Lammers GJ, Pijl H, Iestra J, et al. Spontaneous food choice in narcolepsy. Sleep 1996;19(1):75–6.

19. Dahmen N, Becht J, Engel A, et al. Prevalence of eating disorders and eating attacks in narcolepsy. Neuropsychiatr Dis Treat 2008;4(1): 257–61.

20. Fronczek R, Overeem S, Reijntjes R, et al. Increased heart rate variability but normal resting metabolic rate in hypocretin/orexin-deficient human narcolepsy. J Clin Sleep Med 2008;4(3):248–54.

21. Ohno K, Sakurai T. Orexin neuronal circuitry: role in the regulation of sleep and wakefulness. Front Neuroendocrinol 2008;29(1):70–87.

22. Longstreth WT Jr, Koepsell TD, Ton TG, et al. The epidemiology of narcolepsy. Sleep 2007;30(1):13–26.

23. Todd JA, Bell JI, McDevitt HO. HLA-DQ beta gene contributes to susceptibility and resistance to insulin-dependent diabetes mellitus. Nature 1987; 329:599–604.

24. Siebold C, Hansen BE, Wyer JR, et al. Crystal structure of HLA-DQ0602 that protects against type 1 diabetes and confers strong susceptibility to narcolepsy. Proc Natl Acad Sci U S A 2004;101(7): 1999–2004.

25. Beitinger PA, Fulda S, Dalal MA, et al. Glucose tolerance in patients with narcolepsy. Sleep 2012;35(2): 231–6.

26. Szklo-Coxe M, Young T, Finn L, et al. Depression: relationships to sleep paralysis and other sleep disturbances in a community sample. J Sleep Res 2007;16(3):297–312.

27. Baldwin DS, Papakostas GI. Symptoms of fatigue and sleepiness in major depressive disorder. J Clin Psychiatry 2006;67(Suppl 6):9–15.

28. Hudson JI, Pope HG Jr. Affective spectrum disorder: does antidepressant response identify a family of disorders with a common pathophysiology? Am J Psychiatry 1990;147(5):552–64.

29. Mamelak M. Narcolepsy and depression and the neurobiology of gammahydroxybutyrate. Prog Neurobiol 2009;89(2):193–219.

30. Sharpless BA, Barber JP. Lifetime prevalence rates of sleep paralysis: a systematic review. Sleep Med Rev 2011;15(5):311–5.

31. Ohayon MM, Zulley J, Guilleminault C, et al. Prevalence and pathologic associations of sleep paralysis in the general population. Neurology 1999;52(6): 1194–200.

32. Mellman TA, Aigbogun N, Graves RE, et al. Sleep paralysis and trauma, psychiatric symptoms and disorders in an adult African American population attending primary medical care. Depress Anxiety 2008;25(5):435–40.

33. Moturi S, Ivanenko A. Complex diagnostic and treatment issues in psychotic symptoms associated with narcolepsy. Psychiatry (Edgmont) 2009;6(6): 38–44.

34. Vourdas A, Shneerson JM, Gregory CA, et al. Narcolepsy and psychopathology: is there an association? Sleep Med 2002;3:353–60.

35. Fortuyn HA, Lappenschaar GA, Nienhuis FJ, et al. Psychotic symptoms in narcolepsy: phenomenology and a comparison with schizophrenia. Gen Hosp Psychiatry 2009;31(2):146–54.

36. Kondziella D, Arlien-Soborg P. Diagnostic and therapeutic challenges in narcolepsy-related psychosis. J Clin Psychiatry 2006;67(11):1817–9.

37. Kishi Y, Konishi S, Koizumi S, et al. Schizophrenia and narcolepsy: a review with a case report. Psychiatry Clin Neurosci 2004;58(2):117–24.

38. Douglass AB, Shipley JE, Haines RF, et al. Schizophrenia, narcolepsy, and HLA-DR15, DQ6. Biol Psychiatry 1993;34(11):773–80.

39. Walterfang M, Upjohn E, Velakoulis D. Is schizophrenia associated with narcolepsy? Cogn Behav Neurol 2005;18(2):113–8.

40. Dahmen N, Querings K, Grun B, et al. Increased frequency of migraine in narcoleptic patients. Neurology 1999;52(6):1291–3.

41. Dahmen N, Kasten M, Wieczorek S, et al. Increased frequency of migraine in narcoleptic patients: a confirmatory study. Cephalalgia 2003;23(1):14–9.

42. Dauvilliers Y, Billiard M, Montplaisir J. Clinical aspects and pathophysiology of narcolepsy. Clin Neurophysiology 2003;114:2000–17.

43. Inamoroato E, Minatti-Hannuch SN, Zuckerman E. The role of sleep in migraine attacks. Arq Neuropsiquiatr 1993;51:429–32.

44. Coelho FM, Pradella-Hallinan M, Abud PC, et al. Prevalence of HLA DQB1*0602 allele in patients with migraine. Arq Neuropsiquiatr 2007;65(4B):1123–5.

45. Nishino S, Okuro M, Kotorii N, et al. Hypocretin/orexin and narcolepsy: new basic and clinical insights. Acta Physiol (Oxf) 2010;198(3):209–22.

46. Migraine and idiopathic narcolepsy—a case-control study. Cephalalgia 2003;23(8):786–9.

47. Alberca R, Botebol G, Boza F, et al. Episodic cluster headache and narcolepsy: a case report. Cephalalgia 1991;11(3):113–5.

48. Overeem S, van Vliet JA, Lammers GJ, et al. The hypothalamus in episodic brain disorders. Lancet Neurol 2002;1(7):437–44.

49. McBeth J, Mulvey MR. Fibromyalgia: mechanisms and potential impact of the ACR 2010 classification criteria. Nat Rev Rheumatol 2012;8(2):108–16.

50. Taiwo OB, Russell IJ, Mignot E, et al. Normal cerebrospinal fluid levels of hypocretin-1 (orexin A) in patients with fibromyalgia syndrome. Sleep Med 2007;8(3):260–5.

51. Wolfe F, Ross K, Anderson J, et al. The prevalence and characteristics of fibromyalgia in the general population. Arthritis Rheum 1995;38:19–28.

52. Prados G, Miro E. Fibromyalgia and sleep: a review. Rev Neurol 2012;54(4):227–40 [in Spanish].

53. Disdier P, Genton P, Bolla G, et al. Clinical screening for narcolepsy/cataplexy in patients with fibromyalgia. Clin Rheumatol 1994;13(1):132–4.

54. Disdier P, Genton P, Milandre C, et al. Fibrositis syndrome and narcolepsy. J Rheumatol 1993; 20(5):888–9.

55. Hudson JI, Goldenberg DL, Pope HG Jr, et al. Comorbidity of fibromyalgia with medical and psychiatric disorders. Am J Med 1992;92:363–7.

56. Yamamoto T, Nozaki-Taguchi N, Chiba T. Analgesic effect of intrathecally administered orexin-A in the rat formalin test and in the rat hot plate test. Br J Pharmacol 2002;137:170–6.

57. Buskila D, Sarzi-Puttini P. Genetic aspects of fibromyalgia. Arthritis Res Ther 2006;8(5):218–22.

58. Ohayon MM, Ferini-Strambi L, Plazzi G, et al. How age influences the expression of narcolepsy. J Psychosom Res 2005;59(6):399–405.

59. Schulz H, Wilde-Frenz J. Symposium: cognitive processes and sleep disturbances: the disturbance of cognitive processes in narcolepsy. J Sleep Res 1995;4(1):10–4.

60. Aguirre M, Broughton R, Stuss D. Does memory impairment exist in narcolepsy-cataplexy? J Clin Exp Neuropsychol 1985;7(1):14–24.

61. Rogers AE, Rosenberg RS. Tests of memory in narcoleptics. Sleep 1990;13(1):42–52.

62. Naumann A, Bellebaum C, Daum I. Cognitive deficits in narcolepsy. J Sleep Res 2006;15(3): 329–38.

63. Raggi A, Plazzi G, Pennisi G, et al. Cognitive evoked potentials in narcolepsy: a review of the literature. Neurosci Biobehav Rev 2011;35(5): 1144–53.

64. Simon V, Ho DD, Abdool Karim Q. HIV/AIDS epidemiology, pathogenesis, prevention, and treatment. Lancet 2006;368(9534):489–504.

65. Hand GA, Phillips KD, Dudgeon WD. Perceived stress in HIV-infected individuals: physiological and psychological correlates. AIDS Care 2006; 18(8):1011–7.

66. Reid S, Dwyer J. Insomnia in HIV infection: a systematic review of prevalence, correlates, and management. Psychosom Med 2005;67(2):260–9.

67. Phillips KD, Sowell RL, Rojas M, et al. Physiological and psychological correlates of fatigue in HIV disease. Biol Res Nurs 2004;6(1):59–74.

68. Adinolfi A. Assessment and treatment of HIV-related fatigue. J Assoc Nurses AIDS Care 2001;12(Suppl): 29–34 [quiz: 5–8].

69. Darko DF, McCutchan JA, Kripke DF, et al. Fatigue, sleep disturbance, disability, and indices of progression of HIV infection. Am J Psychiatry 1992;149(4): 514–20.

70. Groopman JE. Fatigue in cancer and HIV/AIDS. Oncology (Williston Park) 1998;12(3):335–44 [discussion: 345–6, 51].

71. Nokes KM, Kendrew J. Sleep quality in people with HIV disease. J Assoc Nurses AIDS Care 1996;7(3): 43–50.

72. Darko DF, Mitler MM, White JL. Sleep disturbance in early HIV infection. Focus 1995;10(11): 5–6.

73. Dafoe ME, Stewart KE. Pain and psychiatric disorders contribute independently to suicidal ideation in HIV-positive persons. Arch Suicide Res 2004; 8(3):215–26.

74. Riley ED, Wu AW, Perry S, et al. Depression and drug use impact health status among marginally housed HIV-infected individuals. AIDS Patient Care STDS 2003;17(8):401–6.

75. Korthuis PT, Zephyrin LC, Fleishman JA, et al. Health-related quality of life in HIV-infected patients: the role of substance use. AIDS Patient Care STDS 2008;22(11):859–67.

76. Chandra PS, Ravi V, Desai A, et al. Anxiety and depression among HIV-infected heterosexuals— a report from India. J Psychosom Res 1998;45(5): 401–9.

77. Diederich N, Karenberg A, Peters UH. Psychopathologic pictures in HIV infection: AIDS lethargy and AIDS dementia. Fortschr Neurol Psychiatr 1988; 56(6):173–85 [in German].

78. Dauvilliers Y, Montplaisir J, Cochen V, et al. Post-H1N1 narcolepsy-cataplexy. Sleep 2010;33(11): 1428–30.

79. Han F, Lin L, Warby SC, et al. Narcolepsy onset is seasonal and increased following the 2009 H1N1 pandemic in China. Ann Neurol 2011; 70(3):410–7.

80. Aran A, Lin L, Nevsimalova S, et al. Elevated anti-streptococcal antibodies in patients with recent narcolepsy onset. Sleep 2009;32(8):979–83.

81. Kornum BR, Faraco J, Mignot E. Narcolepsy with hypocretin/orexin deficiency, infections and autoimmunity of the brain. Curr Opin Neurobiol 2011;21(6): 897–903.

82. Arnulf I, Lin L, Gadoth N, et al. Kleine-Levin syndrome: a systematic study of 108 patients. Ann Neurol 2008;63(4):482–93.

83. Arnulf I, Lecendreux M, Franco P, et al. Kleine-Levin syndrome: state of the art. Rev Neurol (Paris) 2008; 164(8–9):658–68 [in Czech].

84. Fernandez JM, Lara I, Gila L, et al. Disturbed hypothalamic-pituitary axis in idiopathic recurring hypersomnia syndrome. Acta Neurol Scand 1990; 82(6):361–3.

85. Reynolds CF 3rd, Black RS, Coble P, et al. Similarities in EEG sleep findings for Kleine-Levin syndrome and unipolar depression. Am J Psychiatry 1980; 137(1):116–8.

86. Jeffries JJ, Lefebvre A. Depression and mania associated with Kleine-Levin-Critchley syndrome. Can Psychiatr Assoc J 1973;18(5):439–44.

87. Loganathan S, Manjunath S, Jhirwal OP, et al. Lithium prophylaxis in Kleine-Levin syndrome. J Neuropsychiatry Clin Neurosci 2009;21(1):107–8.

88. Poppe M, Friebel D, Reuner U, et al. The Kleine-Levin syndrome—effects of treatment with lithium. Neuropediatrics 2003;34(3):113–9.

89. Muratori F, Bertini N, Masi G. Efficacy of lithium treatment in Kleine-Levin syndrome. Eur Psychiatry 2002; 17(4):232–3.

90. Hart EJ. Kleine-Levin syndrome: normal CSF monoamines and response to lithium therapy. Neurology 1985;35(9):1395–6.

91. Goldberg MA. The treatment of Kleine-Levin syndrome with lithium. Can J Psychiatry 1983; 28(6):491–3.

92. Roth B, Smolik P, Soucek K. Kleine-Levin syndrome—lithium prophylaxis. Cesk Psychiatr 1980;76(3):156–62 [in Czech].

Kleine-Levin Syndrome

Michel Billiard, MD

KEYWORDS

- Kleine-Levin syndrome • Kleine-Levin syndrome without compulsive eating
- Menstrual-related hypersomnia • Recurrent hypersomnia • Compulsive eating
- Disinhibited sexuality • Odd behaviors

KEY POINTS

- Kleine-Levin syndrome is potentially rich in behavioral, cognitive, and mental symptoms, but the number of expressed symptoms varies between patients and even within a single patient from one episode to the other.
- 3% to 4% of cases run in families.
- Infectious triggers are found in approximately 60% of cases, but the agents responsible for the infections are rarely identified.
- Pathophysiology is still unknown. However, single-photon emission computed tomography, functional magnetic resonance imaging, and neuroanatomic studies look promising in identifying involved neuroanatomic areas. Cerebrospinal fluid (CSF) hypocretin-1 measurement during both symptomatic episodes and asymptomatic intervals should be performed to search for a possible dysfunction of the hypocretin system, and CSF screening for the presence of autoantibodies directed against neurons is warranted to check for a possible autoimmune mechanism.
- Multicenter, randomized, double-blind, placebo-controlled trials of present and additional drugs are warranted.

Kleine-Levin syndrome (KLS) is a rare sleep disorder, first described in 1925,[1] which is remarkable for recurrent attacks of hypersomnia associated with a variety of behavioral, cognitive, and mental symptoms, lasting from 1 to 2 days to several weeks. The limits of the syndrome are not totally delineated, and diagnostic criteria for the syndrome have not been listed in the *International Classification of Sleep Disorders* (2nd edition).[2]

This article considers the evolution of the concept of KLS since its origin, describes the different symptoms and physical signs of the syndrome, lists and comments on the clinical variants, discusses the pathophysiology, and reviews the available treatments.

HISTORICAL NOTE

The first descriptions of patients with recurrent periods of sleepiness and pathologic hunger date back to Kleine in Germany,[1] Lewis[3] and Levin[4] in the United States. In 1936 Levin rewrote his original case report, and made for the first time specific mention of "a syndrome of periodic somnolence and morbid hunger" as a new entity in pathology.[5] He detailed the clinical features and put forward the hypothesis that this syndrome was the expression of exhaustion of centers lying within the frontal lobes, with an actual structural alteration of the component cells. Six years later, Critchley and Hoffman reported 2 more cases of periodic somnolence and morbid hunger, discussed Levin's views as the cause of the syndrome, and coined the term Kleine-Levin syndrome.[6] It was only 20 years later, in 1962, that Critchley published a founding article referred to as "Periodic hypersomnia and megaphagia in adolescent males," in which he collected 15 "genuine" instances from the literature and 11 cases of his own, described in depth these

The author has nothing to disclose.
Department of Neurology, Gui de Chauliac Hospital, 80 Avenue Augustin Fliche, 34295 Montpellier cedex 5, France
E-mail address: mbilliard@wanadoo.fr

26 cases, and gave the definition of "a syndrome composed of recurring episodes of undue sleepiness lasting some days, associated with an inordinate intake of food, and often with abnormal behavior."[7] In addition he emphasized 4 hallmarks:

1. Sex incidence whereby males are preponderantly if not wholly affected
2. Onset in adolescence
3. Spontaneous eventual disappearance of the syndrome
4. The possibility that the megaphagia is in the nature of compulsive eating, rather than bulimia.

From this time on, new case reports and reviews have been published. However, in 1960 Alfandary published 4 cases of *hypnolepsie des adolescents*, which matched KLS except for the absence of compulsive eating.[8] In 1968, Bonkalo suggested the term *forme fruste* of KLS for a patient whose food intake was classed from "poor" to "good" but did not show compulsive eating.[9] From that time on, patients with recurrent excessive daytime sleepiness but no compulsive eating have been improperly included in KLS, introducing an unfortunate bias into the concept.

In 2005 the second edition of the *International Classification of Sleep Disorders* was published with diagnostic criteria for recurrent hypersomnia,[2] but only a mention of those cases deserving a diagnosis of KLS, namely "cases in which recurrent episodes of hypersomnia are clearly associated with behavioral abnormalities. These may include binge eating; hypersexuality; abnormal behavior such as irritability, aggression, and odd behavior; and cognitive abnormalities such as feeling of unreality, confusion and hallucinations."

The same year Arnulf and colleagues[10] conducted a thorough review of 186 patients with KLS in the world literature, without distinguishing the full-blown cases and the forms without compulsive eating. This review was followed by a cross-sectional, systematic evaluation of 108 new cases and comparison with matched control subjects, which was of value for the identification of novel predisposing factors including increased birth and developmental problems, and the findings of a disease course longer in men, in patients with disinhibited sexuality, and when onset was after age 20 years.[11] Eventually a recent study, based on the review of 339 cases of recurrent hypersomnia, identified and statistically compared 4 clinical forms, namely KLS (239 cases), KLS without compulsive eating (54 cases), menstrual-related hypersomnia (18 cases), and recurrent hypersomnia with comorbidity (28 cases).[12]

DEMOGRAPHICS

KLS is a rare condition. Two hundred thirty-nine cases collected from 31 different countries have been published in the aforementioned review.[12] The male to female ratio was about 4:1. The median age of onset was 15 in both males (n = 169) and females (n = 45), with a range 4 to 80 in males and 4 to 69 in females. An overrepresentation of Jewish patients has been underlined: one-sixth of the patients in the review by Arnulf and colleagues,[10] and 6 times more than expected, based on the United States population ($P<.033$), all Ashkenazi, in the systematic study and comparison with controls by the same group.[11]

Familial cases are not exceptional: 9 cases of 239 (3.7%) in the series by the author's group,[12] including 2 with more than 2 affected relatives,[13,14] and 5 cases of 104 (4.8%) in the Arnulf series.[11] In addition, one case of Spanish monozygotic twins concordant for KLS has just been reported, raising the possibility of genuine genetic forms of KLS.[15]

PREDISPOSING AND PRECIPITATING FACTORS

By analogy with narcolepsy, an association with human leukocyte antigen (HLA) has been looked for. In a multicenter study based on the analysis of gene polymorphism of HLA-DQB1 in 30 unrelated patients with KLS (25 with full-blown KLS and 5 with KLS without compulsive eating), an HLA-DQB1*0201 allele frequency of 28.3% in patients and 12.5% in controls ($\chi^2 = 4.82$, $P<.03$) was found.[16] However, in the prospective study by Arnulf and colleagues[11] involving 108 patients and 108 matched controls, HLA DR and DQ alleles did not differ between patients and controls.

On the other hand, factors precipitating the first episode are mentioned in all series, in 16 of 34 patients (47%),[17] 23 of 33 patients (77%),[14] 102 of 168 patients (60%),[10] and 159 of 239 patients (66%).[12] These factors consist in upper airway infection, flulike illness, febrile illness in most cases, and in a few cases emotional stress, alcohol intake, summer outing, sunstroke, anesthesia, and head traumatism. Factors triggering subsequent episodes are much less frequent.

CLINICAL FEATURES

Features include behavioral, cognitive, and mental symptoms, and in some cases physical signs (**Table 1**). Various transient symptoms may be observed at the end of episodes followed by an apparent total recovery until the next episode. All possible symptoms are generally not combined in a single patient; one symptom may be

Table 1
Compared frequency of the various symptoms and physical signs during hypersomniac episodes, in a population of 239 subjects (192 males and 47 females) with the Kleine-Levin syndrome

Symptoms and Physical Signs	Males (%)	Females (%)	P Value
Hypersomnia	100	100	NA
Compulsive eating	100	100	NA
Disinhibited sexuality	48.4	27.6	.0035
Odd behavior	29.7	36.1	.39
Confusion	41.6	25.5	.11
Feeling of unreality	37.5	36.1	.85
Delusions/hallucinations	17.2	21.3	.78
Depression	19.8	40.4	NA
Anxiety	12.0	12.8	NA
Signs of autonomic dysfunction	18.2	19.1	.56
Weight gain	9.9	44.6	<.0001

Abbreviation: NA, not applicable.
 Data from Billiard M, Jaussent I, Dauvilliers Y, et al. Recurrent hypersomnias: a review of 339 cases. Sleep Med Rev 2011;15:247–57.

present during one episode and absent during the following one, and in a few cases one symptom such as insomnia or compulsive eating may be replaced by its opposite, insomnia or anorexia, during one or several episodes.

Onset of Episodes

The episodes begin within a few hours, or gradually over 1 or 2 days, with patients becoming extremely tired or complaining of headache.

Behavioral Symptoms

Hypersomnia is the first major symptom. Patients lie in their bed, sometimes with restlessness and untidiness. Vivid dreams may occur. Usual sleep duration during episodes ranges from 12 to 18 hours. Patients wake up spontaneously to void and eat, but are irritable or even aggressive when awakened or prevented from sleep.

Compulsive eating is the second major symptom, even if it is not systematically present during all episodes and sometimes during one episode only from the beginning to the end. A preference for sweets is common. Patients do not necessarily look for food, but cannot refrain from eating food within reach, in a compulsive manner, as in the case of an 18-year-old ordinary seaman (case 3 in Critchley's series) "who ate about a dozen large helpings of suet pudding (in addition to his own heavy meal), the pudding having been rejected by the majority of sailors as being underdone and too stodgy for consumption."[7] Increased

drinking is sometimes associated but never observed alone.

Sexual disinhibition can take the form of overt masturbation, obscene language, sexual advances, shamelessly expressed sexual fantasies, and so forth. It is present in 48.5% of males and in 27.5% of females.[12] However, sexual disinhibition in females could assume a less visible expression such as a fantasy of being "chatted up" by men or experiencing love affairs.

Odd behaviors are diverse and totally awkward. They include talking in a childish manner, singing loudly, playing a CD over and over, talking on the phone without dialing first, making a handstand on the bed, writing on walls, or stripping down wallpaper.

Cognitive Symptoms

These symptoms include dramatic ones such as altered perception (people and objects seem distorted, unreal, dreamlike), which seems to be one of the most typical, confusion, fragmentary delusions, and visual and auditory hallucinations, which are observed in 20% to 40% of patients.[12] In comparison, less severe symptoms such as apathy, impaired speech, concentration, and memory are observed in a majority of patients.[11]

Mental Symptoms

Depression during the episode is more frequent in females than in males. Some patients may report suicidal thoughts. Anxiety is less frequent than depression.

Physical Signs

Absence of neurologic signs is remarkable. Signs of autonomic dysfunction including profuse sweating, reddish, congestive, or puffy face, hypertension and/or bradycardia, and nauseating body, hair, or urine are found in about 20% of patients.[12] Weight gain of a few kilograms may be observed during the attacks, and are much more frequent in females than in males.

End of Episodes

The episodes of hypersomnia may end abruptly or insidiously over a few days. It is not uncommon for an episode to be followed by amnesia of the past events, manic behavior with insomnia as if the subject was trying to catch up for lost time, and depression lasting for 1 or 2 days.

LABORATORY TESTS

The diagnosis of KLS is purely clinical. Laboratory investigations serve mainly at eliminating epilepsy (electroencephalography), focal brain lesions (brain imaging), and meningitis or encephalitis (cerebrospinal fluid [CSF] analysis). However, most patients undergo a series of tests before being suspected of having KLS (Table 2).

Routine blood tests including blood count, plasma electrolytes, urea, creatinine, and hepatic function are normal. Baseline levels of the main anterior pituitary hormones, growth hormone, prolactin, thyroid-stimulating hormone, testosterone, and cortisol are normal. The same applies to levels obtained after stimulation tests.

Agents responsible for upper airway infection, flulike illness, or other infections are rarely identified, and when identified differ from one patient to the other.

CSF white blood cell counts and protein levels are normal in all patients, ruling out infectious meningitis. Immunoelectrophoresis is also normal in the few cases where it has been performed.

Electroencephalography is most often remarkable for a general slowing of the background activity, sometimes with bursts of bisynchronous, generalized, moderate to high-voltage, 5- to 7-Hz waves, 0.5 to 2 seconds in duration.[18,19]

Nocturnal polysomnography is not easy to perform within the short duration of the episode. An important reduction in stage 3 during the first half of the symptomatic period, with progressive return to normal during the second half, has been reported as well as a decrease of rapid eye movement (REM) sleep during the second half of the symptomatic period.[20] Sleep efficiency is poor during the symptomatic period (Fig. 1). Sleep-onset REM periods are common. Results of the multiple sleep latency test are highly dependent on the subject's willingness to comply with the procedure. Nevertheless, a reduced mean sleep latency and sleep-onset REM periods have been reported. In practice, it is more instructive to carry out a continuous polysomnographic recording for 24 hours, providing indications on total sleep time over 24 hours and possible sleep-onset REM periods.

Computed tomography and magnetic resonance imaging (MRI) of the brain show no abnormality.

Psychological interview and testing should always be performed when the episode is over to ensure that there is no background personality disorder or that the subject is not expecting some benefit from the symptomatic episode.

COURSE

KLS is characterized by episodes lasting a median of 8 to 9 days, with a cycle length (time from onset of one episode to the onset of the next episode) of 60 to 100 days and normal functioning between episodes.[12] A disease course longer in females (9 ± 8.7 years) than in males (5.4 ± 5.6 years, $P = .01$) is indicated by Arnulf and colleagues[10] in those patients with a known reported termination

---

Table 2
Laboratory tests in Kleine-Levin syndrome

Of Limited Interest	Of Diagnostic Value	Of Potential Pathophysiologic Value
Routine blood tests	EEG	SPECT
Hormonal tests (static and dynamic)	Brain imaging (CT, MRI) CSF analysis (white blood cell count, glucose, protein) Psychological testing	fMRI Polysomnography CSF hypocretin-1 measurement Immunohistochemical screening of serum and CSF for autoantibodies against neurons

Abbreviations: CSF, cerebrospinal fluid; CT, computed tomography; EEG, electroencephalography; fMRI, functional MRI; MRI, magnetic resonance imaging; SPECT, single-photon emission computed tomography.

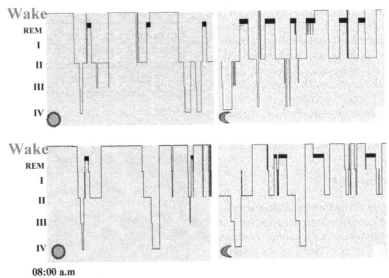

Fig. 1. Forty-eight-hour polysomnographic recording from 8 AM on day one to 8 AM on day three, in a 22-year-old man with Kleine-Levin syndrome. Total sleep time was 16 hours 12 minutes during the first 24 hours, and 12 hours 14 minutes during the second 24 hours. Note the poor sleep efficiency and the presence of sleep-onset REM periods.

of the disorder (no more episode for more than twice the mean interepisode length), whereas Billiard and colleagues[12] found a disease course longer in males (median 3.6 years [3 weeks–33.5 years]) than in females (median 2.0 years [2 weeks–18.2 years]) in those cases when the duration of the follow-up was at least 1 year after the last episode. Although it is common to say that episodes decrease in frequency, severity, and duration, a decrease in frequency was documented in only 25.9% of cases, a decrease in severity in only 21.3% of cases, and a decrease in duration in only 15.9% of cases.[12] Complications are mainly social and occupational. In exceptional cases subjects have been reported to choke while eating voraciously during the episode.[21,22]

Between episodes patients are described as normal in most cases.

CLINICAL VARIANTS

KLS without compulsive eating is a *forme fruste* of KLS. According to the review by the author's group, all symptoms and physical signs are found in a lesser percentage of patients with KLS without compulsive eating than in patients with full-blown KLS, except for the feeling of unreality observed in the same proportion of patients in both conditions.[12] Considering the number of reported cases in the world literature (54 vs 239 cases of KLS in Ref.[12]), the condition may be less frequent than KLS. However, it is possible that cases with isolated recurrent hypersomnia are less published than cases of full-blown KLS.

Menstrual-related hypersomnia is characterized by episodes of hypersomnia, plus or minus other symptoms and physical signs of KLS, which occur in association with the menstrual cycle and sometimes with puerperium. The condition occurs for the first time within the first months after menarche or later. Episodes generally last about 1 week, with resolution at the time of menses (**Fig. 2**). Menstrual-related hypersomnia is a very rare disease, with only 18 cases in recent review.[12]

KLS, KLS without compulsive eating, and menstrual-related hypersomnia may be secondary

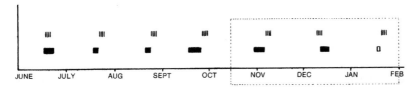

Fig. 2. Menstrual-related hypersomnia in a 14-year-old girl. Vertical bars represent menstruations and shaded boxes episodes of hypersomnia. Note the temporal relationship between hypersomniac episodes and menstruations. The unshaded box on the far right refers to an episode with hostility but no hypersomnia. (*From* Billiard M, Guilleminault C, Dement WC. A menstruation-linked periodic hypersomnia. Neurology 1975;25:437; with permission.)

to physical diseases including tumor, head traumatism, stroke, viral encephalitis, and genetic disease. In favor of causality are a late age of onset, an initial severe head injury, neurologic signs persisting between episodes, abnormal neuroimaging, and an unfavorable outcome. Cases associated with mild head traumatism or pervasive developmental disorder (autistic disorder, Asperger syndrome) may not be secondary to the associated condition.

DIFFERENTIAL DIAGNOSIS

Recurrent episodes of hypersomnia plus or minus significant weight gain or increase in appetite are reported in the context of psychiatric disorders, such as recurrent major depressive disorder, bipolar I disorder, and bipolar II disorder.

PATHOPHYSIOLOGY

Knowledge of the pathophysiology of KLS is still in its infancy. However, several approaches deserve consideration.

Contribution of Neuroimaging Studies

Single-photon emission computed tomography (SPECT) studies performed during symptomatic periods and/or asymptomatic intervals have evidenced decreased tracer perfusion in as many regions as basal ganglia, thalamus, hypothalamus, and frontal, parietal, temporal, or occipital lobes, during symptomatic periods, and a partial normalization during asymptomatic intervals.[20,23–34] These regions have extensive connectivity to each other and to limbic structures through neuroanatomic circuits that are organized in parallel, so that lesions in one part can result in a malfunction in other areas.

Functional spectroscopic MRI (fMRI) has been performed in two patients. In a first one, a 19-year-old with typical KLS, a lower concentration ratio of N-acetylaspartate (NAA), a marker of neuronal integrity, and a higher concentration ratio of glutamate/glutamine (Glu-Gln), which plays an important role in excitatory neurotransmission and mitochondrial metabolism, were observed in the right and left thalami during the symptomatic period in comparison with the asymptomatic interval.[35] In the second patient, a 20-year-old woman with KLS without compulsive eating, an increase in glutamine metabolites was observed in the left thalamus and basal ganglia during the symptomatic episodes in comparison with the asymptomatic intervals.[36]

Neuropathologic Data

Neuropathologic examinations have been performed in 3 cases of typical KLS[21,22,37] and in 1 case of KLS secondary to a presumptive brain tumor (**Table 3**).[38] These examinations have shown various abnormalities in different locations of the brain.

Role of Hypocretins

Given the role of hypocretin neuropeptides in both sleep-wake regulation and feeding, hypocretins seem good candidates to be involved in the functional abnormality of KLS; hence the assessment of CSF hypocretin-1 performed in a few patients with KLS. To date 11 patients with KLS have been investigated, 4 during symptomatic periods only,[31,37,39,40] 5 during asymptomatic intervals only,[39,41] and 2 during both symptomatic periods and asymptomatic intervals (**Table 4**).[41,42] In these 2 patients a decrease of CSF hypocretin-1 was demonstrated, from a normal level during an asymptomatic interval to an intermediate level during a symptomatic period in the first one, and from a normal level to a normal level in the second one. Although of potential interest, these results are far too limited to draw any conclusion.

Recurrence

Surprisingly enough, the issue of recurrence of abnormal episodes has only been recently considered. Based on the generally young age at onset, the recurrence of symptoms, the frequent infectious trigger, and a significantly increased frequency of the HLA-DQB1* allele in a multicenter group of 30 unrelated patients with KLS and KLS without compulsive eating, an autoimmune etiology for KLS has been suggested.[16] However, no direct evidence for this putative autoimmune process has so far been reported.

KLS and Mood Disorder

There are some analogies between KLS and bipolar disorders even if the former differ by the sudden occurrence of the episodes, their transient duration and overnight disappearance.

KLS reoccurs just as mood disorders do. A few cases of KLS are remarkable for an alternation between hypersomniac episodes and manic-depressive episodes.[43,44] Odd behaviors have a distinct psychiatric flavor, frequently in the direction of dissociative disorder. Depression, sometimes with suicidal thoughts, is a symptom of hypersomniac episodes in a substantial percentage of patients, up to 40.4% of women and 20% of men with KLS and 35.3% of women

Table 3
Neuropathologic findings in 3 cases of primary Kleine-Levin syndrome and 1 case of secondary Kleine-Levin syndrome

	Kleine-Levin Syndrome			Secondary Kleine-Levin Syndrome
Authors	Carpenter et al[21]	Koerber et al[22]	Fenzi et al[35]	Takrani and Cronin[38]
Sex	Male	Male	Female	Female
Age of onset (y)	39	11	8	48
Behavioral symptoms	Hypersomnia, compulsive eating, disinhibited sexuality	Hypersomnia, compulsive eating, disinhibited sexuality	Hypersomnia, compulsive eating	Hypersomnia, compulsive eating, disinhibited sexuality
Physical signs	None	Dysautonomic signs	Upward-gaze palsy, mild ptosis +10 kg	None
Neuroimaging	CT: normal	CT: prominent ventricles, otherwise normal	CT: normal	CT: normal
Cause of death	Choked on meat, sudden death 9 d later	Episode of compulsive eating, cardiopulmonary arrest next morning	Fracture of humerus, 10 d later developed left femoroiliac thrombophlebitis complicated by a pulmonary embolism that caused sudden death	Lapsed into a coma and died (presumptive cerebral tumor)
Autopsy	Abundant infiltrates of inflammatory cells, cuffing of veins and venules, gliosis and focal calcifications, virtually limited to the thalami	Mild hypopigmentation of the substantia nigra	Perivascular lymphomonocyte infiltration in the medial and intralaminar thalamic nuclei and in the hypothalamus, particularly on the floor of the third ventricle	Lymphocyting, cuffing in the small vessels in the hypothalamus, amygdaloid nuclei, and in the anterior medial gray matter of the temporal lobes Microglial nodules in the periaqueductal gray region and in oculomotor nerve nuclei

with menstruation-related hypersomnia.[12] Elation occurs in 13% of men on emergence from hypersomniac episodes.[12] Mood stabilizers such as carbamazepine, lithium carbonate, and sodium valproate are prophylactic against the recurrence of episodes in some cases.

Moreover, there are distinct similarities between KLS and 2 mood-disorder specifiers, "depression with atypical features" and "seasonal affective disorders," for example, the already mentioned possibility of hypersomnia, increase in appetite, and weight gain. Thus, one can speculate on a possible congruence between the neuroanatomic circuits of KLS and those of bipolar disorders.

TREATMENT

A recent Cochrane Database Systematic Review, aimed at evaluating whether pharmacologic treatments for KLS are effective and safe, did not find any randomized controlled trials (RCTs) and quasi-RCTs.[45] Therefore one is left with individual

Table 4
Cerebrospinal fluid hypocretin-1 measurement in patients with Kleine-Levin syndrome

Authors	No. of Subjects	Symptomatic Period (pg/mL)	Asymptomatic Interval (pg/mL)
Katz and Ropper[40]	1	>200	—
Mignot et al[39]	3	194 (extracted (assay))	—
		—	290
		—	360
Dauvilliers et al[41]	4	—	897
		—	453
		—	268
		111	221
Podesta et al[42]	1	282	282
Poryazova et al[35]	1	530	—
Itokawa et al[31]	1	>200	—

cases or small series in which one or several drugs have been administered and clinically evaluated by patients' doctors.

There are 2 types of treatment for recurrent hypersomnia: symptomatic and prophylactic. Symptomatic treatments are mainly based on stimulants (amphetamine and methylphenidate) and on the wake-promoting drug modafinil. However, proper evaluation of these drugs is somewhat unreliable because of the spontaneous eventual disappearance of the symptoms after a few days of evolution. In contrast to symptomatic treatments, prophylactic treatments based on mood stabilizers (lithium and antiepileptic drugs) are easy to evaluate, based on the recurrence (or not) of hypersomniac episodes. The proposed shared mechanism of these drugs is sodium-channel antagonism.[46,47] According to a recent review by the author's group (M. Billiard, unpublished data, 2011), a positive response rate is found in 25.9% to 39% of cases according to the use of different drugs.

Of note, a very recent letter to *Sleep Medicine* mentions a 24-year-old man experiencing recurrent episodes of hypersomnia sometimes associated with compulsive eating and disinhibited sexuality, occurring several times a year since the age of 13. This patient was treated with 4 g of sodium oxybate per night and has remained asymptomatic after 30 months of treatment.[48]

In the case of menstrual-related hypersomnia, estroprogestative drugs are active in a majority of cases.

SUMMARY

Interest in Kleine-Levin syndrome has been recently rejuvenated with the use of SPECT studies and the reports of familial cases including 2 multiplex families and of one case of monozygotic twins concordant for Kleine-Levin syndrome. Next steps should be linkage analysis and the new generation exome sequencing to identify a potential mutation, CSF hypocretin-1 measurements during both symptomatic periods and asymptomatic intervals, and, in view of the autoimmune hypothesis, the screening of CSF for the presence of autoantibodies directed against neurons in presumed affected neuroanatomical regions.

REFERENCES

1. Kleine W. Periodische Schlafsucht. Mschr Psychiat Neurol 1925;57:285–320 [in German].
2. American Academy of Sleep Medicine. International classification of sleep disorders. Diagnostic and coding manual. 2nd edition. Westchester (IL): American Academy of Sleep Medicine; 2005.
3. Lewis ND. The psychoanalytic approach to the problem of children under twelve years of age. Psychoanal Rev 1926;13:424–43.
4. Levin M. Narcolepsy (Gelineau's syndrome) and other varieties of morbid somnolence. Arch Neurol Psychiatr (Chicago) 1929;22:1172–200.
5. Levin M. Periodic somnolence and morbid hunger. A new syndrome. Brain 1936;59:494–504.
6. Critchley M, Hoffman HL. The syndrome of periodic somnolence and morbid hunger (Kleine-Levin syndrome). Br Med J 1942;1:137–9.
7. Critchley M. Periodic hypersomnia and megaphagia in adolescent males. Brain 1962;85:627–56.
8. Alfandary I. Hypnolepsy in adolescents with psychomotor disorders. Rev Neurol (Paris) 1960;102:684–9 [in French].

9. Bonkalo A. Hypersomnia: a discussion of psychiatric implications based on three cases. Br J Psychiatry 1968;114:69–75.

10. Arnulf I, Zeitzer JM, File J, et al. Kleine-Levin syndrome: a systematic review of 186 cases in the literature. Brain 2005;128:2763–76.

11. Arnulf I, Lin L, Gadoth N, et al. Kleine-Levin syndrome: a systematic study of 108 patients. Ann Neurol 2008;63:482–92.

12. Billiard M, Jaussent I, Dauvilliers Y, et al. Recurrent hypersomnias: a review of 339 cases. Sleep Med Rev 2011;15:247–57.

13. Suwa K, Toru M. A case of periodic somnolence whose sleep was induced by glucose. Folia Psychiatr Neurol Jpn 1969;23:253–62.

14. BaHammam AS, GadElRab MO, Owais SM, et al. Clinical characteristics and HLA typing of a family with Kleine-Levin syndrome. Sleep Med 2008;9:575–8.

15. Peraita-Adrados R, Vicario JL, Garcia de Leon M, et al. Monozygotic twins affected with Kleine-Levin syndrome. Sleep 2012;35:1–2.

16. Dauvilliers Y, Mayer G, Lecendreux M, et al. Kleine-Levin syndrome. An autoimmune hypothesis based on clinical and genetic analyses. Neurology 2002;59:1739–45.

17. Gadoth N, Kesler A, Vainstein G, et al. Clinical and polysomnographic characteristics of 34 patients with Kleine-Levin syndrome. J Sleep Res 2001;10:337–41.

18. Thacore VR, Ahmed M, Oswald I. The EEG in a case of periodic hypersomnia. Electroencephalogr Clin Neurophysiol 1969;27:605–6.

19. Smirne S, Castellotti V, Passerini D, et al. Studio EEG in un caso di sindrome di Kleine-Levin. Riv di Neurologia 1970;40:357–65 [in Italian].

20. Huang YS, Guilleminault C, Kao PF, et al. SPECT findings in the Kleine-Levin syndrome. Sleep 2005;28:955–60.

21. Carpenter S, Yassa R, Ochs R. A pathologic basis for Kleine-Levin syndrome. Arch Neurol 1982;39:25–8.

22. Koerber RK, Torkelson ER, Haven G, et al. Increased cerebrospinal fluid 5-hydroxytryptamine and 5-hydroxyindoleacetic acid in Kleine-Levin syndrome. Neurology 1984;34:1597–600.

23. Lu ML, Liu HC, Chen CH, et al. Kleine-Levin syndrome and psychosis: observation from an unusual case. Neuropsychiatry Neuropsychol Behav Neurol 2000;13:140–2.

24. Landtblom AM, Dige N, Schwerdt K, et al. A case of Kleine-Levin syndrome examined with SPECT and neuropsychological testing. Acta Neurol Scand 2002;105:318–21.

25. Landtblom AM, Dige N, Schwerdt K, et al. Short-term memory dysfunction in Kleine-Levin syndrome. Acta Neurol Scand 2003;108:363–7.

26. Arias M, Crespo-Iglesias JM, Pérez J, et al. Syndrome de Kleine-Levin: aportacion diagnostica de la SPECT cerebral. Rev Neurol 2002;35:531–3 [in Spanish].

27. Nose I, Ookawa T, Tanaka J, et al. Decreased blood flow of the left thalamus during somnolent episodes in a case of recurrent hypersomnia. Psychiatry Clin Neurosci 2002;56:277–8.

28. Portilla P, Durand E, Chalvon A, et al. Hypoperfusion temporomésiale gauche en TEMP dans un syndrome de Kleine-Levin. Rev Neurol (Paris) 2002;158:593–5 [in French].

29. Saignes X. Syndrome de Kleine-Levin, à propos de deux cas. Thèse [medical thesis]. Université de Paris VI, Pierre et Marie Curie, Faculté de Médecine de Saint-Antoine, 2002 [in French].

30. Hong SB, Joo EY, Tae WS, et al. Episodic diencephalic hypoperfusion in Kleine-Levin syndrome. Sleep 2006;29:1091–3.

31. Itokawa K, Fukui M, Ninomiya M, et al. Gabapentine for Kleine-Levin syndrome. Intern Med 2009;48:1183–5.

32. Hsieh CF, Lai CI, Lan SH, et al. Modafinil-associated vivid visual hallucination in a patient with Kleine-Levin syndrome: case report. J Clin Psychopharmacol 2010;30:347–50.

33. Hoexter MQ, Shih MC, Felicio AC, et al. Greater reduction of striatal dopamine transporter availability during the symptomatic than asymptomatic phase of Kleine-Levin syndrome. Sleep Med 2010;11:959.

34. Huang YS, Guilleminault C, Lin KL, et al. Relationship between Kleine-Levin syndrome and upper respiratory infection in Taiwan. Sleep 2012;35:123–9.

35. Poryazova R, Schnepf B, Boesiger P, et al. Magnetic resonance spectroscopy in a patient with Kleine-Levin syndrome. J Neurol 2007;254:1445–6.

36. Billings ME, Watson NF, Keogh BP. Dynamic fMRI changes in Kleine-Levin syndrome. Sleep Med 2011;12:532.

37. Fenzi F, Simonati A, Crosato F, et al. Clinical features of Kleine-Levin syndrome with localized encephalitis. Neuropediatrics 1993;24:292–5.

38. Takrani LB, Cronin D. Kleine-Levin syndrome in a female patient. Can Psychiatr Assoc J 1976;21:315–8.

39. Mignot E, Lammers GJ, Ripley B, et al. The role of cerebrospinal fluid hypocretin measurement in the diagnosis of narcolepsy and other hypersomnias. Arch Neurol 2002;59:1553–62.

40. Katz JD, Ropper AH. Familial Kleine-Levin syndrome. Arch Neurol 2002;59:1959–61.

41. Dauvilliers Y, Baumann CR, Carlander B, et al. CSF hypocretin-1 levels in narcolepsy, Kleine-Levin syndrome, and other hypersomnias and

neurological conditions. J Neurol Neurosurg Psychiatry 2003;74:1667–73.

42. Podesta C, Ferreras M, Mozzi M, et al. Kleine-Levin syndrome in a 14-year-old girl: CSF hypocretin-1 measurements. Sleep Med 2006;7:649–51.

43. Wilder J. A case of atypical Kleine-Levin syndrome. J Nerv Ment Dis 1972;154:69–72.

44. Jeffries JJ, Lefebvre A. Depression and mania associated with Kleine-Levin-Critchley syndrome. Can Psychiatr Assoc J 1973;18:439–44.

45. Oliveira MM, Conti C, Saconato H, et al. Pharmacological treatment for Kleine-Levin syndrome. Cochrane Database Syst Rev 2009;2:CD006685. 1–12.

46. Bourin M, Chenu F, Hascoët M. The role of sodium channels in the mechanism of action of antidepressants and mood stabilizers. Curr Drug Targets 2009;10:1052–60.

47. Huang X, Lei Z, El-Mallakh RS. Lithium normalizes elevated cellular sodium. Bipolar Disord 2007;9: 298–300.

48. Ortega-Albas JJ, Lopez-Bernabé R, Vera JF, et al. Treatment of Kleine-Levin syndrome with sodium oxybate. Sleep Med 2011;12:730.

Behaviorally Induced Insufficient Sleep

Christer Hublin, MD, PhD[a,b,*], Mikael Sallinen, PhD[a,c]

KEYWORDS

- Sleep • Insufficient sleep • Neurobehavioral function • Work • Behavior

KEY POINTS

- Behaviorally induced insufficient sleep (BIIS) is a common and often long-lasting condition but it is ill-defined.
- BIIS can profoundly affect individual's neurobehavioral and physiological functions and safety.
- There are no established methods for management except the recommendation to sleep more.

The inability to obtain sufficient sleep is a common condition, and its causes are various, ranging from sleep disorders and other medical conditions, irregular and/or extended working hours, to social activities and domestic responsibilities. When the condition lasts for a long period, it leads to chronic sleep deprivation, increasing sleepiness and impairing cognitive function to a degree comparable to acute total sleep deprivation. For various reasons, people with behaviorally induced insufficient sleep (BIIS), who have no difficulties with their sleep as such, voluntarily sleep less than their natural sleep requirement. When BIIS is long lasting (≥ 3 months), it may meet the diagnostic criteria of BIIS syndrome (BIISS), defined by the International Classification of Sleep Disorders (ICSD-2).[1] This review is focused on BIIS in adults, with a special emphasis on work-related aspects.

WHEN IS SLEEP SUFFICIENT AND WHEN IS IT INSUFFICIENT

Sleep duration is highly individual in all age groups, and it is clearly dependent on age. In population-based studies, the mean sleep length has usually been 7 to 8 hours among adults, and there is a U-shaped relationship between age and average sleep time, with the minimum being in middle-aged individuals. In both extremes of the continuum, there are people with sleep disorders, such as insomnia among short sleepers and hypersomnia among long sleepers, but also healthy individuals, because a few percentage of population are so-called natural short sleepers or natural long sleepers.[2] In addition, there seem to be differences between countries. For example, a study by Steptoe and colleagues[3] that was based on data from 24 countries showed that sleep duration was shortest (6.0-6.5 hours) among Japanese and Taiwanese students and longest (about 8 hours) among Bulgarian, Greek, Romanian, and Spanish students.

It has been claimed that the sleep length has generally shortened during the last decades, but there are so far few population-based studies to support this view. In the most recent UK survey, the mean sleep duration was 7.04 hours,[4] and it has changed little over the last 50 years.[5] In a re-analysis of self-reported sleep duration (>440,000 persons) in population-based surveys in Finland from 1972 to 2005, only a minor decrease

Funding: None.

Conflicts of interest: The authors have no conflicts of interest.

[a] Centre of Expertise for Human Factors at Work, Finnish Institute of Occupational Health, Topeliuksenkatu 41 a A, FIN-00250 Helsinki, Finland; [b] Department of Clinical Neurosciences, Helsinki University, PB 22, FIN-00014 Helsinki, Finland; [c] Agora Center, University of Jyväskylä, PB 35, FIN-40014 Jyväskylä, Finland

* Corresponding author. Centre of Expertise for Human Factors at Work, Finnish Institute of Occupational Health, Topeliuksenkatu 41 a A, FIN-00250 Helsinki, Finland.

E-mail address: christer.hublin@ttl.fi

Sleep Med Clin 7 (2012) 313–323

doi:10.1016/j.jsmc.2012.03.008

(18.3 minutes or about 4% to 7.3 hours) was observed.[6] In this study, sleep was shortest in middle-aged employees. However, there may be substantial differences in the development of sleep duration over decades between countries. In the United States, the self-reported modal sleep duration in the 1960s was about 8 hours,[7] but, in more recent Gallup surveys, the estimates have been 7 hours or even less (National Sleep Foundation 2005). In a large population-based survey in the United States, 28.3% of adults slept 6 hours or less per day.[8] This amount of sleep per 24 hours may considerably decrease alertness, as a reduction of total sleep time for one night by 1.0 to 1.5 hours in normal young adults shortens their mean sleep latencies on the Multiple Sleep Latency Test (MSLT) by up to one-third.[9]

In addition to the mean length of sleep, it is essential to take into consideration its day-to-day variation, for example, over a workweek, when assessing BIIS and its consequences. American Time Use Surveys revealed that the average sleep time was longer on Sundays (9.59 hours) and Saturdays (8.97 hours) than on the weekdays, in which case it gradually decreased from Monday (8.41 hours) to Friday (8.03 hours).[10] Similarly, in an actigraphic study, the daily standard deviation was more than an hour for both sleep duration and time in bed, meaning that the day-to-day variation within individuals was greater than the variation between their mean sleep durations.[11] Thus, although a mean sleep length for a longer period can be usual (around the norm of 7–8 hours of sleep per day), a substantial part of it can be spent in a condition of insufficient sleep that compromises alertness and cognitive function (see section "Consequences of Sleep Deprivation").

In population-based studies, the assessment of sleep length is practically always based on self-reports because use of objective methods such as polysomnography has so far been too laborious and expensive for this purpose. It is, however, probable that individuals differ in terms of how accurately they are able to assess their sleep length. Based on clinical experience, those with fragmented sleep (eg, individuals with insomnia) are more inclined to more often report unexpectedly short sleep length than those with consolidated sleep. In true insufficient sleep, as in BIIS, sleep should be consolidated, and therefore self-reports probably are more reliable. Even though the occurrence of insufficient sleep seems to be strongly dependent on sleep length, it is also important to take into account individual sleep need when assessing BIIS.[12,13] Thus, it is important to take into account both self-reported sleep length and sleep need, when assessing sleep sufficiency.

One additional problem is that there are no exact and generally accepted definitions of and methods to measure either sleep need or sleep sufficiency. Broman and colleagues[12] suggested using the amount of habitual sleep to the amount of estimated need for sleep (sleep sufficiency index [SSI]) ratio. To delineate subjects with a substantial chronic sleep loss, a condition termed persistent insufficient sleep (PIS) was operationally defined as SSI less than 80% and having an experience of getting too little sleep at least 3 times per week during the last 3 months. This cutoff at 80% is arbitrary but corresponds rather well to about 6.5 hours of sleep in the average individual whose self-estimated daily sleep need is about 8 hours.[12] Despite the obvious need to operationalize the condition of insufficient sleep, the authors are unaware of any later publication using this definition or its modifications.

Generally speaking, there are 2 major views on the phenomenon of insufficient sleep and its consequences and significance. The first argues that there are no data to show any such decrease in sleep length during the last decades that would result in large-scale and severe increases in sleep deprivation or excessive daytime sleepiness.[5] In addition, it has been pointed out that human adults probably are capable of biologically adapting to various sleep durations if the range of variation remains between 6 and 9 hours per day.[5,14] The other major view underlines the gradual decrease in sleep length and the increase of sleep deprivation in adult population and also cognitive deficits caused by these trends. In experimental studies, cognitive deficits have been shown to exacerbate over days of sleep restriction, even though sleep-deprived individuals may not be aware of the cumulative deficits.[15,16]

BIISS

ICSD-2[1] includes a description and diagnostic criteria of BIISS (**Box 1**). BIISS occurs when an individual persistently fails to obtain the amount of sleep required to maintain normal levels of alertness and wakefulness. The ability to initiate and maintain sleep is unimpaired or above average, with little or no psychopathology and no medical explanation for the patient's sleepiness. There is a substantial disparity between the need for sleep and the amount actually obtained. A markedly extended sleep time on weekend nights or during holidays compared with weekday nights is suggestive of this disorder. In addition to sleepiness, patients may develop irritability, concentration and attention deficits, reduced motivation, dysphoria, fatigue, incoordination, and restlessness.[1]

A. The patient has a complaint of excessive sleepiness or, in prepubertal children, a complaint of behavioral abnormalities suggesting sleepiness. The abnormal sleep pattern is present almost daily for at least 3 months.

B. The patient's habitual sleep episode, established using history, a sleep log, or actigraphy, is usually shorter than expected from age-adjusted normative data. (Note: in the case of individuals with long sleep time, habitual sleep periods may be normal, based on age-adjusted normative data. However, these sleep periods may be insufficient for this population.)

C. When habitual sleep schedule is not maintained (weekends or vacation time), patients sleep considerably longer than usual.

D. If diagnostic polysomnography is performed (not required for diagnosis), sleep latency is less than 10 minutes and sleep efficiency greater than 90%. During the MSLT, a short mean sleep latency of less than 8 minutes (with or without multiple sleep-onset rapid eye movement period) may be observed.

E. The hypersomnia is not better explained by another sleep disorder, medical or neurologic disorder, mental disorder, or medication use or substance use disorder.

Data from ICSD-2. International classification of sleep disorders, 2nd edition. Diagnostic and coding manual. American Academy of Sleep Medicine; 2005.

The differential diagnosis of BIISS includes other causes of excessive daytime sleepiness or shortening of nocturnal sleep.[1] The diagnosis may be especially difficult to make in subjects who are natural long sleepers (see later). There are descriptions of cases in which BIISS has incorrectly been diagnosed as narcolepsy without cataplexy with typical findings on sleep registrations in the sleep-deprived condition.[17]

EPIDEMIOLOGY OF INSUFFICIENT SLEEP

Sleeping difficulties are common, about one-third of the general population is affected by transient insomnia and about one-tenth by severe and/or chronic insomnia,[2] and these difficulties can be assumed to be a major cause of insufficient sleep. However, other causes also seem to be prevalent. In a Swedish population sample aged 30 to 65 years, 28% of women and 21% of men experienced too little sleep, but only about one-third of them had concomitant symptoms suggesting insomnia.[18] In a telephone survey done in Australia, insufficient sleep was reported by 28%, and about three-quarters of these respondents related it to external factors and the remaining quarter to internal factors.[19]

In another Swedish questionnaire study based on a population sample aged 20 to 64 years, PIS (defined earlier) was found in 12% of the subjects.[12] One-half of the subjects with PIS also reported concomitant sleeping difficulties, and, in the remaining, the most conspicuous causes were work-related factors and simply too little time for sleep. Thus, behavioral causes of insufficient sleep seemed to be as common as symptoms indicating possible sleep disorder. The following consequences of insufficient sleep were reported by the respondents: cognitive/behavioral fatigue, somatic symptoms, sleepiness, swelling, headache, and dysphoric mood. Insufficient sleep decreased with age.[12]

A Finnish population-based study, in which insufficient sleep was determined as a difference of 1 hour or more between the self-reports of the need of sleep and the actual length of sleep, found that the prevalence among 33- to 60-year-old subjects was 20.4% (16.2% in men and 23.9% in women).[13] In the same base population, the corresponding figure was 3.6% among men and 6.7% among women after excluding regular nappers and insomniacs.[20] The occurrence of insufficient sleep was strongly dependent on sleep length.[13] Insufficient sleep was reported by 37% of men and 54% of women who slept for 6 hours or less but only by 3.5% of men and 4.3% of women who slept for 9 hours or more. Similarly, 49% of men and women reporting need of sleep for 9 hours or more had insufficient sleep in contrast with 3.3% of men and 5.2% of women with need of sleep of 7 hours or less. There was a significant age effect, a self-report of insufficient sleep being more common in younger age groups in both genders. The strongest significantly positively associated factors were daytime sleepiness (odds ratio, about 4), insomnia (odds ratio, 2.5–3.0), not able to sleep without disturbance (odds ratio, 2.0–2.5), and evening type (odds ratio, about 2). Among men, weekly working hours of 75 or more were also strongly associated with insufficient sleep (odds ratio, about 3), and not working was a protective factor against it in both genders (odds ratio, about 0.7). Insufficient sleep was measured twice with a 9-year interval in the authors' sample and showed considerable stability: 44% of those with insufficient sleep in 1981 also had it 9 years later. Thus, insufficient sleep seems to be a long-standing condition in a large part of the population.[13]

In another Finnish population study, the prevalence of similarly defined insufficient sleep was even higher (36%), being about one-third more common in women than in men (31% vs 41%).[21] There was also a significant age effect: insufficient sleep was twice as prevalent in the youngest compared with the oldest individuals (age range, 24–65 years). The association with work status was also similar to the results of the earlier-mentioned Finnish study. Also in the Finnish studies, behavioral causes (including work-related factors) of insufficient sleep were found to be prevalent.

In a large-scale telephone survey of noninstitutionalized US population aged 18 years or more, frequent ($\geq$14 days in the past 30 days) insufficient sleep was reported by 26%.[22] It was significantly more common in women, adults younger than 55 years, persons employed or unable to work or students (vs retired), and those with fair/poor general health. Insufficient sleep was significantly more likely if frequent physical or mental distress, activity limitations, anxiety, pain, or depressive symptoms were also present. Additional examples in which insufficient sleep are more significantly common include smoking, physical inactivity, obesity, and heavy alcohol use in men.[22]

There are few epidemiologic studies on BIISS. ICSD-2[1] states that this condition affects both sexes across the life span. It may be more frequent in adolescence when sleep need is high, but social pressure and tendency to delayed sleep phase often lead to chronic restricted sleep. In a Japanese study including more than 1200 patients referred to an outpatient clinic for complaint of excessive daytime sleepiness, the rate of BIISS was 7.1%, with BIISS being the fourth most common cause after obstructive sleep apnea, idiopathic hypersomnia, and narcolepsy.[23] In this patient series with polysomnographically verified diagnosis, the male to female ratio was 7:3, the median age of symptom onset was 28.6 years, and the average sleep length during weeknights was 5.5 and 7.9 hours on weekends. The mean Epworth Sleepiness Scale score before treatment was 13.6.[23]

In a Norwegian questionnaire study, the estimated prevalence of BIISS was 10.4% among a representative sample of nearly 1300 high-school students aged 16 to 19 years.[24] A diagnosis of BIISS was given if the following 3 criteria were met: (1) excessive daytime sleepiness was present, (2) total sleep time on weekdays was less than 7 hours, and (3) sleep duration was at least 2 hours longer on weekends/vacations than on weekdays. Use of alcohol and living in an urban area were positively related to BIISS, and it was also associated with poor grades and symptoms of anxiety and depression.[24]

Insufficient sleep is common in the general population, but there is considerable variation in the reported frequencies, ranging from 12% to 36%. This is explained at least partly by differences in definition of insufficiency and other methodological aspects. Insufficient sleep seems to decrease with age. Some studies indicate that one-quarter to one-half of the subjects with insufficient sleep have no simultaneous symptoms suggesting insomnia or other sleep disorder. This indicates that behavioral factors are common causes of insufficient sleep.

CONSEQUENCES OF SLEEP DEPRIVATION

Many earlier reports suggested that human adults are highly adaptable to chronic sleep restriction down to 4 to 5 hours per day, but most of these studies were performed outside laboratory settings, with little or no control over potentially confusing factors such as napping, actual length of sleep periods, use of stimulants (caffeine and nicotine), and physical activity.[16] The later well-controlled studies conducted under standardized laboratory conditions with continuous behavioral, physiologic, and medical monitoring have shown many significant disadvantageous changes due to cumulative sleep restriction over several consecutive days. The results from these studies are discussed in the next section.

Sleep Architecture and Physiologic Sleepiness

Although timing and duration of sleep and the number of days with restricted sleep affect sleep architecture, the general feature is the conservation of slow wave sleep and the reduction of the other non–rapid eye movement sleep stages and rapid eye movement sleep.[25–27] There is also an increase in slow wave activity during and after a period of sleep restriction.[16,25,27]

The MSLT is a well-documented objective measure of sleepiness, showing a significant negative correlation between total sleep time at night and sleep latency on the following day.[28] In a large population-based study including more than 600 subjects, a significant association was found between self-reported sleep duration and the risk of falling asleep on the MSLT; compared with those reporting more than 7.50 hours of sleep a day, individuals reporting 6.75 to 7.50 hours and less than 6.75 hours of sleep a day had a 27% and 73% increase in risk for falling asleep on the test, respectively.[29]

Neurobehavioral Effects

Studies on the neurobehavioral effects of cumulative sleep restriction have shown performance impairments on various mental tasks. These include, for example, measures of sustained attention (eg, vigilance and reaction time tasks), information processing speed (eg, serial addition/subtraction tasks), working memory (eg, digit symbol substitution task), and dynamic allocation of attention between multiple tasks (multitasks consisting of multiple simultaneously active subtasks).[26,27,30-33] Until now, the study by Balkin and colleagues[34] is the only one that has focused on the question which of the neurobehavioral tasks are the most sensitive to cumulative sleep restriction. In this study, participants were daily presented with 11 mental tasks while being subjected to 3, 5, 7, or 9 hours time in bed per night for a week. The Psychomotor Vigilance Task proved to be the most sensitive to sleep restriction, whereas a logical reasoning task showed least sensitivity. The differences in sensitivity to the sleep restriction were quite large between the mental tasks, suggesting that the type of the task is of considerable importance when assessing the neurobehavioral consequences of cumulative sleep restriction.

Besides the cognitive demands of a task, task duration seems to be an important factor. This was particularly demonstrated in the study by Haavisto and colleagues[33] that examined multitasking performance in the condition of cumulative sleep restriction (4 hours time in bed) over a period of 5 days. The investigators found that the deterioration of performance within 50-minute task sessions (so-called time-on-task effect) became intensified during the course of the experiment in the group of sleep-restricted individuals but not in the group of controls permitted to sleep 8 hours each night. This finding emphasizes the importance of task duration when assessing risks caused by insufficient sleep.

Another question of interest is how severely neurobehavioral functions are compromised by cumulative sleep restriction compared with the effects of total sleep loss. Until now, only the study by Van Dongen and colleagues[27] has explicitly investigated this issue. The investigators found that performance on all 3 tasks that measured vigilance, working memory, and information processing speed deteriorated under 2 weeks of cumulative sleep restriction (4 or 6 hours time in bed per night) similarly to what was observed following 1 to 2 days of total sleep loss. Another interesting finding was that self-reported sleepiness did not show such a pattern. It reached its maximum after already 2 days with the 4- or 6-hour sleep opportunity per night. This level of self-reported sleepiness was equivalent to the level that was observed following one night without any sleep. The investigators analyzed, using the data from both conditions (total sleep loss and cumulative sleep restriction), whether the neurobehavioral effects were better explained by the cumulative loss of sleep time or by cumulative wake extension. They concluded that the latter was the primary cause of progressively impaired vigilance performance. This observation of the importance of excess wakefulness is useful when trying to compare different conditions resulting in insufficient sleep in the real world.

Also, it is important to know which factors are the strongest modifiers of the neurobehavioral consequences of cumulative sleep restriction. The current body of research evidences that these factors include (1) amount of sleep per night,[26,27] (2) excess wakefulness,[27] (3) the number of sleep restriction days,[26,27,30,31,33] (4) time of day,[35] and (5) the amount of sleep before the beginning of a sleep restriction regimen.[31] The importance of the last factor was demonstrated by Rupp and colleagues[31] who subjected healthy volunteers to either habitual sleep length (about 7 hours that may not have been totally sufficient for all participants) or extended sleep (10 hours time in bed) for a week before the sleep restriction regimen (3 hours time in bed for 7 days). In practice, the sleep extension group obtained approximately 2 hours more sleep than the habitual sleep group. During the days of sleep restriction, the sleep extension group showed less severe impairments in their vigilance performance and better ability to maintain wakefulness than the habitual sleep group, suggesting a protective effect from the prior additional sleep. This observation may encourage people to sleep longer than habitually before a sleep restriction period if it is possible to anticipate the occurrence of the period.

Recovery from cumulative sleep restriction has been under intense examination since the study by Belenky and colleagues[26] in 2003, which was the first study that properly investigated this issue. In light of the results of total sleep deprivation studies, the investigators somewhat surprisingly found that the decrements in vigilance performance observed during the course of sleep restriction (3 or 5 hours time in bed for 7 days) did not completely recover after 3 days of normal sleep (8 hours time in bed). The investigators suggested that the brain adapts to cumulative sleep restriction, which makes sleep-restricted individuals inclined to make performance errors, not only during a period of sleep restriction but also during several ensuing days.

A later study by Banks and colleagues[32] was the first to systematically examine the dose-response effect of recovery sleep following a sleep restriction regimen. In this experiment, 142 healthy adults were first subjected to 5 days of sleep restriction (4 hours time in bed per night), and, following this, they were allocated to 1 of 6 recovery sleep groups (0, 2, 4, 6, 8, or 10 hours time in bed for 1 night). The study revealed that recovery of vigilance performance and subjective sleepiness followed by the sleep restriction was strongly dependent on the amount of sleep on the recovery night; the greater the amount of recovery sleep, the better the level of recovery. In addition, the 2-hour increase in the recovery sleep opportunity was more valuable among the short recovery sleep groups (ie, 0, 2, and 4 hours) than among the longer groups (ie, 6, 8, and 10 hours). However, not even the longest recovery sleep yielded a full recovery. On the other hand, performance on 2 other tasks (a modified version of the Maintenance of Wakefulness Test and on the Digit Symbol Substitution Task) recovered in a linear manner and showed a full recovery after either the 8-hour or the 10-hour recovery sleep opportunity. These findings suggest that the recovery process of neurobehavioral functions following cumulative sleep restriction takes more time than the corresponding process following total sleep loss, although the level of performance deterioration caused by these 2 types of sleep loss would be equal.[32]

The earlier-mentioned studies show that when individuals with 7 to 9 hours of daily sleep restrict their daily sleep dose to 4 to 6 hours per night for at least 5 days, many of the individuals' neurobehavioral functions become impaired to the extent that it is comparable to 1 to 2 days of total sleep loss. In addition, the studies show that the recovery process takes several days. Although these main findings are of importance when evaluating neurobehavioral consequences of BIIS (and also BIISS), they do not provide a practical basis for the clinical evaluation of these conditions. In addition, there are at least 2 main theoretical questions that are still open: are the neurobehavioral consequences of cumulative sleep restriction found among mostly young healthy men in the studies described earlier similar to that in other pertinent groups of people (eg, in the elderly and in women) and what happens when individuals are subjected to periods of cumulative sleep restriction and following recovery opportunities repeatedly. A study by Everson and Szabo[36] showed that rats exposed to recurrent periods of cumulative sleep restriction developed marked behavioral changes in food and water intake, leading to weight loss and structural changes in the small intestine and adipocytes.

Risk of Accidents

One important outcome of insufficient sleep is increased risk of accidents.[37] Most of the studies in this field deal with traffic, and up to 20% of all traffic accidents in industrial societies are sleep and vigilance related.[38] Insufficient sleep among drivers is common. For example, half of 2196 randomly stopped French drivers had decreased their total sleep time in the 24 hours before the interview compared with their regular self-reported sleep time.[39] About 12.5% had a sleep debt greater than 180 minutes, and 2.7% had a sleep debt greater than 300 minutes. Being young, commuting to work, driving long distances, starting the trip at night, being an "evening" person, being a long sleeper during the week, and sleeping in on the weekend were risk factors significantly associated with sleep debt.[39] In a sample of American truck drivers actigraphically measured, mean sleep of 1 week was less than 6 hours in 34%, and short sleep was significantly associated with decreased performance.[40]

The data on sleep-related accidents in other fields (eg, industry and health care) are scarce compared with traffic. One reason may be that the overall accident risk in these sectors is lower than in the transport sector, where, for example, a single perceptual error may be fatal.[37] In a population-based study by Akerstedt and colleagues,[41] it was found that disturbed sleep and shift work were associated with a 50% increased risk of fatal occupational accidents.

Physiologic Effects

There is increasing evidence of associations between sleep length and different health outcomes in population. However, the mediating mechanisms are still incompletely understood, although studies have found detrimental effects of sleep loss on endocrine, metabolic, immune, and inflammatory functions.[42,43] For example, the link between insufficient sleep and insulin resistance can be explained by several plausible mechanisms: (1) increased release of counterregulatory hormones, including epinephrine and cortisol; (2) increased sympathetic nervous activity with elevated levels of norepinephrine; (3) inflammation, with elevations of interleukin 1β, tumor necrosis factor α, interleukin 6, and C-reactive protein; (4) increased risk of weight gain and obesity, a major risk factor for insulin resistance.[44] Failure to obtain adequate amounts of sleep promotes low-level systemic inflammation, and, although the physiologic mechanisms underlying the links between sleep deprivation and these immune and inflammatory responses remain largely unknown, neuroendocrine-dependent, autonomic vascular stress–dependent, and slow wave sleep hormone–dependent changes are likely involved.[45]

Most of the population studies assessing health risk associated with sleep length do not include detailed information of factors affecting the length, that is, whether self-reported short sleep is a result of insufficient sleep (either behavioral or other cause), of insomnia, or of being a natural short sleeper. Although the occurrence of insufficient sleep cannot directly be assessed from sleep length solely, it seems to be clearly more common in short sleepers.[13] There is a significant U-shaped association between sleep length and subsequent mortality, showing that those sleeping 7 hours had the lowest risk of mortality.[46] In addition, it has been shown that there is a significant association between short sleep and obesity especially in younger people[47] and somatic diseases or disorders such as type 2 diabetes[48] and cardiovascular disease.[49]

FACTORS AFFECTING RISK OF AND ADAPTATION TO INSUFFICIENT SLEEP

Insufficient sleep is significantly associated with diurnal type (also called chronotype), which in turn is strongly genetically determined; about one-half of the interindividual variability in adults is explained by genetic effects.[50] Insufficient sleep, defined as a difference of at least 1 hour between the self-reports of the need of sleep and the actual length of sleep, was reported by 12% among morning types (29% in this population-based adult sample), and it had an increasing trend toward the evening types (10% of the sample), 28% of whom reported it.[50] Some of those who evaluate themselves as extreme evening-type individuals actually suffer from delayed sleep phase syndrome, which is characterized by habitual sleep-wake times that are delayed usually several hours relative to conventional times.[1] This condition is more common among adolescents and young adults.

Other studies have shown that evening type is clearly associated with poor sleep hygiene. Compared with morning types, evening types more often show a considerable sleep debt on work days, consume more caffeine and alcohol, and are more often habitual smokers.[51,52] The concept of "social jet lag" has been proposed because so many people in the present society shift their sleep and activity times several hours between the workweek and the weekend in a way comparable with genuine jetlag.[52] Thus, many behavioral aspects may contribute to insufficient sleep, especially in evening-type people.

ICSD-2[1] includes under the heading "Isolated Symptoms, Apparently Normal Variants and Unresolved Issues" the entity "Long Sleeper" (also called healthy hypersomnia or extreme high end of normal sleep duration continuum). The diagnostic criteria include daily total sleep time of 10 hours or more (documented by a sleep log over a minimum of 7 days), excessive daytime sleepiness following less than 10 hours of sleep, and having had that particular sleep pattern since childhood. The prevalence of long sleep is poorly known because the numerous studies on sleep length and different health outcomes have not separated it from other causes of long sleep (about 2% of the population sleeps at least 10 hours per night) such as untreated sleep apnea.[1] However, it can be assumed that natural long sleepers are especially at risk for BIIS (and also BIISS) as exemplified by the case described earlier.

It is well known that individuals differ considerably in their response to insufficient sleep caused by shift work or extended working hours. Age, sex, diurnal type, physical fitness, and domestic and personality factors explain only a minor part of the variation.[53] A study by Van Dongen and colleagues[54] suggested that these individual differences constitute a trait. In their study, 21 healthy young adults were monitored for wakefulness during 3 separate laboratory visits, each of which included 36 hours of total sleep deprivation and neurobehavioral testing at 2-hour intervals. During the week prior to the sessions, the participants' daily sleep opportunity was either restricted to 6 hours (prior sleep restriction condition) or extended to 12 hours (prior sleep extension condition). The main findings of the study showed that (1) there are substantial individual differences in sleepiness and performance impairment due to sleep deprivation, (2) these individual differences are highly replicable over repeated exposures to sleep deprivation, and (3) the individual differences in response to sleep deprivation were not predicted by prior sleep history, circadian rhythm parameters, age, or sex or psychosocial factors. From these findings, it was concluded that vulnerability to performance impairment due to sleep deprivation constitutes a trait.[54,55] Later studies have suggested that genes involved in the adenosinergic and circadian regulation (PER3 polymorphism) of sleep are possible candidate predictors of individuals' resistance or vulnerability to performance impairments under sleep deprivation,[56,57] even though negative findings have also been reported.[58]

The abruptness of sleep restriction plays a role in the adaptation process. Drake and coworkers[59] assessed alertness, memory, and performance following 3 schedules of approximately 8 hours of sleep loss (slow, intermediate, and rapid accumulation) in comparison with an 8-hour time in bed sleep schedule. Twelve young healthy adults completed each of 4 conditions: no sleep loss (8-hours for 4 nights) and slow (6 hours for 4 nights), intermediate (4 hours for 2 nights), and rapid (0 hours in bed for 1 night) sleep loss. The rapid sleep loss produced significantly more severe impairments on tests of alertness, memory, and performance than the slow accumulation of a comparable amount of sleep loss. The impairing effects of sleep loss vary as a function of rate, suggesting the presence of a compensatory adaptive mechanism operating in conjunction with the accumulation of a sleep debt.[59]

MANAGEMENT

Despite the relatively high prevalence of BIIS and its possible health and neurobehavioral consequences, there are no established ways of treating this condition, except the recommendation of extending sleeping time to better satisfy the individual's sleep need. To the best of the authors' knowledge, there are no studies assessing the effect of treatment of BIIS or BIISS. The need for effective and innovative treatments is emphasized by results indicating that insufficient sleep may be quite long lasting (stable in 44% over a period of 9 years, see earlier),[13] and therefore it may also be quite resistant to general recommendations to extend sleep time. The long-lasting nature of BIIS is also suggested by an early study by Friedmann and colleagues.[60] They described 4 young adult collegiate couples who gradually restricted their sleep down to about 5 hours per night over a period of 6 to 8 months (measured using sleep log). At the end of an additional 12-month follow-up, total sleep time was still 1.0 to 2.5 hours below baseline,[60] indicating a long-lasting change in sleep-wake behavior.

Because BIIS is behaviorally induced by definition, it is obvious that pharmacologic treatment such as sleep-promoting medication is not among the first-line choices. The behavioral component is strongly present in many other sleep disturbances also, such as in insomnia and sleep apnea. Ruminative thoughts at bedtime making sleep initiation difficult and compliance with use of the continuous positive airway pressure (CPAP) device are examples of the behavioral component involved in sleep disturbances. Cognitive behavioral treatments are most effective in management of different forms of insomnia,[61] and it is probable that similar techniques could also be useful in the management of BIIS and BIISS.

Given the origin of BIIS, it is possible to equate it with other unhealthy behaviors, such as physical inactivity, smoking, or heavy alcohol consumption. There are a few influential theories that have been applied to unhealthy behaviors until now. An example of these is the Transtheoretical Model of Behavior Change (TTM).[62,63] The basic idea underlying this model is that individuals differ significantly in terms of their readiness to change their unhealthy behavior. Individuals can be categorized into one of the following stages: (1) precontemplation stage in which there is no intention to change the behavior, probably because of unawareness of the need to change; (2) contemplation stage in which there is awareness of the problem but no readiness to do anything concrete, probably because of not being sure if the pros outweigh the cons; (3) preparation stage in which there are plans to take action in the near future but also worries of failure; (4) action stage in which individuals do something concrete but worry about the need to work hard to maintain the new behavior; or (5) maintenance stage in which individuals try to prevent relapse into the old unhealthy behavior, particularly in stressful situations. It is apparent that treatment of these different groups requires different approaches. For example in BIIS or BIISS, those at the precontemplation stage would need an awakening to the unhealthiness of their sleep-wake behavior, whereas those at the preparation stage would need support to take action to increase their sleep length and/or to have more regular sleeping habits.

Treatments applying TTM have been shown to be effective in reducing stress,[64] improving medication adherence,[65,66] and facilitating smoking cessation[67] and weight loss.[68] There is some evidence of the usefulness of the TTM in identifying patients with obstructive sleep apnea syndrome who have low or high adherence to CPAP therapy and low or high intention to exercise.[69–71] On the other hand, there has also been criticism regarding the effectiveness of the TTM in facilitating changes in health behavior.[72–74] Whether TTM-based approaches could be effective in treating BIISS remains to be investigated.

Among adults, long working hours and shift work are often associated with insufficient sleep.[13,75,76] In such cases, attention should be paid not only to sleep but also to the duration and arrangement of working hours, to ensure about 8 hours time in bed per day.

SUMMARY

BIIS, both as a phenomenon and as a syndrome, is a common condition. It is well documented that the detrimental effects of chronic sleep deprivation on well-being, performance, and safety are comparable to those caused by acute total sleep deprivation lasting 1 to 2 days. As insufficient sleep is common among short sleepers, it is possible that chronic sleep deprivation plays a significant role in the associations shown between short sleep and many common diseases. There are observations indicating that insufficient sleep may be long lasting and can therefore also be resistant to treatments based on recommendations only. Thus, it is important to investigate cost-effective preventive and treatment methods for it. Assessment of sleep sufficiency should be one focus in health care system, especially when dealing with adolescents, young adults, and employees (particularly having shift work, extended working hours, and safety critical jobs).

REFERENCES

1. ICSD-2. International classification of sleep disorders. Diagnostic and coding manual. 2nd edition. Westchester (IL): American Academy of Sleep Medicine; 2005.
2. Partinen M, Hublin C. Epidemiology of sleep disorders. In: Kryger M, Roth T, Dement WC, editors. Principles and practice of sleep medicine. 5th edition. St Louis (MO): Elsevier Saunders; 2011. p. 694–715.
3. Steptoe A, Peacey V, Wardle J. Sleep duration and health in young adults. Arch Intern Med 2006;166: 1689–92.
4. Groeger JA, Zijlstra FR, Dijk DJ. Sleep quantity, sleep difficulties and their perceived consequences in a representative sample of some 2000 British adults. J Sleep Res 2004;13:359–71.
5. Horne J. The end of sleep: 'sleep debt' versus biological adaptation of human sleep to waking needs. Biol Psychol 2011;7:1–14.
6. Kronholm E, Partonen T, Laatikainen T, et al. Trends in self-reported sleep duration and insomnia-related symptoms in Finland from 1972 to 2005: a comparative review and re-analysis of Finnish population samples. J Sleep Res 2008;17:54–62.
7. Kripke DF, Simons RN, Garfinkel L, et al. Short and long sleep and sleeping pills. Is increased mortality associated? Arch Gen Psychiatry 1979;36:103–16.
8. Krueger PM, Friedman EM. Sleep duration in the United States: a cross-sectional population-based study. Am J Epidemiol 2009;169:1052–63.
9. Bonnet MH, Arand DL. We are chronically sleep deprived. Sleep 1995;18:908–11.
10. Basner M, Fomberstein KM, Razavi FM, et al. American time use survey: sleep time and its relationship to waking activities. Sleep 2007;30:1085–95.
11. Knutson KL, Rathouz PJ, Yan LL, et al. Intra-individual daily and yearly variability in actigraphically

recorded sleep measures: the CARDIA study. Sleep 2007;30:793–6.
12. Broman JE, Lundh LG, Hetta J. Insufficient sleep in the general population. Neurophysiol Clin 1996;26:30–9.
13. Hublin C, Kaprio J, Partinen M, et al. Insufficient sleep: a population based study in adults. Sleep 2001;24:392–400.
14. Horne J. Is there a sleep debt? Sleep 2004;27:1047–9.
15. Dinges DF. Sleep debt and scientific evidence. Sleep 2004;27:1050–2.
16. Banks S, Dinges DF. Chronic sleep deprivation. In: Kryger M, Roth T, Dement WC, editors. Principles and practice of sleep medicine. 5th edition. St Louis (MO): Elsevier Saunders; 2011. p. 67–75.
17. Janjua T, Samp T, Cramer-Bornemann M, et al. Clinical caveat: prior sleep deprivation can affect the MSLT for days. Sleep Med 2003;4:69–72.
18. Liljenberg B, Almqvist M, Hetta J, et al. The prevalence of insomnia: the importance of operationally defined criteria. Ann Clin Res 1988;20:393–8.
19. Lack L, Miller W, Turner D. A survey on sleeping difficulties in an Australian population. Community Health Stud 1988;12:200–7.
20. Hublin C, Kaprio J, Partinen M, et al. Daytime sleepiness in an adult Finnish population. J Intern Med 1996;239:417–23.
21. Sallinen M, Härmä M, Kalimo R, et al. The prevalence of sleep debt and its association with fatigue, performance and accidents in the modern society. In: Rantanen J, Lehtinen S, Saarela KL, editors. Proceedings of the European Conference on Safety in the Modern Society, 15–17 September 1999. Helsinki (Finland): Finnish Institute of Occupational Health; 2000. p. 140–3.
22. Strine TW, Chapman DP. Associations of frequent sleep insufficiency with health-related quality of life and health behaviors. Sleep Med 2005;6:23–7.
23. Komada Y, Inoue Y, Hayashida K, et al. Clinical significance and correlates of behaviorally induced insufficient sleep syndrome. Sleep Med 2008;9: 851–6.
24. Pallesen S, Saxvig IW, Molde H, et al. Brief report: behaviorally induced insufficient sleep syndrome in older adolescents: prevalence and correlates. J Adolesc 2011;34:391–5.
25. Brunner DP, Dijk DJ, Borbély AA. Repeated partial sleep deprivation progressively changes in EEG during sleep and wakefulness. Sleep 1993;16:100–13.
26. Belenky G, Wesensten NJ, Thorne DR, et al. Patterns of performance degradation and restoration during sleep restriction and subsequent recovery: a sleep dose-response study. J Sleep Res 2003;12:1–12.
27. Van Dongen HP, Maislin G, Mullington JM, et al. The cumulative cost of additional wakefulness: dose-response effects on neurobehavioral functions and sleep physiology from chronic sleep restriction and total sleep deprivation. Sleep 2003;26:117–26.

28. Arand D, Bonnet M, Hurwitz T, et al. The clinical use of the MSLT and MWT. Sleep 2005;28:123–44.

29. Punjabi NM, Bandeen-Roche K, Young T. Predictors of objective sleep tendency in the general population. Sleep 2003;26:678–83.

30. Axelsson J, Kecklund G, Akerstedt T, et al. Sleepiness and performance in response to repeated sleep restriction and subsequent recovery during semi-laboratory conditions. Chronobiol Int 2008;25:297–308.

31. Rupp TL, Wesensten NJ, Bliese BD, et al. Banking sleep: realization of benefits during subsequent sleep restriction and recovery. Sleep 2009;32:311–21.

32. Banks S, Van Dongen HP, Maislin G, et al. Neurobehavioral dynamics following chronic sleep restriction: dose-response effects of one night for recovery. Sleep 2010;33:1013–26.

33. Haavisto ML, Porkka-Heiskanen T, Hublin C, et al. Sleep restriction for the duration of a work week impairs multitasking performance. J Sleep Res 2010;19:444–54.

34. Balkin TJ, Bliese PD, Belenky G, et al. Comparative utility of instruments for monitoring sleepiness-related performance decrements in the operational environment. J Sleep Res 2004;13:219–27.

35. Mollicone DJ, Van Dongen HP, Rogers NL, et al. Time of day effects on neurobehavioral performance during chronic sleep restriction. Aviat Space Environ Med 2010;81:735–44.

36. Everson CA, Szabo A. Recurrent restriction of sleep and inadequate recuperation induce both adaptive changes and pathological outcomes. Am J Physiol Regul Integr Comp Physiol 2009;297:R1430–40.

37. Akerstedt T, Philip P, Capelli A, et al. Sleep loss and accidents—work hours, life style, and sleep pathology. Prog Brain Res 2011;190:169–88.

38. Philip P, Sagaspe P, Taillard J. Drowsy driving. In: Kryger M, Roth T, Dement WC, editors. Principles and practice of sleep medicine. 5th edition. St Louis (MO): Elsevier Saunders; 2011. p. 769–74.

39. Philip P, Taillard J, Guilleminault C, et al. Long distance driving and self-induced sleep deprivation among automobile drivers. Sleep 1999;22:475–80.

40. Pack AI, Maislin G, Staley B, et al. Impaired performance in commercial drivers: role of sleep apnea and short sleep duration. Am J Respir Crit Care Med 2006;174:446–54.

41. Akerstedt T, Fredlund P, Gillberg M, et al. A prospective study of fatal occupational accidents—relationship to sleeping difficulties and occupational factors. J Sleep Res 2002;11:69–71.

42. Grandner MA, Drummond SP. Who are the long sleepers? Towards an understanding of the mortality relationship. Sleep Med Rev 2007;11:341–60.

43. Grandner MA, Hale L, Moore M, et al. Mortality associated with short sleep duration: the evidence, the possible mechanisms, and the future. Sleep Med Rev 2010;14:191–203.

44. Van Cauter E. Sleep disturbances and insulin resistance. Diabet Med 2011;28:1455–62.

45. Faraut B, Boudjeltia KZ, Vanhamme L, et al. Immune, inflammatory and cardiovascular consequences of sleep restriction and recovery. Sleep Med Rev 2012;16(2):137–49.

46. Gallicchio L, Kalesan B. Sleep duration and mortality: a systematic review and meta-analysis. J Sleep Res 2009;18:148–58.

47. Nielsen LS, Danielsen KV, Sørensen TI. Short sleep duration as a possible cause of obesity: critical analysis of the epidemiological evidence. Obes Rev 2011;12:78–92.

48. Cappuccio FP, D'Elia L, Strazzullo P, et al. Quantity and quality of sleep and incidence of type 2 diabetes: a systematic review and meta-analysis. Diabetes Care 2010;33:414–20.

49. Kronholm E, Laatikainen T, Peltonen M, et al. Self-reported sleep duration, all-cause mortality, cardiovascular mortality and morbidity in Finland. Sleep Med 2011;12:215–21.

50. Koskenvuo M, Hublin C, Partinen M, et al. Heritability of diurnal types: a nationwide study of 9212 adult twin pairs. J Sleep Res 2007;16:156–62.

51. Taillard J, Philip P, Bioulac B. Morningness/eveningness and the need for sleep. J Sleep Res 1999;8:291–5.

52. Wittmann M, Dinich J, Merrow M, et al. Social jetlag: misalignment of biological and social time. Chronobiol Int 2006;23:497–509.

53. Härmä M. Sleepiness and shiftwork: individual differences. J Sleep Res 1995;4(Suppl 2):57–61.

54. Van Dongen HP, Baynard MD, Maislin G, et al. Systematic interindividual differences in neurobehavioral impairment from sleep loss: evidence of trait-like differential vulnerability. Sleep 2004;27:423–33.

55. Van Dongen HP, Belenky G. Individual differences in vulnerability to sleep loss in the work environment. Ind Health 2009;47:518–26.

56. Viola AU, Archer SN, James LM, et al. PER3 polymorphism predicts sleep structure and waking performance. Curr Biol 2007;17:613–8.

57. Landolt HP. Sleep homeostasis: a role for adenosine in humans? Biochem Pharmacol 2008;75:2070–9.

58. Goel N, Banks S, Mignot E, et al. PER3 polymorphism predicts cumulative sleep homeostatic but not neurobehavioral changes to chronic partial sleep deprivation. PLoS One 2009;4:e5874.

59. Drake CL, Roehrs TA, Burduvali E, et al. Effects of rapid versus slow accumulation of eight hours of sleep loss. Psychophysiology 2001;38:979–87.

60. Freidmann J, Globus G, Huntley A, et al. Performance and mood during and after gradual sleep reduction. Psychophysiology 1977;14:245–50.

61. Morin CM, Bootzin RR, Buysse DJ, et al. Psychological and behavioral treatment of insomnia: update of the recent evidence (1998-2004). Sleep 2006;29:1398–414.

62. Prochaska JO, DiClemente CC. Stages and processes of self-change of smoking: toward an integrative model of change. J Consult Clin Psychol 1983;51:390–5.

63. Prochaska JO. Decision making in the transtheoretical model of behavior change. Med Decis Making 2008;28:845–9.

64. Evers KE, Prochaska JO, Johnson JL, et al. A randomized clinical trial of a population- and transtheoretical model-based stress-management intervention. Health Psychol 2006;25:521–9.

65. Johnson SS, Driskell MM, Johnson JL, et al. Transtheoretical model intervention for adherence to lipid-lowering drugs. Dis Manag 2006;9:102–14.

66. Johnson SS, Driskell MM, Johnson JL, et al. Efficacy of a transtheoretical model-based expert system for antihypertensive adherence. Dis Manag 2006;9: 291–301.

67. Velicer WF, Redding CA, Sun X, et al. Demographic variables, smoking variables, and outcome across five studies. Health Psychol 2007;26:278–87.

68. Johnson SS, Paiva AL, Cummins CO, et al. Transtheoretical model-based multiple behavior intervention for weight management: effectiveness on a population basis. Prev Med 2008;46:238–46.

69. Stepnowsky CJ, Marler MR, Palau J, et al. Social-cognitive correlates of CPAP adherence in experienced users. Sleep Med 2006;7:350–6.

70. Aloia MS, Arnedt JT, Stepnowsky C, et al. Predicting treatment adherence in obstructive sleep apnea using principles of behavior change. J Clin Sleep Med 2005;1:346–53.

71. Smith SS, Doyle G, Pascoe T, et al. Intention to exercise in patients with obstructive sleep apnea. J Clin Sleep Med 2007;3:689–94.

72. Riemsma RP, Pattenden J, Bridle C, et al. Systematic review of the effectiveness of stage based interventions to promote smoking cessation. BMJ 2003;326: 1175–7.

73. Bridle C, Riemsma RP, Pattenden J, et al. Systematic review of the effectiveness of health behavior interventions based on the transtheoretical model. Psychol Health 2005;20:283–301.

74. Aveyard P, Lawrence T, Cheng KK, et al. A randomized controlled trial of smoking cessation for pregnant women to test the effect of a transtheoretical model-based intervention on movement in stage and interaction with baseline stage. Br J Health Psychol 2006;11(Pt 2):263–78.

75. Virtanen M, Ferrie JE, Vahtera J, et al. Long working hours and sleep disturbances: the Whitehall II prospective cohort study. Sleep 2009;32:737–45.

76. Sallinen M, Kecklund G. Shift work, sleep, and sleepiness—differences between shift schedules and systems. Scand J Work Environ Health 2010; 36:121–33.

Behavioral Management of Hypersomnia

Deirdre A. Conroy, PhD, CBSM*, Danielle M. Novick, PhD,
Leslie M. Swanson, PhD

KEYWORDS

- Sleepiness • Behavioral • Non-pharmacologic options • Treatment

KEY POINTS

- Ensuring that the patient practices adequate sleep hygiene can be an initial step in managing hypersomnolence.
- Many healthy adults who are experiencing hypersomnolence can benefit from a short, 15- to 30-minute nap, but the nap should be timed in the mid-afternoon to prevent sleep disruption.
- In young adults, who are often sleep deprived because of psychosocial influences, a regular sleep-wake schedule may help to improve daytime alertness.

Stimulants and other psychotropics are the first-line and gold standard treatment for many of the hypersomnias, including narcolepsy. Many patients with hypersomnia, however, only achieve moderate improvements in alertness with pharmacotherapy alone.[1] Thus, to attain the best possible outcomes for patients with hypersomnia, a comprehensive treatment approach involving both medication and behavioral components may be needed. This article details some behavioral and psychological approaches that might be useful as independent interventions or adjunctive therapies for the management of for hypersomnia.

BEHAVIORAL AND PSYCHOLOGICAL OPTIONS FOR THE TREATMENT OF HYPERSOMNOLENCE

There are several reasons a clinician may choose to initiate behavioral or psychological treatments in their patients. The most common are described in **Box 1**. These include patient's nonadherence to pharmacotherapy, inadequate response to pharmacotherapy, and preference. In some cases, patients with hypersomnolence may have difficulty adhering to their medication regimen, which may be because of the dose schedule, type of medication, or amount of medication. For example, multiple dosing schedules may interfere with class or work schedules. Behavioral and psychological options may also help when persistent hypersomnolence is present despite the use of stimulant medications.- Some patients may even prefer to adopt adjunctive strategies to maintain wakefulness. Some behavioral strategies are discussed below.

Sleep Diaries

Sleep diaries help both the patient and clinician to understand daily sleep patterns, quality of nocturnal sleep, substances that may interfere with sleep, and daily napping patterns. The utility of the diary for a sleepy patient depends on the ability to use the information from the diary to help schedule prophylactic napping.[2]

Exercise

Patients with hypersomnolence typically acknowledge the potential benefits of exercise but are often caught in a cycle of persistent sleepiness that

The authors have nothing to disclose.
Behavioral Sleep Medicine Program, University of Michigan Hospital and Health Systems, Ann Arbor, MI, USA
* Corresponding author. Department of Psychiatry, University of Michigan, 4250 Plymouth Road, Ann Arbor, MI 48109.
E-mail address: daconroy@umich.edu

Sleep Med Clin 7 (2012) 325–331
doi:10.1016/j.jsmc.2012.03.005

<table>
<tr><td>

Box 1
Rational for behavioral interventions

1. Limited adherence to stimulants
2. Persistent sleepiness despite stimulants
3. Patient preference

</td><td>

Box 2
Sleep hygiene recommendations

1. Make the last hour before bed a wind-down time. Have a light carbohydrate snack (eg, crackers, bread, cereal) during this time.
2. Eat regular meals every day.
3. Limit liquid consumption to 8 to 10 oz in the evening.
4. Avoid caffeinated products and stimulants (eg, nicotine) for several hours before bedtime.
5. Do not consume alcohol too close to bedtime.
6. Maintain the temperature of bedroom at a comfortable and cool side (around 65°F).
7. Make sure that the bed is comfortable and bedroom should be dark and quiet.
8. Exercise regularly, but do not engage in activities that increase body temperature (eg, warm baths, aerobic activity) within 1.5 hours of bedtime.

</td></tr>
</table>

affects motivation, energy, and, in some cases, fewer waking hours available to prioritize exercise. Sleepiness has been shown to interfere with exercising. A secondary analysis of questionnaire data from approximately 1500 respondents to the National Sleep Foundation Sleep in America Poll, confirmed that daytime sleepiness predicted infrequent exercise and impaired physical function even after controlling for age, BMI, income, and many comorbid conditions.[3] Animal studies suggest that despite the neurobiological differences associated with narcolepsy (eg, orexin deficiency), exercise can help to increase wakefulness. When orexin knockout mice were given the opportunity for spontaneous wheel running, they experienced a 20% increase in wakefulness, albeit in the presence of more cataplectic attacks.[4]

Distracting Techniques

Several studies have been conducted on whether chewing gum is an effective way to moderate alertness. In a recent reanalysis, Johnson and colleagues[5] 2011 confirmed previous findings that chewing gum was effective in increasing alertness following a stressor.

Sleep Hygiene

Good sleep hygiene is an important basic treatment element for hypersomnia, regardless of the cause. Education on sleep hygiene (outlined in **Box 2**) provides patients with information about lifestyle and environmental factors that may affect sleep. Sleep hygiene provides an essential foundation for other management approaches but is not an adequate treatment for hypersomnia on its own.

Napping

Prophylactic napping can be an effective adjunctive treatment for patients who experience daytime sleepiness while using a stimulant or for patients who are taking a break from stimulant use. A discussion with the patient about opportune times for napping is helpful. In addition, a consistent sleep-wake schedule helps to regularize circadian rhythms and is important for symptom management.

AGE CONSIDERATIONS IN THE BEHAVIORAL MANAGEMENT OF HYPERSOMNOLENCE
Young Adults

Many young adults curtail nighttime sleep to meet school, work, and social demands, which can result in sleep deprivation and excessive daytime sleepiness. Adequate sleep is essential for good cognitive functioning and performance. The primary treatment strategy for individuals who are experiencing hypersomnia due to insufficient time devoted to sleep is educating the patient regarding the importance of adequate sleep, and collaborating with the patient to extend their nocturnal sleep window to a sufficient duration. Regularizing the sleep-wake schedule is also important; a study of college students showed that maintaining consistent bed and wake times resulted in improved alertness, even though subjects were only sleeping for 7.5 hours.[6]

For young adults who are experiencing acute sleep deprivation, very short (15 minute) naps in the mid-afternoon can increase alertness and performance.[7] Ingestion of a moderate dose of caffeine can also alleviate sleepiness caused by sleep deprivation.[8] The combination of a short nap and a moderate dose of caffeine produces greater reductions in sleepiness than those in napping or caffeine alone.[9]

Older Adults

Sleep changes dramatically as age increases. Excessive daytime sleepiness is a common concern among older individuals. Brief (up to 30 minutes) appropriately timed (before 15:00 hour) sleep may improve daytime alertness in older adults without disrupting nocturnal sleep or shifting circadian rhythms.[10]

TREATING HYPERSOMNOLENCE IN THE CONTEXT OF THE PARENT DISORDER
Narcolepsy

Although stimulant medications are likely to be the most effective treatments for hypersomnia, few patients use stimulant monotherapy, and 50% of patients use behavioral monotherapy.[11] Although rarely effective individually, napping and sleep-scheduling strategies are important in managing the symptoms of patients with narcolepsy.

Although an adequate period of nocturnal sleep is imperative for patients with narcolepsy, sleeping ad libitum or greatly extending nocturnal sleep is only minimally effective at increasing sleep latency on the Multiple sleep latency test (MSLT) although it reduces subjective sleepiness.[12] In addition to showing little benefit, sleep extension can be difficult for many patients to accommodate in their daily schedules.

Maintenance of a regular sleep-wake schedule has been shown to improve the severity of narcolepsy symptoms but does not reduce the amount of unscheduled daytime sleep episodes.[13] Scheduled napping can improve alertness and aid in symptom management, particularly when used with a stimulant. Individuals with narcolepsy show a greater propensity to nap earlier in the day than healthy controls, and may derive greater benefit from naps taken earlier in the day (ie, before the typical mid-afternoon circadian dip).

Stimulant therapy with a consistent sleep-wake schedule may have added benefit on napping. Both short and long naps have been found to be helpful in patients with narcolepsy. Two regularly scheduled 15-minute naps per day have been shown to reduce unscheduled daytime sleep bouts and improve narcolepsy symptoms.[13] Longer naps, for example, 2 hours, have also been shown to be more effective than several short naps in patients with narcolepsy.[14] A long nap taken in the midday has been shown to improve reaction time through the evening hours in patients who are not using a stimulant medication.[14] When considering scheduled napping for individuals with narcolepsy, the alerting effects of a long nap typically dissipate within a few hours in patients who are not using stimulant medications.[15] Therefore, nap opportunities should be scheduled at regular intervals.

Idiopathic Hypersomnia

Patients with idiopathic hypersomnia may respond only minimally to sleep hygiene. Nevertheless, patients should be counseled to maintain good sleep habits. In contrast to patients with narcolepsy, naps are typically unrefreshing to patients with idiopathic hypersomnia, and many experience sleep drunkenness or severe sleep inertia after napping. Similarly, sleep extension may offer little benefit.

Continuous Positive Airway Pressure Management for Sleep Apnea

Sleep apnea can be associated with hypersomnolence. Even patients who are treated with continuous positive airway pressure (CPAP) and who use it regularly can experience residual sleepiness.[16,17] Approximately 22% of patients who use CPAP more than 6 hours had excessive sleepiness documented by MSLT.[16] Although modafinil has been found to be helpful in patients with residual sleepiness despite CPAP,[18] behavioral interventions geared toward CPAP adherence may also help. Once the patient has received adequate instruction on how to use the device as well as a proper mask fit, behavioral management of CPAP adherence, including a combination of systematic desensitization to the mask and motivational enhancement therapy[19,20] toward the use of CPAP, can be implemented. Resurgence of hypersomnolence that occurs after many years of adequate CPAP usage may require a CPAP retitration study to ensure that the patient's CPAP is still controlling the respiratory events.

Circadian Rhythm Sleep Disorders

Hypersomnolence can be one of the clinical characteristic of circadian rhythm sleep disorders such as jet lag, free-running, and shift work sleep disorder.[21] These disorders are often the result of a misalignment of the individual's circadian sleep propensity and their social and/or physical environment. A well-established treatment of circadian rhythm sleep disorders is the use of phototherapy. The goal of phototherapy is to align the timing of the main sleep period to the maximum circadian sleep propensity.

Appropriately timed light exposure serves as the zeitgeber (time giver), which provides information about the time of day to the endogenous circadian clock.[22] A thorough assessment of the patient's intrinsic sleep schedule (typically via sleep diaries or 24-hour sleep logs in the clinic) and the patient's preferred schedule is needed to determine the timing of the exposure to light therapy. The utility of phototherapy on the endogenous circadian pacemaker has been characterized[23] and tested for the purposes of jet lag,[24] shift work,[25] and several other circadian disorders.[26] The mechanisms underlying the alerting properties of light seem to be in the suppression of endogenous melatonin, a primary output of the suprachiasmatic nucleus. The alerting effects are not only reported subjectively but also have been captured in the objective EEG changes and reduction in slow rolling eye movements.[27] Wavelength of light has also been found to be important. Receptors involved in synchronizing the circadian clock seem to be more sensitive to light in the short, 460-nm wavelength, which is experienced as blue light.[28] Blue-enriched light also appears to be better for decreasing subjective sleepiness ratings[29] in healthy young adults.

Unipolar and Bipolar Depression

Hypersomnia often occurs in the context of a major depressive episode (MDE).[30,31] Approximately 16% to 20% of depressed individuals report hypersomnia (for review see[32]), and 25% of individuals with bipolar disorder (BP) experience hypersomnia during the inter-episode period.[33,34] Higher rates are found among women, adolescents and young adults, individuals with a family loading of BP, and individuals with underlying or overt BP.[35–37] When hypersomnia is present, individuals are at increased risk for the onset of an MDE, recurrence of an MDE, and a protracted or treatment-resistant MDE. Hypersomnia may be less responsive to treatment than other depressive symptoms and may persist past remission of an MDE.[34]

In the Diagnostic and Statistical Manual of Mental Disorders, 4th Edition, Text Revision, Mood Disorders, hypersomnia is one of the secondary diagnostic criteria for an MDE, and one of the primary diagnostic criteria for applying the parenthetic modifier of atypical depression to an MDE.[38] In addition to the presence of hypersomnia, atypical depressions are characterized by mood reactivity, rejection sensitivity, and other neurovegetative symptoms, including increased appetite or weight gain, leaden paralysis, and anxious or irritable mood.[39]

Few therapies exist specifically to address hypersomnia in the context of depression, save for morning bright-light therapy; a treatment of seasonal affective disorder.[40] This therapy targets the circadian delay, which is thought to underlie seasonal affective disorder.[41] Another intervention called interpersonal social rhythm therapy (IPSRT) may be of benefit for patients with hypersomnia

and BP. IPSRT is a psychosocial acute and maintenance intervention based on interpersonal psychotherapy and behavioral principles.[42] IPSRT was developed based on the belief that regular and stable social routines and interpersonal relationships have a protective effect. Accordingly, although psychological in nature, IPSRT is theorized to exert therapeutic effects, in part, by directly or indirectly shifting, resetting, or stabilizing biologic systems implicated in mood disorders. Typically, a course of IPSRT includes 16 to 20 acute sessions followed by monthly booster sessions for 1 year. IPSRT is conceptualized as an adjunctive treatment to pharmacotherapy for bipolar I disorder and as either an adjunctive or monotherapy for other disorders, including bipolar II and bipolar spectrum disorders.[43]

Box 3 describes steps involved IPSRT. Treatment is conceptualized as including an initial, intermediate, maintenance, and termination phase. The initial phase focuses on the extent to which disruptions in the individual's social routines, interpersonal relationships, or social roles precipitated new episodes or symptom exacerbations. The individual completes a social rhythm metric (SRM), which provides information about the regularity of the individual's social routines. The SRM is a self-report diary of mood and specified activities, such as going to bed or eating dinner.[44] The activities are thought to have a relatively strong influence

---

Box 3
Components of Frank's IPSRT

1. Evaluation for pharmacotherapy

2. Assessment of illness course and the extent to which disruptions in social routines, interpersonal problems, or social role transitions were associated with illness episodes

3. Psychoeducation

4. Assessment of the quality of interpersonal relationships

5. Assessment of the regularity of social routines with the SRM

6. Selection of an interpersonal problem area: grief for the lost healthy self, role transitions, interpersonal role disputes, interpersonal deficits, or unresolved grief

7. Stabilization of social rhythms

8. Resolution of selected interpersonal problem area

9. Maintenance of good interpersonal and social role functioning

on circadian rhythms, and were, during instrument development, selected from a larger set of possible zeitgebers based on results from factor analysis. Clinicians may focus on interpersonal problem areas, which may become a primary focus of treatment. Possible problem areas include grief for the lost healthy self, role transitions, interpersonal role disputes, interpersonal deficits, and unresolved grief. During the intermediate phase of treatment, the clinician helps the individual regularize his or her social rhythms and resolve the interpersonal problem area. The maintenance phase of treatment involves helping the individual maintain good interpersonal relationships and regular social routines, anticipate possible disruptions, and minimize such disruptions.

COGNITIVE-BEHAVIORAL INTERVENTION FOR HYPERSOMNIA

The authors are aware of only one empirical report detailing initial efforts to develop a specific treatment for hypersomnia.[34] Cognitive-behavioral intervention for hypersomnia (CB-H) is a multicomponent 4- to 8-session treatment. This intervention is in the early stages of treatment development, refinement, and efficacy testing. Kaplan and Harvey[34] (2009) are developing this treatment to target psychological mechanisms contributing to the maintenance of hypersomnia and functional impairment resulting from hypersomnia.

In CB-H, the clinician uses interviews and information from standard sleep diaries with supplemental questions to uncover psychological and contextual

---

Box 4
Components of Kaplan and Harvey hypersomnia intervention

1. Functional analysis
2. Motivational interviewing
3. Goal setting
4. Psychoeducation
5. Sleep-wake scheduling
6. Behavioral experimentation
7. Relapse prevention

---

variables that may contribute to the individual's hypersomnia. With motivational interviewing, the clinician explores the individual's reasons for and against undergoing treatment and managing his or her hypersomnia. Initially, with goal setting, the clinician helps the individual determine sleep and life goals and delineate small steps, and solutions to possible obstacles, toward the goals. Later, with psychoeducation and sleep scheduling, the clinician teaches the individual about circadian rhythms, sleep inertia, and the importance of sleep-wake routines and regularity. Behavioral experimentation allows the clinician to help the individual devise experiments to test his or her beliefs about sleep. Finally, at treatment termination, the clinician helps the individual review his or her treatment gains, and explores ways the individual may maintain such gains and prevent a relapse of his or her hypersomnia (**Box 4**).

Table 1
Causes of hypersomnia

Causes	Suggested Non-Pharmacologic Treatment

Narcolepsy	• Maintenance of regular sleep-wake schedule
	• Regularly scheduled napping
	    ◦ Short (15-min) naps early in the day or
	    ◦ Longer (2-h) naps midday
	• CB-H

Idiopathic hypersomnolence	• Maintenance of regular sleep-wake schedule • CB-H
Hypersomnolence despite CPAP therapy	• Systematic desensitization • Motivational enhancement therapy • CPAP re-titration • CB-H
Circadian rhythm sleep disorder	• Appropriately timed light exposure • CB-H
Unipolar and bipolar depression	• Interpersonal social rhythm therapy • CB-H

SUMMARY

Depending on the clinical history and patient characteristics, behavioral therapies may be a beneficial supplement to the ongoing pharmacologic management. An appreciation of patient preferences regarding medication use, lifestyle, and whether there are other comorbid conditions helps the clinician choose the behavioral strategies that may be most feasible. Ensuring that the patient practices adequate sleep hygiene (see **Box 2**) can be an initial step in managing hypersomnolence. Many healthy adults who are experiencing hypersomnolence can benefit from a short, 15- to 30-minute nap, but the nap should be timed in the mid-afternoon to prevent sleep disruption. Patients who are not using a stimulant medication or are on a drug holiday may benefit from longer naps scheduled in the late morning. In young adults, who are often sleep deprived due to psychosocial influences, a regular sleep-wake schedule may help to improve daytime alertness.

The specific behavioral management strategy the clinician choses to use may vary depending on the parent disorder (**Table 1**). Adding behavioral treatments to stimulant regimens is common in patients with narcolepsy. Regularizing the sleep-wake schedule and scheduled brief naps may be helpful. Longer naps can improve daytime symptoms, but this improvement may dissipate after only a few hours in the absence of a stimulant medication. Extension of the nocturnal sleep period has not been shown to be beneficial in narcolepsy or idiopathic hypersomnolence. Patients with sleep apnea may still experience hypersomnolence despite CPAP usage; therefore napping, sleep scheduling, desensitization to CPAP mask, or a CPAP re-titration study may be considered. Hypersomnolence in circadian rhythm sleep disorder may benefit from phototherapy, which realigns the individual's internal biologic clock to the external social environment. In unipolar depression, hypersomnolence can occur in up to 30% of patients. IPSRT (see **Box 3**) is a psychological treatment that may help with hypersomnolence in BP because it uses an SRM that is thought to have a strong influence on circadian rhythms. At present, there is only 1 psychological treatment specifically developed to target hypersomnia. CB-H (see **Box 4**) is a treatment provided in the early stages of development. Randomized clinical trials are needed for CB-H and other non-pharmacologic strategies for managing hypersomnolence.

REFERENCES

1. Wise MS. Treatment of narcolepsy and other hypersomnias of central origin. Sleep 2007;30(12):1712–27.
2. Rogers AE. Scheduled sleep periods as an adjuvant treatment for narcolepsy. In: Perlis ML, Aloia MS, Kuhn B, editors. Behavioral treatments for sleep disorders: a comprehensive primer of behavioral sleep medicine interventions, vol. 1. London: Academic Press; 2011. p. 237–9.
3. Chasens E, Sereika S, Weaver T, et al. Daytime sleepiness, exercise, and physical function in older adults. J Sleep Res 2007;16(1):60–5.
4. Espana R, McCormack S, Mochizuki T, et al. Running promotes wakefulness and increases cataplexy in orexin knockout mice. Sleep 2007;30(11):1417–25.
5. Johnson A, Jenks R, Miles C, et al. Chewing gum moderates multi-task induced shifts in stress, mood, and alertness. A re-examination. Appetite 2011;56(2):408–11.
6. Manber R. The effects of regularizing sleep-wake schedules on daytime sleepiness. Sleep 1996;19(5):432–41.
7. Takahashi M. Maintenance of alertness and performance by a brief nap after lunch under prior sleep deficit. Sleep 2000;23(6):813–9.
8. Wesensten NJ. Maintaining alertness and performance during sleep deprivation: modafinil versus caffeine. Psychopharmacology (Berl) 2002;159(3):238–47.
9. Reyner LA. Suppression of sleepiness in drivers: combination of caffeine with a short nap. Psychophysiology 1997;34(6):721–5.
10. Takahashi M. The role of prescribed napping in sleep medicine. Sleep Med Rev 2003;7(3):227–35.
11. Cohen FL. Symptom description and management in narcolepsy. Holist Nurs Pract 1996;10(4):44–53.
12. Uchiyama M, Mayer G, Meier-Ewert K. Differential effects of extended sleep in narcoleptic patients. Electroencephalogr Clin Neurophysiol 1994;91(3):212–8.
13. Rogers AE. A comparison of three different sleep schedules for reducing daytime sleepiness in narcolepsy. Sleep 2001;24(4):385–91.
14. Mullington J, Broughton R. Scheduled naps in the management of daytime sleepiness in narcolepsy-cataplexy. Sleep 1993;16:444–56.
15. Helmus T. The alerting effects of short and long naps in narcoleptic, sleep deprived, and alert individuals. Sleep 1997;20(4):251–7.
16. Weaver T, Maislin G, Dinges D, et al. Relationship between hours of CPAP use and achieving normal levels of sleepiness and daily functioning. Sleep 2007;30(6):711–9.

17. Santamaria J, Iranzo A, Ma Montserrat J, et al. Persistent sleepiness in CPAP treated obstructive sleep apnea patients: evaluation and treatment. Sleep Med Rev 2007;11:195–207.

18. Weaver T, Chasens E, Arora S. Modafinil improves functional outcomes in patients with residual excessive sleepiness associated with CPAP treatment. J Clin Sleep Med 2009;5(6):499–505.

19. Aloia M, Arnedt J, Stepnowsky C, et al. Predicting treatment adherence in obstructive sleep apnea using principles of behavior change. J Clin Sleep Med 2007;1(4):346–53.

20. Aloia M, Smith K, Arnedt J, et al. Brief behavioral therapies reduce early positive airway pressure discontinuation rates in sleep apnea syndrome: preliminary findings. Behav Sleep Med 2007;5(2): 89–104.

21. Morgenthaler T, Lee-Chiong T, Alessi C, et al. Practice parameters for the clinical evaluation and treatment of circadian rhythm sleep disorders: an American Academy of Sleep Medicine Report. Sleep 2007;30(11):1445–59.

22. Cajochen C. Alerting effects of light. Sleep Med Rev 2007;11:453–64.

23. Zeitzer J, Khalsa S, Boivin D, et al. Temporal dynamics of late-night photic stimulation of the human circadian timing system. Am J Physiol Regul Integr Comp Physiol 2005;289(3):R839–44.

24. Parry B. Jet lag: minimizing it's effects with critically timed bright light and melatonin administration. J Mol Microbiol Biotechnol 2002;4(5):463–4.

25. Horowitz T, Cade B, Wolfe J, et al. Efficacy of bright light and sleep/darkness scheduling in alleviating circadian maladaptation to night work. Am J Physiol Endocrinol Metab 2001;281(2):E384–91.

26. Gooley J. Treatment of circadian rhythm sleep disorders with light. Ann Acad Med Singapore 2008; 37(8):669–76.

27. Cajochen C, Krauchi K, Danilenko K, et al. Evening administration of melatonin and bright light: interactions on the EEG during sleep and wakefulness. J Sleep Res 1998;7:145–57.

28. Revell V, Arendt J, Fogg L, et al. Alerting effects of light are sensitive to very short wavelengths. Neurosci Lett 2006;399:96–100.

29. Chellappa S, Steiner R, Blattner P, et al. Non-visual effects of light on melatonin, alertness, and cognitive performance: can blue-enriched light keep us alert? PLoS One 2011;6(1):e16429.

30. Germain A, Kupfer D. Circadian rhythm disturbances in depression. Hum Psychopharmacol 2008;23:571–85.

31. Parker G, Hadzi-Pavlovic D, Tully L. Distinguishing bipolar and unipolar disorders: an isomer model. J Affect Disord 2006;96:67–73.

32. Tsuno N, Besset A, Ritchie K. Sleep and depression. J Clin Psychiatry 2005;66(10):1254–69.

33. Kaplan K, Gruber J, Eidelman P, et al. Hypersomnia in inter-episode bipolar disorder: does it have prognostic significance? J Affect Disord 2011;132:438–44.

34. Kaplan K, Harvey A. Hypersomnia across mood disorders: a review and synthesis. Sleep Med Rev 2009;13:275–85.

35. Akiskal H, Kilzieh N, Maser J, et al. The distinct temperament profiles of bipolar I, bipolar II, and unipolar patients. J Affect Disord 2006;92:19–33.

36. Armitage R. Sleep and circadian rhythms in mood disorders. Acta Psychiatr Scand Suppl 2007;433: 104–15.

37. Hasler G, Buysse D, Gamma A, et al. Excessive daytime sleepiness in young adults: a 20-year prospective community study. J Clin Psychiatry 2005;66:519–21.

38. American Psychiatric Association. Diagnostic and statistical manual of mental disorders (4th edition, text rev.). Washington, DC: Author; 2000.

39. Parker G, Roy K, Mitchell P, et al. Atypical depression: a reappraisal. Am J Psychiatry 2002;159(9):1480–1.

40. Lewy A, Bauer V, Cutler N. Morning vs evening light treatment of patients with winter depression. Arch Gen Psychiatry 1998;55:890–6.

41. Lewy A, Sack R, Miller L. Antidepressant and circadian phase-shifting effects of light. Science 1987; 235:352–4.

42. Frank E. Treating bipolar disorder: a clinician's guide to interpersonal and social rhythm therapy. New York: Guilford Press; 2005.

43. Swartz H, Novick D, Frank E. Psychotherapy as monotherapy for the treatment of bipolar II depression: a proof of concept study. Bipolar Disord 2009;11:89–94.

44. Monk T, Frank E, Potts J, et al. A simple way to measure daily lifestyle regularity. J Sleep Res 2002;11:183–90.

Pharmacotherapy of Excessive Sleepiness

Thomas Roth, PhD

KEYWORDS

- Pharmacotherpay • Stimulants • Excessive daytime sleepiness • Sleepiness

KEY POINTS

- Stimulants are effective in the management of excessive sleepiness, primarily through inhibition of dopamine reuptake.
- The use of any medication, especially when one is dealing with symptomatic management, is a trade-off between efficacy and safety.
- Large-scale clinical trials and multiple doses measuring the relative efficacy and safety profile of the different classes of these stimulants are necessary.

Stimulants refer to drugs that enhance alertness, improve cognitive functioning, and improve mood (**Tables 1** and **2**). These drugs historically have been used to combat fatigue and enhance waking function. Amphetamine, the most widely recognized stimulant, was developed as a synthetic substitute for ephedrine. It was cheaper to produce, and it was felt to be safer in terms of frequency and severity of adverse reactions and the development of tolerance. Stimulants were used widely by the military during World War II for soldiers in combat. In Japan, it was used to enhance the productivity in munition workers, and as a result many young people became dependent on the drug.[1]

The first medical use for stimulants was narcolepsy. Doyle and Daniels in 1931 first reported on the efficacy of ephedrine in treating narcolepsy.[2] Since that time stimulants have been the standard for the treatment of narcolepsy, and other stimulants such as methypheindate and modafinil have also become used for the treatment of sleepiness in narcolepsy. In addition, stimulants have been used in other sleep disorders as well as other medical and psychiatric conditions, albeit off label.

This history clearly points to some of the issues associated with the use stimulants. A very important question relates to the role of these drugs for medical conditions versus life style issues.

Given that these drugs target symptoms rather than disorders, there is the temptation to use these medications in a variety of medical as well as societal contexts. Also the safety of these medications is an issue as the same receptor systems, which mediate alertness, potentially cause serious cardiovascular and other side effects. Also, at least among individuals vulnerable to substance abuse, these drugs have high abuse potential. Thus the question arises as to whether the safety concerns (eg, cardiovascular, abuse liability) of stimulants require a narrow indication for use.

INDICATIONS

It is critical to recognize that stimulants are drugs that enhance alertness and improve functions that are compromised by elevated levels of sleepiness. Thus, these medications are meant for symptomatic management not disease modification or prevention. The first US Food and Drug Administration (FDA)-approved indication for stimulants was the excessive sleepiness (ES) associated with narcolepsyVarious amphetamine-related products as well as modafinil-related products have been approved for sleepiness associated with narcolepsy. It is important to remember that narcolepsy is a disorder that has a constellation of symptoms including cataplexy,

Henry Ford Hospital Sleep Center, 2799 West Grand Boulevard, CFP-3, Detroit, MI 48202, USA
E-mail address: troth1@hfhs.org

Sleep Med Clin 7 (2012) 333–340
doi:10.1016/j.jsmc.2012.03.002
1556-407X/12/$ – see front matter © 2012 Elsevier Inc. All rights reserved.

Table 1
Commonly used pharmacologic compounds for excessive daytime sleepiness

Stimulant Compound	Usual Daily Doses	$T_{1/2}$ (h)
Amphetamine and Amphetamine-like Central Nervous System Stimulants		
D-Amphetamine sulfate	5–60 mg (15 mg, 100 mg)	$T_{1/2}$ 16–30
Methamphetamine HCl	5–60 mg (15 mg, 80 mg)	$T_{1/2}$ 9–15
Methylphenidate HCl	10–60 mg (30 mg, 100 mg)	$T_{1/2}$ 3
Pemoline	20–115 mg (37.5 mg, 150 mg)	$T_{1/2}$ 11–13
Dopamine or Norepinephrine Uptake Inhibitor		
Mazindol	2–6 mg	$T_{1/2}$ 10–13
Other Agents for Treatment of Excessive Daytime Sleepiness		
Modafinil	100–400 mg	$T_{1/2}$ 9–14
Armodafinil	150–250 mg	$T_{1/2}$ 10–15
Sodium oxybate	4.5–9 mg per night	$T_{1/2}$ 30–60 min
Monoamine Oxidase Inhibitor with Alerting Effect		
Selegiline	5–40 mg	$T_{1/2}$ 2
Xanthine Derivative		
Caffeine	100–200 mg	$T_{1/2}$ 3–7

hypnogogic hallucinations, and sleep paralysis.[3] Stimulants have no effects on these symptoms. A final symptom associated with narcolepsy is disturbed nocturnal sleep. Stimulants depending on dose and time of ingestion have the potential to further disturb sleep thereby further compromising alertness. There is one drug indicated for the treatment of narcolepsy, sodium oxybate, which has as an indication for both sleepiness and cataplexy and has been shown to improve disturbed sleep.[4]

More recently, modafinil and its isomer have been studied and approved for refractory sleepiness associated with obstructive sleep apnea (OSA) as well as shift work disorder (SWD).[5,6] It is important to clarify that these medications do not improve the OSA per se or the circadian mismatch seen in SWD; they merely improve the sleepiness produced by these disorders. This improvement in alertness is important from the point of improving safety and productivity and overall quality of life. However, sleepiness is typically the major symptom of concern for the patient. Given that the medications improve this symptom, the clinician needs to monitor the continued adherence to treatment for the primary disorder. The demonstrated efficacy of modafinil and armoafinil in these 3 specific conditions reflects the fact that stimulants seem to work for sleepiness arising from different etiologies. In the case of narcolepsy, the sleepiness is due to a central nervous system (CNS) pathology (ie, orexin deficiency), while for OSA, it is due to sleep fragmentation, which is functionally the same as sleep deprivation. Finally in SWD, the sleepiness is due

to circadian factors in that shift workers, who fail to adjust their circadian cycle to night work and are trying to maintain wakefulness and function during the down part of their circadian cycle.

The other stimulants have not been studied in OSA and SWD, and hence not approved for these 2 indications. Given that other stimulants are effective for treating sleepiness in narcolepsy, one might infer that they can be used for these other indications as well. This is not the case. First given the cardiovascular effects of the traditional stimulants, their use safety in an OSA population, in whom there is an increased prevalence of hypertension and other cardiovascular disorders, is of concern. Similarly to the extent that the duration of action of a stimulant impinges on the sleep period, there is the potential to disturb sleep which is already present in SWD.[7] In addition, the dose of medication needed to treat the level of sleepiness seen in different conditions needs to be empirically determined. In the case of both modafinil as well as rmodafinil, the dose shown to be effective and hence the FDA-approved dose in SWD, is lower than that indicated for narcolepsy. Thus until the dose-related efficacy and safety of a given drug in various ES populations are determined, their off-label use is ill advised.

Aside from these indications, stimulants, and especially the more recently developed ones, are used off label for sleepiness due to other sleep disorders such as Kelin Levine syndrome, idiopathic CNS hypersomnolence, sleepiness due to neurologic disorders such as Parkinson disease, multiple sclerosis, closed head injury,

Table 2
Safety of commonly used pharmacologic compounds for excessive daytime sleepiness

Stimulant Compound	Schedule	Adverse Events	Special Comments
Amphetamine and Amphetamine-like Central Nervous System Stimulants			
D-Amphetamine sulfate	II	Irriitability, mood changes, headaches, palpitations, tremors, excessive sweating, insomnia	Black box warning regarding high potential for abuse
Methamphetamine HCl	II	Same as D-amphetamine	Same as D-amphetamine
Methylphenidate HCl	II	Same as D-amphetamine	Same as D-amphetamine
Pemoline	IV	Less sympathomimetic effect; occasionally produces liver toxicity	Has been withdrawn form the US market
Dopamine or Norepinephrine Uptake Inhibitor			
Mazindol	IV	Dry mouth, irritability, headaches, gastrointestinal symptoms	
Other Agents for Treatment of Excessive Daytime Sleepiness			
Modafinil	IV	Headaches, nausea, anxiety, insomnia, nervousness	
Armodafinil	IV	Same as Modafinil;	
Sodium oxybate	II	hallucinations or severe confusion; shallow breathing; sleepwalking; or walking and confused behavior at night; agitation or paranoia; depression	Black box warning
Monoamine Oxidase Inhibitor with Alerting Effect			
Selegiline		Dizziness, dry mouth, light-headedness, nausea, stomach pain, vivid dreams	
Xanthine Derivative			
Caffeine		Palpitations, hypertension	

and sleepiness associated with psychiatric disorders such as bipolar disorder, atypical depression and seasonal affective disorder.[7–9] Finally, these medications have been used to treat sleepiness and fatigue in patients undergoing chemotherapy.[10] It must be recognized that while there are individual published studies of the use of stimulants, typically modafinil, in these populations, there are no large-scale clinical trials defining the appropriate dose or the safety of the medication in that specific population. While the ability to enhance alertness and improve waking function seems to be present in different populations, safety may not be the same. Thus, cardiovascular side effects would be a bigger issue in OSA patients. Similarly, in bipolar patients, the possibility of increased alertness driving a manic episode is a possible concern. Finally, there are uses of stimulants that inherently seem

inappropriate. A clear example of where stimulants are inappropriate is chronic insufficient sleep.[11] Stimulants are intended in conditions where sleepiness, while excessive in severity, is stable. Thus using appropriate dose–response studies, it can be determined what is the appropriate therapeutic dose for this level if sleepiness. However, in the case of chronic insufficient sleep, the level of sleepiness is not stable, but rather is increasing as a function of accumulating sleep drive necessitating progressively higher doses to maintain a constant level of alertness. This is the experience of many individuals using the stimulant caffeine.

MEASURING EFFICACY OF STIMULANTS

Given that the therapeutic action of stimulant medications is the alleviation of sleepiness, rather than a disease-altering effect, the question arises as to how to measure the efficacy of any stimulant medication. It is important recognize that sleepiness is a symptom (patient-reported outcome) that can also be quantified objectively and results in declines in various aspects of neurocognitive functioning and quality of life. As a result, there are multiple assays that are used to evaluate the efficacy of stimulants. The earliest measures of sleepiness were introspective in nature. Sleepiness is a sensation experienced by all individuals and to a greater degree among patients with disorders of ES. The primary differences between sleepiness in normal patients and ES patients is intensity and chronicity. The sensation of sleepiness is a homeostatic signal of a sleep deficit; as a result, performance (eg, driving, studying) is suboptimal, and it may be counterproductive or even dangerous to continue with the activity. The universality of this experience is seen by the presence of a sleepiness/fatigue/vigor scale on virtually all mood scales. For example, the vigor scale on the Profile of Mood States is sensitive to manipulation of sleepiness alertness. With the recognition of sleep disorders and their treatment, scales intended to specifically measure sleepiness were developed. The first of these developed and validated was the Stanford Sleepiness Scale (SSS) in 1972.[12] It is a 7-point scale, with each point having several terms describing the perceived level of sleepiness at a point in time. While it was a useful tool for experimental research, especially repeated measure studies, it was not very effective in clinical populations as it did not differentiate differing levels of sleepiness among ES patients. The Karolinska Sleepiness Scale (KSS) is similar to the ESS in that it is a validated introspective measure of sleepiness at a point in time to be able to identify changes in sleepiness over time.[13] The scale consists of 9 statements ranging from extremely alert to extremely sleepy. However, like the SSS and other introspective measures, its sensitivity declines as various factors obscure the perceived level of sleepiness. These are referred to as masking factors and include variables such as motivation, activity, and environmental stimulation. In an attempt to overcome these masking factors, a patient/subject-reported measure was developed that was based on the individual's judgment about probability of falling asleep in certain situations over a specified period of time. The Epworth Sleepiness Scale (ESS) asks individuals to judge likelihood of falling asleep in 8 different situations, which are felt to unmask sleepiness.[14] The ESS is the most widely used patient reported measure to quantify the level of sleepiness in various patient populations and to define the efficacy of stimulants. A limitation of this measure is that unlike the ESS and KSS, it does not provide for an estimate of sleepiness at a specific point in time.

While the SSS overcame some of the objections, there remain concerns about subjective measures including masking effects and differentiating the experiences of sleepiness from that of fatigue. In an attempt to overcome the subjective nature of sleepiness, many different physiologic assays of sleepiness were developed. However, the most widely accepted measure of sleepiness is the Multiple Sleep Latency Test (MSLT). It was developed by Carskadon and Dement.[15] This test has a single assumption that if one is sleepy, he or she will fall asleep rapidly. The MSLT measures sleep latency on several nap opportunities during the day. The standardized version of the test requires 4 to 5 nap opportunities at 2-hour intervals starting 2 hours after arising. The nap opportunities optimize sleep onset by using a methodology that negates all masking factors. Subjects are in a dark room quiet room; they are lying down and are told to try to fall asleep.[16] Several investigators have speculated that the efficacy of alerting drugs and other interventions should be determined by the ability to stay awake rather than to fall asleep.[17,18] Thus the MWT was developed in an attempt to measure ability to stay awake. Again the subjects have 4 to 5 nap opportunities across the day, but the subjects are not lying down. The room is not dark, and importantly subjects are told to stay awake. However, it is important to note the primary endpoint of both test sleep latency on multiple naps across the day. Currently the MSLT is considered the gold standard of measuring sleepiness/alertness as it has been more broadly validated, standardized, and has more normative data than the MWT.

Finally, the efficacy of stimulants is measured with tests of neurocognitive performance. Test of sustained attention show impairments in ES patients and improvements with the use of stimulants. The tests most sensitive to this are ones that are long, monotonous, and do not pride feedback as to level of performance. The most commonly used test is the psychomotor vigilance test (PVT), which measures reaction time to a continuous series of lights.[19] The sleepiness-related impairments are felt to be best characterized by brief periods of nonresponsivity (termed lapses). These lapses were felt to represent brief periods or microsleeps. That is, individuals with ES can in fact function normally much of the time; however, they experience minisleep episodes when they cease to function for brief periods of time. More recently, it has been observed that beyond isolated lapses in performance, the entire performance output is shifted in the direction of impaired performance. Thus, the impairment does not simply reflect infrequent microsleeeps, but rather state instability. That is, individuals who are sleepy experience a state of consciousness that is unstable. An example of a long, boring monotonous task is driving. Individuals and patient populations with ES have an increased frequency of car accidents. The standard measure of driving ability is the standard deviation of lateral position.[20] The increased variability in lateral position of the car on the highway can be thought of reflecting the state instability associated with ES.

All 3 of these measures of sleepiness/alertness have been shown to improve with the use of stimulants. In addition, while these measures are intercorrelated, the correlations are statistically significant but modest in the amount of variance accounted for (and are in the range of 0.30% to 0.50% of variance). As a result, it is thought that they reflect different aspects of sleepiness/alertness, and all should be used to quantify benefits of stimulants.

AMPHETAMINES

Amphetamine is the basic structural element in a number of stimulants that are collectively referred to as psychostimulants. The amphetamines approved for narcolepsy include dextroamphetamine, reacemic amphetamine, and several combinations of the two. Methaamphetamine has also been studied for the treatment of narcolepsy and is often used off label for this purpose. Amphetamines increase alertness, inhibit sleep activity, and improve mood and neurocognitive performance. These drugs increase alertness primarily by inhibiting the dopamine reuptake transporter and in some cases by increasing dopamine release, as well as by inhibition of adrenergic uptake. Amphetamine increases catecholamine (dopamine [DA] and norepinephrine [NE]) release and inhibits reuptake from presynaptic terminals, thereby enhancing postsynaptic stimulation. Amphetamine derivatives also work by inhibiting the DA and NE transporters. At higher doses, monoamine oxidase inhibition and reuptake blockade occur, with the potency of this activity varying among the various amphetamine derivatives.[1]

Amphetamine is rapidly absorbed from the gastrointestinal (GI) tract, reaching peak plasma within 1 to 3 hours. It is rapidly metabolized through liver enzymes, with a half-life of 10 to 12 hours. The half-life of methamphetamine is 4 to 5 hours.[21]

The amphetamines have been shown to be effective in enhancing alertness associated with several causes. The only sleep-related indication for amphetamine is narcolepsy. The wake-enhancing properties of the amphetamines are dose-related; therefore in clinical use, the dose is gradually titrated until the desired therapeutic effect is achieved. The limiting factors for dose are adverse effects and abuse liability. Even at clinical doses, amphetamine is associated with headache, disturbed sleep, jitteriness, GI disturbance, weight loss, and increased heart rate. Physiologically, increases in heart rate, blood pressure brochodilation, and vasoconstriction have been found.[22]

At high doses, in animal studies, neurotoxicity in brain dopamine and seretonin neurons occurs. In human studies, methamphetamine has been shown to lead to loss of brain dopamine transporters, at least temporarily.[23]

Tolerance is common during long-term administration of amphetamine and methamphetamine. Abuse has also been reported with these drugs. Importantly these problems are not commonly encountered in appropriately diagnosed narcolepsy patients using appropriate therapeutic doses.

METYLPHENIDATE

Methylphenidate is another stimulant that is approved for sleepiness associated with narcolepsy. Methylphenidate resembles amphetamine structurally and is in the peperidine class of compounds. The mechanism of action is primarily by binding to the norepinephrine transporter and dopamine active transporter (DAT), thereby increasing catecholamine levels. Unlike amphetamine, it does not have a major effect of presynaptic release. It is almost totally absorbed after oral ingestion, reaching peak plasma concentration within 2 hours. Additionally, it has a short duration of action with a half-life of about 3 hours. Like the amphetamines, the limitations of methylphenidate are adverse effects. However, unlike the amphetamines, it does not produce neurotoxicity, and it is generally considered to have less abuse liability than the amphetamines.[24]

MODAFINIL AND ARMODAFINIL

Modafinil is available as a racemic mixture, r and s modafinil, both of which are active, as well as the r isomer only. The R-entiomer has a half-life of 10 to 14 hours, while the S-entiomer has a half-life of 3 to 4 hours.[25] This difference in half-lives may explain why modafinil needs to be taken twice a day for maximum therapeutic benefit, at least initially while the drug is reaching steady-state. Also, the half-life of the racemate and the R-entiomer blood level of armoafinil are higher late in the day as compared with modafinil. This is attributable to the monophasic decline in plasma concentrations of armodafinil as compared with the biphasic decline seen with modafinil. Both drugs are rapidly absorbed, with peak levels being reached in about 2 hours. Both compounds have high protein binding. They are metabolized in the liver primarily by CYP3A4.

Modafinil and armodafinil are indicated for sleepiness associated with narcolepsy as well as refractory sleepiness of OSA and SWD. Because it is felt that modafinil is safer and has less abuse liability than classical stimulants, studies have been performed in a variety of off-label populations including Parkinson disease, multiple sclerosis, closed head injury, depression, bipolar disorder, and chronic fatigue syndrome.[26]

The most common adverse effects of modafinil are headache and nausea. Other, less frequently reported adverse effects include dizziness and insomnia.[25] There have been cases of rare but serious rashes reported. Finally, there have been reports of increases in blood pressure in the OSA trials and of mania and suicidal ideation in some of the psychiatric trials.[27] Because of drug interactions, women on oral contraceptives should be cautioned to use additional or alternative methods of contraception while on modafinil and for several moths after discontinuation.

While the mechanism of action of modafinil is highly debated, it is at least in part mediated by inhibition of DAT not unlike the classic stimulants. The most supportive evidence of this is the fact that modafinil effects on alertness are entirely abolished in DAT knockout mice and in mice lacking D1 and D2 receptors.[28] However, the adverse effect profile and abuse liability are lower than the other DAT inhibitors, leading many to conclude that it does not have potent effects on dopamine, and other transmitter systems are involved in its alerting producing properties. Modafinil's action appears to be mediated through multiple neurotransmitter systems including dopamine with certainty, and possibly norepinephrine, histamine, orexin, and serotonin.[25]

Modafinil is an attractive alternative to amphetamine-like stimulants because of decreased risk of abuse liability and few effects on the neuroendocine system (prolactine, cortisol and elatonin). Additionally, at therapeutic doses, it has fewer effects on the cardiovascular system.

Modafinil and armodafinil have been recommended by the American Academy of Sleep Medicine as the standard therapy for the treatment of sleepiness associated with narcolepsy and refractory sleepiness associated with OSA and SWD.

CAFFEINE

Caffeine is the most commonly used stimulant in the United States as well as the rest of the world. Caffeine is found in coffee, foods, and in energy drinks. Typically a cup of coffee contains 50 to 150 mg of caffeine, but some Starbucks coffees contain 350 mg of caffeine. Tea, chocolate and cola drinks also contain 25–50 mg of caffeine. Recently, energy drinks have become popular. The caffeine content of these varies (eg, Red Bull 100 mg, 5 hour energy drink 207 mg). Finally, there are over-the-counter products (No Doz 100 g and Vivarin 200 mg).

Caffeine is a xanthine derivative. The mechanism of action is adenosine receptor antagonism. Adenosine is thought to be the basis of the sleep hemostat accumulating during wakefulness and dissipating during sleep.[29] Population-based data show that sleep duration relates to caffeine consumption.

Caffeine has been shown to increase alertness and improve reaction time, reversing the effects of sleep deprivation and of sedative drugs, The side effects include palpitations; increased blood pressure, gastric secretions and urine production; and sleep disturbance. At high doses, it produces agitation, anxiety, tremors, and increased respiratory rate.

Caffeine is rapidly absorbed and has a relatively short half-life (3 to 5 hours). With repetitive use, the stimulatory effects of caffeine are substantially reduced over time. Tolerance develops quickly to some (but not all) effects of caffeine, especially among heavy coffee and energy drink users Withdrawal symptoms include headache, irritability, inability to concentrate, drowsiness, and insomnia, which appear within 12 to 24 hours after discontinuation of heavy caffeine use.

SUMMARY

There is no question that there are stimulants that are effective in the management of ES.[30] Virtually all currently available medications that are used to treat ES act, at least in part, through inhibition of dopamine reuptake. As such, all of these medications have efficacy but hypothesized differential safety and abuse liability. The use of any medication, especially when one is dealing with symptomatic management, is a tradeoff between efficacy and safety. One of the limitations of comparing the safety profile of these medications is that one does not know what the equally efficient doses of the different stimulant drugs are. Thus, large-scale clinical trials are needed measuring the relative efficacy and safety profile of the different classes of these stimulants at multiple doses.

Finally as more is learned about the control of sleep wake, research is needed on the wake-enhancing properties of other transmitter systems. Currently research is being done on the orexin and the histamine systems in terms of their ability to more safely produce increased alertness. Finally, the FDA-approved indications for stimulants covers only a small part of the clinical population with ES. Even within sleep disorders, most ES patients fall outside the current indications. There are no indications for ES associated with neurologic, psychiatric, or other medical disorders. Large-scale clinical trials measuring both safety and efficacy are needed in these populations. As this article clearly demonstrates, there is significant morbidity associated with ES. The role of stimulants in alleviating this morbidity needs to be more specifically defined.

REFERENCES

1. Kryger M, Roth T, Dement WC. Wake-promoting medications: basic mechanism and pharmacology. In: Kryger MH, Roth T, Dement WC, editors. Principles and practice of sleep medicine. St Louis (MO): Elsevier; 2011. p. 510–26.
2. Doyle JB, Daniels LE. Symptomatic treatment for narcolepsy. JAMA 1931;96:1370–2.
3. Mignot E. Narcolepsy: pathophysiology and genetic predisposition. In: Kryger MH, Roth T, Dement WC, editors. Principles and practice of sleep medicine. St Louis (MO): Elsevier; 2011. p. 510–26.
4. The Xyrem International Study Group. A double-blind placeo controlled study demonstrates sodium oxybate is effective for the treatment of excessive daytime sleepiness in narcolepsy. J Clin Sleep Med 2005;1:391–7.
5. Schwartz J, Hirshkowtiz M, Erman M, et al. Modafinil as adjunct therapy for daytime sleepiness in obstructive sleep apnea. Chest 2003;124:2192–9.
6. Czeisler C, Walsh J, Wesnes K, et al. Armodafinil for treatment of excessive sleepiness associated with shift work disorder: a randomized controlled study. Mayo Clin Proc 2009;11:958–72.
7. Drake CL, Roehrs T, Richardson G, et al. Shift work sleep disorder: prevalence and consequences beyond that of symptomatic day workers. Sleep 2004;27(8):1–10.
8. Chellappa SL, Cajochen C. Depression and sleepiness: a chronobiological approach. In: Thorpy MJ, Billiard M, editors. Sleepiness causes, consequences and treatment. Cambridge (UK): University Press; 2011. p. 279–91.
9. Rye DB. Excessive daytime sleepiness in Parkinson's disease. In: Thorpy MJ, Billiard M, editors. Sleepiness causes, consequences and treatment. Cambridge (UK): University Press; 2011. p. 301–15.
10. Jean-Pierre P, Marrow GR, Roscoe JA, et al. A phase III randomized, placebo-controlled, double-blind clinical trial of the effect of modafinil on cancer-related fatigue among 631 patients receiving chemotherapy: a URCC CCOP research base study. Cancer 2010;116:3513–20.
11. Roehrs T, Zorick F, Sicklesteel J, et al. Excessive Daytime Sleepiness Associated With Insufficient Sleep. Sleep 1983;6:319–25.
12. Hoddes E, Zarcone V, Smythe H, et al. Quantification of sleppiness: a new approach. Psychophysiology 1973;10:431–6.
13. Horne JA, Baulk SD. Awareness of sleepiness when driving. Psychophysiology 2004;41:161–5.
14. Johns MW. Reliability and factor analysis of the Epworth Sleepiness Scale. Sleep 1992;15:376–81.
15. Carskadon MA, Dement WC. Effects of total sleep loss on sleep tendency. Percept Mot Skills 1979; 48:495–506.
16. Carskadon M, Dement WC, Mitler MM, et al. Guidelines for the multiple sleep latency test (MSLT): a standard measure of sleepiness. Sleep 1986;9:519–24.
17. Hartse KM, Roth T, Piccione PM, et al. Rebound insomnia. Science 1980;208:423.
18. Mitler M, Gujavarty K, Browman CP. Maintenance of wakeful test: a polysomnographic technique for evaluating treatment in patients with excessive somnolence. Electroencephalogr Clin Neurophysiol 1982;153:658–61.
19. Doran SM, Van Dongen HP, Dinges DF. Sustained attention performance during sleep deprivation: evidence of state instability. Arch Ital Biol 2001; 139:253–67.
20. Verster JC, Roth T. Standard operation procedures for conducting the on-the-road driving test, and measurement of the standard deviation of lateral position (SDLP). Int J Gen Med 2011;4:359–71.
21. Mignot E, Nishino S. Pathophysiological and pharmacologic aspects of the sleep disorder narcolepsy. In: Davis KL, Charney D, Cole JT, et-al, editors. Neuropsychopharmacology: the fifth generation of progress. Philadelphia: Lippincott, Williams and Wilkins; 2022. p. 1907–22.
22. Miller MA, Huges AL. Epidemiology of amphentamine use in the United States. In: Cha AK, Segal DS, editors. Amphetamine and its analogs: psychopharmacology, toxicology and abuse. New York: Academic Press; 1994. p. 439–57.
23. Seiden LS, Fischman MW, Schuster CR. Long-term methamphetamine induced changes in brain catecholamines in tolerant rhesus monkeys. Drug Alcohol Depend 1976;1:215–9.
24. McCann UD. Amphetamines, methylphenidate and excessive sleepiness. In: Thorpy MJ, Billiard M, editors. Sleepiness causes, consequences and treatment. Cambridge (UK): University Press; 2011. p. 401–7.

25. Nuvigil (armodafinil) tables prescribing information. (tables prescribing information, 2009). Available at: http://www.nuvigil.com/media/full-prescribing-information.pdf. Accessed March 3, 2012.

26. Monderer R, Thorpy MJ. Modafinil/armodafinil in the treatment of excessive daytime sleepiness. In: Thorpy MJ, Billiard M, editors. Sleepiness causes, consequences and treatment. Cambridge (UK): University Press; 2011. p. 408–20.

27. DeBattista C, Dogramji M, Menza M, et al. Adjunct modafinil for short-term treatment of fatigue and sleepiness in patients with major depressive disorder: a preliminary double-blind, placebo-controlled study. J Clin Psychiatry 2003;64:1057–64.

28. Wisor JP, Nishino S, Sora I, et al. Dopaminergic role in stimulant-induced wakefulness. J Neurosci 2001; 21:1787–94.

29. Porkka-Heiskanen T, Strecker RE, Thakkar M, et al. Adenosine: a mediator of the sleep-inducing effects of prolonged wakefulness. Science 1997; 276:1265–8.

30. Wise MS, Arand DL, Auger RR, et al. Treatment of narcolepsy and other hypersomnia of central origin. Sleep 2007;30:1712–27.

Quality of Life in Narcolepsy

Meeta Goswami, BDS, MPH, PhD

KEYWORDS

- Narcolepsy • Health-related quality of life in narcolepsy • Psychosocial management of narcolepsy
- Non-pharmacologic management of narcolepsy

KEY POINTS

- Hypersomnia in narcolepsy greatly affects the psychosocial and economic burden to the patient and society, pointing to the importance of early diagnosis and biopsychosocial management.
- Educational programs must be directed toward professionals and the public to create greater sensitivity to the wide-ranging effects of hypersomnolence on the lives of patients and their families.
- A multidisciplinary team, with the patient as a team member, pursuing a person-centered and family-centered approach, including a monitoring strategy to identify patients' perceived barriers to accessing treatment and adhering to treatment plan, contributes to optimal delivery of health care and improves the quality of life in patients.

With a steady increase in the aging population and a rise in chronic illnesses, mortality and morbidity statistics are not sufficient to determine the effects of health interventions; hence, quality of life (QOL) indicators have gained significance in evaluating outcomes. Most patients would like to reduce the levels of discomfort and disability associated with illness and increase general satisfaction with their lives. Data gathered from QOL studies could be useful in the national health surveillance system[1] and in channeling resources according to the expressed needs of the population. Planning and policy would be affected. Studies on QOL are important in evaluating health programs, justifying funding, and making appropriate changes in program development. Health agencies can consider collaboration with health partners, including social service agencies, community planners, and business groups.[2] This approach has the added benefit of reducing duplication and overuse of services, thus lowering costs.

From patients' point of views, most of them would like their physicians to go beyond the physiopathologic level of health services and care for them from a total patient perspective. They would like to be seen as individuals first and not as disease entities; so comprehensive therapy can be tailored to patients' needs by incorporating results from QOL studies, preventive measures can be instituted to avert serious consequences of the disorder/condition or health behavior, the treatment may have to be modified, appropriate referral to a health or social agency can be made, and follow-up monitoring programs may be instituted. Furthermore, results of such studies could be valuable for family members in understanding the patient's disability and in providing an effective support system.[3] Whereas clinicians tend to focus on symptoms as indicators of severity or absence of disease, patients, on the other hand, may be more concerned about the symptoms as they affect their social functioning. They may learn to live with their disorder if reasonable functioning is possible. Biomedical effectiveness of treatment may not be acceptable to patients if the side reactions or long-term effects of medications impinge

The author has received grants from Cephalon Inc. and Jazz Pharmaceuticals Inc. There is no conflict of interest.
Narcolepsy Institute, Sleep-Wake Disorders Center, Montefiore Medical Center, Department of Neurology, Albert Einstein College of Medicine, 111 East 210 Street, Bronx, NY 10467, USA
E-mail address: mgoswami@aol.com

on their social roles. For instance, certain stimulants, especially amphetamines, in the treatment of excessive daytime sleepiness may cause irritability, hyperactivity, sweating, tremors, mood changes,[4] and dyskinesias[5]; the adverse effects of some tricyclic antidepressants for cataplexy on erectile dysfunction have been noted.[6,7] These adverse effects diminish the QOL of patients and reduce compliance with treatment regimen. Thus, QOL studies generate data that may be applied to improve overall quality of care in patients.

THEORETICAL CONSIDERATIONS IN DEVELOPING QOL INDICATORS

The physical, mental, social, and spiritual facets of health are important considerations in a paradigm that examines the construct of QOL in terms of one's aspirations of finding a purpose and meaning to life. How can the facilitators and barriers to fulfillment of human potential be studied scientifically? An approach is to narrow the gap between the person's expectations and reality by enhancing function with treatment and accepting limitations with appropriate counseling.[8–10]

Generally, 5 dimensions of health are considered in defining health-related QOL (HRQOL), that is, physical health (including pain), emotional state (including concentration and memory), intellectual function, performance of social roles, and general feelings of well-being or life satisfaction.[11–13] Others have proposed subjective well-being, health, and welfare. Subjective well-being refers to individuals' perceptions of their life situations. Health is a subjective as well as an objective evaluation of physical and mental status, and welfare reflects the objective environmental factors.[14] Subjective well-being[15] and the social dimension of treatment-related subjective health, such as social performance and social well-being, the role of social support, and implications of social adjustment,[16] are important considerations in developing meaningful QOL indicators. In most QOL measuring instruments, professionals select the domains and generally measure function. However, some individuals with disabilities adapt to their compromised health status and are quite happy. How can scientists capture the factor that determines this differential response to disability? How can we measure the saliency of different areas of life that are meaningful to the individual? To address this question, the Individual Quality of Life Interview and The Duggan-Dijkers Approach are among several instruments that incorporate individuals' choices of domains and aspirations that are meaningful to them.[17]

The World Health Organization defines QOL as individuals' "perception of their position in life in the context of the culture and value systems in which they live, and in relation to their goals, expectations, standards and concerns."[18] Following this definition, satisfaction with life is based on individual perception and is culturally influenced. The role of sociocultural environment and spirituality on one's perception of life, health, and disability has been discussed[19] and studied, and questionnaires have been developed to include items that measure these determinants of health and well-being.[20–22] Spiritual QOL is most closely associated with the psychological domain, particularly hope, optimism, and inner peace, and "makes a significant and distinctive contribution to QOL assessment in health."[23]

MEASUREMENT OF QOL

Instruments measuring QOL may be generic or disease specific. Generic measures are generally longer than disease-specific ones, have a wider scope, and combine into global or overall scores. They are useful in making comparisons between different health conditions and in elucidating differences across demographic and cultural groups. They are used to formulate policy and allocate resources. Listed below are selected generic measures that provide a health profile for certain components of HRQOL and some disease-specific measures:

Generic measures

- Sickness Impact Profile (SIP)[24]
- Nottingham Health Profile[25]
- McMaster Health Index[26]
- Quality of Well-Being scale[27]
- Medical Outcomes Study–Short Form.[28]

Disease-specific measures

- Clinical Interview for Depression[29]
- Arthritis Impact Measurement Scales[30]
- Quality of Life Index (cancer)[31]
- Diabetes Control and Complications Trial Questionnaire[32]
- Functional Outcomes of Sleep Questionnaire (FOSQ).[33]

Disease-specific instruments are suitable for assessing clinically important changes of health interventions in specific conditions or diagnostic categories or in special populations. A combination of both types of measures (generic and disease specific) would ensure comprehensiveness and scope.[19] Incorporating objective and subjective measures is another method of producing a comprehensive instrument. The QOL instrument should have sensitivity to changes over time with high discriminative power, be easy to administer, and be clear to the respondent to increase the response rate. The instrument should be reliable, that is, reproducible and stable, and have high internal consistency or validity.[19,34,35] Selection biases, method of recruiting subjects, training of interviewers, the type of instrument and method of administration, the year when the study was conducted, and the order of items in the questionnaire affect the quality of data gathered and the response rate. The instrument should have high external validity (generalizability) and must be pretested on the population under study. Confounding variables such as sociodemographic variables, stressful life events, multiple diseases, and medications for other diseases must be considered in interpreting results. For instance, age may be related to depression, sleep disorders, and memory problems. Gender may be related to social roles and physiology. The questionnaire must be user friendly from the respondent's perspective. Certain items may "produce emotional upset...researchers and clinicians should understand how an instrument's theoretical focus will have influenced domains, items, and scoring."[36]

SELECTED HRQOL INSTRUMENTS

The 36-Item Short Form Health Survey (SF-36) is a comprehensive generic measure with high reliability and validity and is the most frequently used instrument to asses HRQOL; its shorter versions are Short Form 12 and Short Form 8,[37,38] and an SF-36 version 2 has improved wording and instructions, better internal consistency and reliability, and reduced floor and ceiling effects compared with the older version.[39,40] The instrument measures 8 dimensions: physical functioning, role functioning-physical, role functioning-emotional, mental health, social functioning, vitality, bodily pain, and general health. It does not ask questions about sleep and uses vitality as a proxy, a term that can be misinterpreted by the respondent. Vitality is included in the mental health summary score but correlates significantly with both mental and physical health.[41]

SIP is a generic measure of functional status of patients with chronic illness with high reliability and validity. It includes 136 items grouped in 12 categories, namely, sleep and rest, alertness behavior, work, mobility, ambulation, body care and movement, eating, recreation and pastimes, home management, communication, social interaction, and emotional behavior.[42] This instrument is more suitable for those with severe disabilities and may not be appropriate for studies of narcolepsy.

The FOSQ is a disease-specific tool that measures activity level, vigilance, intimacy and sexual relationships, general productivity, and social outcome. Its 35 items assess the impact of excessive daytime sleepiness in physical, mental, and social functioning in daily activities. The instrument has good reliability and validity, construct validity with the Epworth Sleepiness Scale, and also concurrent validity with the SIP and SF-36.[33]

The World Health Organization Quality of Life Assessment (WHOQOL-100) is a cross-cultural validated instrument of HRQOL developed collaboratively in some 4500 respondents in 15 cultural settings and has 100 items to assess QOL. The instrument produces a multidimensional profile of scores across 6 domains and 24 subdomains or facets of QOL. It is organized into 6 broad domains of QOL: (1) physical, (2) psychological, (3) level of independence, (4) social relationships, (5) environment, and (6) spirituality/religion/personal beliefs.[43,44] It has been validated across different countries and illnesses or conditions.[45] The WHOQOL-BREF is a 26-item version of the WHOQOL-100 questionnaire developed in the context of 4 domains related to QOL: physical health, psychological health, social relationships, and environment. It also includes one facet on overall QOL and general health. Cross-sectional data were gathered from 23 countries (n = 11,830) and analyzed. It was determined to have good reliability and validity as indicated by analyses of internal consistency, item-total correlations, discriminant validity, and construct validity.[43,46] Recently, the WHOQOL-BREF was found to be a high-quality patient-centered generic tool suited to individual assessment in clinics and for research and audit.[47] Its validity and reliability have been established in many countries and across different illnesses. It is a useful generic tool for cross-cultural comparisons and comprehensive evaluation and for conducting epidemiologic studies.[48–51] Its strengths lie in sound conceptual and methodical design, sensitivity to the meaning of different aspects of life to the patient, and its relative ease of administration in generating a profile of 4 domains with a smaller set of 26 items compared with the WHOQOL-100.[52]

REVIEW OF STUDIES ON NARCOLEPSY AND QOL

Several publications have discussed the negative psychosocial effects of narcolepsy on work, education, recreation, personality, interpersonal relations, marital life, and intimacy.[53–59] Although most persons with narcolepsy (PWN) (61%) were employed full-time or part-time in one survey, the unemployment rate was higher (13%) than the national US average (7.5%).[60] Hypersomnolence is a risk factor for automobile accidents,[61,62] and PWN have poor driving records.[63] In one study, patients with sleep apnea and narcolepsy accounted for 71% of all sleep-related accidents, and the rate of sleep-related accidents was highest in the narcolepsy group.[64] Compared with matched controls, drivers involved in automobile accidents show significantly more sleepiness, slower reaction times, and a trend for greater objective sleepiness.[65] Among the patients reporting driving habits in Japan, an Epworth Sleepiness Score (ESS) of 16 or more was positively associated with the experience of automobile accidents.[66] Other accidents reported by patients include falls, burns from objects and cigarettes, burning food while cooking, dropping things, and walking into a glass door.

Frequently, 10 to 15 years elapse from inception of symptoms to obtaining a correct diagnosis because of denial, misdiagnosis, and misunderstanding of symptoms and complaints by the patient. During this period, the individual is unable to fulfill role obligations, feels isolated, develops low self-esteem, and develops defense mechanisms to cope with illness. In support groups and conferences for patients, they often complain about lack of understanding from family, co-workers, and friends. Procrastination, undertaking and completing assignments, punctuality, planning and organizing time, issues with memory and concentration, low levels of motivation, and decision making are areas of concern to many patients.[3] Patients present concerns about traveling alone and the social stigma of having narcolepsy.[67] Fatigue is a major hindrance to executing activities of daily living. Recently, a study demonstrated lack of perseverance and a selective reduced performance on decision making under ambiguity in narcolepsy with cataplexy in contrast to normal decision making under explicit conditions; patients with narcolepsy-cataplexy may opt for choices with higher immediate emotional rewards, regardless of higher future punishment, to compensate for their reduced reactivity to emotional stimuli.[68]

Contrary to findings that depression is a common feature in narcolepsy[69–71] with rates ranging from 25% in Italy[72] to 55.1% in France[73] and to 56.9% in the UK[74] and 49% versus 9% to 31% of the normal population in the United States,[75] a study in the United Kingdom found that narcolepsy is neither associated with psychiatric disorders nor with diagnosable depressive disorders. Variance in sample size and characteristics, lack of

standardized measures of symptoms, selection bias, variable effects of medications (from amphetamines to modafinil [Provigil]), and confusing hypnagogic hallucinations of narcolepsy, especially auditory hallucinations, with schizophrenia could explain some of these differences in results.[76] There were no differences in the depression rates between narcolepsy with cataplexy and narcolepsy without cataplexy.[77] Negative effects on mental health[78] and neurocognitive deficits are observed in narcolepsy.[79] Reduced vigilance, attention, and execution with slower response time in PWN compared with healthy controls are reported.[80,81] Hypnagogic hallucinations are very bothersome to some patients and can be very frightening when they occur simultaneously with cataplexy or sleep paralysis.[60]

In the United States, in a national randomized and controlled investigation of HRQOL in narcolepsy,[82] the SF-36 and supplemental narcolepsy-specific scales were pretested in 2 sleep centers before administration.[83] The survey compared scores for patients with narcolepsy with scores for those with epilepsy and Parkinson disease and for the general population. Patients with narcolepsy reported significant role limitations caused by physical problems, lower vitality, lower social functioning, and role limitations due to emotional problems. The data revealed that SF-46 scores on overall impairment parameters, including physical function, role limitation, physical function, bodily pain, general health, social function, vitality, and mental health, for PWN were similar to those for patients with Parkinson disease and even greater than those for patients with epilepsy (except bodily pain) (**Fig. 1**).

In the United Kingdom, treated PWN had significantly lower SF-36 scores than those treated for obstructive sleep apnea–hypopnea syndrome (OSAHS) for mental health and general health, and no significant differences were observed between patients who were treated for narcolepsy and patients with OSAHS who were not treated. PWN had difficulties in relation to leisure activities; subjects reported falling asleep in class (50%), at work (67%), and when losing or leaving a job because of narcolepsy (52%).[71] Similarly, in a mailed questionnaire survey of 305 members of the United Kingdom Association of Narcolepsy, respondents scored significantly lower on all domains of the SF-36 compared with age-matched and sex-matched normative data, with more pronounced differences in the physical, energy/vitality, and social functioning domains. The psychosocial questions developed for this study showed that narcolepsy affected education, work, relationships, activities of daily living, and

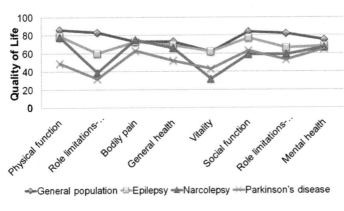

Fig. 1. HRQOL in narcolepsy data. (*Data from* Beusterien KM, Rogers AE, Walsleben JA, et al. Health-related quality of life effects of modafinil for treatment of narcolepsy. Sleep 1999;22(6):757.)

leisure activities. There was no difference among groups receiving different medications, suggesting the inadequacy of the pharmacologic management of narcolepsy.[74]

In Italy, the SF-36 was self-administered, and PWN were compared with patients with idiopathic hypersomnia and sleep apnea. All domains, except bodily pain, scored lower than the Italian norm. Some of the variance was explained by excessive daytime sleepiness (inverse relation) and disease duration (direct relation, possibly due to adaptation).[84] In a 5-year prospective survey of 54 patients in Italy, there was no significant difference between the assessments of SF-36 (self-administered) and the Zung depression scale (ZDS) in 1998 and 2003. ZDS score (inversely) and duration of disease (directly) explained a percentage of variance of role physical, vitality, social functioning (SF), and role emotional. Self-reported diabetes frequency doubled after 5 years (from 7% to 17%).[72] Despite the clinical consensus recommending antidepressants for cataplexy, the evidence that antidepressants have a positive effect on cataplexy is scant.[85]

A survey of 129 members of the Australian Narcolepsy Support Group, using the Psychosocial Adjustment of Illness Subscale—Self Report total score, reported more adjustment problems in comparison to patients with cardiac problems, mixed cancers, and diabetes.[86] These results are difficult to compare with other studies because of different measuring instruments and a self-selected sample.

In a cross-sectional study of members of the Norwegian Association for Sleep Disorder ([NASD] n = 77), with the exception of vitality, people with narcolepsy and cataplexy had significantly lower scores on all domains of the scale of the SF-36 (mailed) when compared with the normal population, and medication status did not affect any domain. It is reported that this difference in results from other studies may be because of a difference in mind-set or public education in Norway or because of membership in the NASD.[87]

In Germany, investigators mailed the SF-36 and the Euro-QOL questionnaires to 75 subjects diagnosed with narcolepsy. Results revealed that the economic costs for patients with narcolepsy were higher than for the normal population and comparable to that for those with diseases such as Parkinson disease, Alzheimer disease, epilepsy, and stroke. Thirty-two subjects in this study reported job loss due to narcolepsy.[88] Furthermore, bivariate and multivariate analyses showed that, compared with the normal German population, HRQOL scores were low, especially in the areas of physical role, vitality, and general health perceptions. The investigators confirmed the role of social factors such as employment status, living with a partner, and professional advancement on HRQOL. Responses to the Euro-QOL revealed that the most frequently affected dimensions of health were usual activity (63.8%), pain/discomfort (61.7%), and anxiety/depression (41.1%).[89] The item including pain/discomfort is a double-barreled question, and it is not clear if patients felt pain and/or discomfort.

HRQOL in narcolepsy was significantly lower than the normal Japanese population as measured by the SF-36 in a study of drug-naive patients (n = 137) with narcolepsy plus cataplexy, narcolepsy without cataplexy, and idiopathic hypersomnia without long sleep time. Disease duration was positively correlated with mental health among all subjects; however, this study did not find significant differences among the 3 diagnostic groups.[66]

A French investigation included 517 (47.6% men, 52.4% women) patients, of whom 82% were cataplexy positive (C+), 13.2% were cataplexy negative (C−), and 4.8% had idiopathic hypersomnolence (IH). Mean ESS and body mass index were higher in C+ patients than in C−/IH patients. C+ patients treated with anticataleptic drugs (38.7%) had higher short version Beck Depression Inventory (S-BDI) and lower SF-36 scores than C+ patients treated with stimulants alone. Of those who had depression, 26.3% had mild, 23.2% had moderate, and 5.6% had severe depressive symptoms. C+ patients had higher S-BDI and Pittsburgh Sleep Quality Index and lower SF-36 scores than C−/IH patients. ESSs were higher in depressed patients than in nondepressed patients, with no difference in age, gender, duration of disease, or multiple sleep latency test parameters.[73]

In a study using the SIP (personal interviews), of the 81 PWN, 62.5% reported severe fatigue with an increase in functional deficits. There was a correlation between increased functional deficits and low QOL as indicated by responses to the SF-36.[90] Another investigation on 226 PWN revealed a total dysfunction score on the SIP (mean = 13.2%), which was higher than the general population score (mean = 3.6%). Dysfunction was observed (mean percentage) in the following areas: sleep and rest (23.6%), alertness behavior (22.6%), recreations and pastimes (20.6%), and work (15.3%). The psychosocial aspect was more dysfunctional (mean = 13.2%) than the physical (mean = 5.0%). Areas of concern to patients included social isolation, reduced sexual activity, and forgetfulness.[91]

Application of the FOSQ in a randomized trial of the effectiveness of sodium oxybate including 285 PWN revealed that sodium oxybate produced significant dose-related improvements in the Total Functional Outcomes of Sleep Questionnaire score from baseline. Similar improvements were observed in the following subscales: activity level, general productivity, vigilance, and social outcomes ($P<.01$); however, the subscales intimacy and sexual relationships were not affected.[92]

In Canada, researchers studied the effects of excessive sleepiness (ES) on HRQOL. The study design included a comparison of 1758 people with obstructive sleep apnea, depression, narcolepsy, multiple sclerosis, and shift work (Group A) with 1977 people without these conditions (Group B). The researchers measured the dependent variables by using the Work Productivity and the Activity Impairment Scale, Short Form 12, Medical Outcomes study 6-item Cognitive Function Scale, and the Toronto Hospital Alertness Test. In both groups, ES was significantly associated with impairments in health status, daily activities, and work productivity for all measures ($P<.0001$), except for absenteeism ($P = .0400$ for group A, $P = .8360$ for group B). The researchers concluded that the incremental negative effect of ES may be measurable above that of obstructive sleep apnea, multiple sclerosis, narcolepsy, depression, or shift work.[93]

In a Brazilian study of 40 PWN, QOL scores measured by the WHOQOL-BREF were lower than that in the control group in the physical, psychological, and social domains ($P<.05$). In the patient group, all areas evaluated in the physical domain were significantly impaired compared with that in controls, including sleep satisfaction ($P<.001$), energy for daily activities ($P = .039$), capacity to perform activities ($P = .001$), and capacity to work ($P = .001$).[94]

The socioeconomic burden of having narcolepsy was significantly higher in PWN than in age-matched and sex-matched randomly selected citizens in the Danish Civil Registration System Statistics ($P<.001$). The income level of employed PWN was lower than that of the employed control subjects, perhaps indicating the effect of having this disorder on promotion at work. Compared with control subjects, PWN showed significantly higher rates of medication use and expenses, as well as higher unemployment rates.[95] Again, in 2010, these investigators reported that patients with hypersomnia when compared with control subjects presented significantly higher health-related contact rate, expenses, and medication use; however, no differences were identified in employment and income possibly because of differential effects of types of hypersomnia. The difference in the annual burden of direct and indirect costs between the 2 groups was significant ($P<.001$).[96]

NONPHARMACOLOGIC MANAGEMENT OF NARCOLEPSY

Although this review of national and international scientifically designed studies vary in their methodologies, a pattern discloses the wide ranging impact of narcolepsy, especially unrelenting hypersomnolence and overwhelming fatigue, on the physical, mental, and social well being of patients. The psychological aspect was more dysfunctional than the physical aspect. Decreased role performance has a direct negative influence on relationships with family, friends, and coworkers. Treated PWN have lower QOL in comparison to patients who were treated for OSAHS. Some patients discontinue treatment either because of the side reactions or because the treatment of ES and cataplexy does not produce optimal results, pointing to the need for improved pharmacologic treatment. Narcolepsy can be a very disabling condition for some; however, there is no consensus among professionals on standards to assess disability status for eligibility to obtain disability benefits or a driver's license, indicating the need for further research in this area.[97] Pharmacologic treatment is necessary but not sufficient in managing the clinical symptoms of this disorder. Improving the QOL and learning to live with a disorder are major concerns for patients. Thus, nonpharmacologic management comprising behavior modification and social support is a crucial component of health care delivery. Successful management of objective and observable clinical features may be affected by other complaints in patients with narcolepsy, such as low level of energy and fatigue, problems with memory and time management, perception of lack of security in the environment, and depressed mood. Furthermore, personality factors, such as a passive dependent personality, may affect mental status and delay medical attention. Also, individuals' perceptions of needs will determine their decision to access health services and elicit support from significant others. Thus, subjective measures play an important role in assessing QOL and providing high quality of care.

Making behavioral and life style changes assists in ameliorating the devastating impact of symptoms on QOL. Sleep and fatigue can be partially allayed, and further progression of the condition may be slowed or prevented by scheduling rest periods or naps and regular sleep-wake hours, engaging in a regular moderately paced exercise program with graded increases, and performing breathing exercises. Clinical observations reveal that a management plan incorporating a balanced diet, regular meal times with small servings that include fresh fruits and vegetables, are beneficial; meals that are high in caloric content, fats, or sugars negatively affect alertness and energy levels. Well-designed controlled studies are needed in this area. Often, patients cannot differentiate between the symptoms of ES, fatigue, cataplexy, sleep paralysis, and automatic behavior, and

hypnagogic hallucinations can be very bothersome to some. Explanation of all symptoms and their management along with written material increase patient collaboration and provide much relief to patients.

Social support and social networking have a positive association with the immune system and general health.[98] Support groups led by a professional provide a forum to discuss shared experiences, exchange information, access resources, and develop self-esteem and self-confidence. Social networking relieves the sense of isolation felt by many patients. On a positive note, patients with narcolepsy do make successful transitions after treatment as they discard the sick role and adapt to normal life; support and counseling can be beneficial during this transitional phase.[99] An appropriate referral for spiritual counseling, if needed, enables some patients to cope with their illness.

PWN could benefit with counseling for making suitable occupational choices because narcolepsy presents obstacles to upward social mobility. A survey showed that PWN were engaged in a wide spectrum of occupations, including professional, management, and administrative positions.[100] Some PWN were self-employed, and others were engaged in sales of computers, real estate, automobiles, hardware, and antiques. Self-selection was an important factor in the occupational choice of some of these patients. PWN should choose work that will allow them to break up long assignments into shorter ones with time flexibility and variability in tasks as well as periods of rest between assignments. Mentally stimulating tasks with some physical mobility have an alerting effect. Tasks that are sedentary and monotonous and occupations involving the use of machinery or equipment that could be hazardous to self or to others must be avoided.

The high rate of accidents in hypersomnolence is another major area of concern. Sleepiness results in negative behavioral consequences, including cognitive deficit, errors, and accidents.[101] Public health measures for prevention of accidents and education of professionals and patients are needed. Patients should be cautioned regarding accidents at home.

Psychosocial care is significant in reducing discomfort in chronic illness and improving the QOL of patients. However, diffusion of this knowledge, of implementing research findings in clinical practice, is hindered due to variable methodologies to assess indicators of HRQOL and low use of novel approaches of disseminating research findings to clinicians. The Internet is one mechanism of providing updated research findings to clinicians.

In addition, a short and simple pretreatment and posttreatment evaluation form to assess changes in levels of the patient's discomfort, distress, and patient satisfaction (an integral component of the US Affordable Health Care Act) will provide pertinent feedback to clinicians, making them aware of deficits in the management plan. Patients' comments are invaluable in guiding both the patients and the staff to make relevant personal as well as institutional changes and facilitate the process of fulfilling the goal to foster high level of quality of care and enhance the QOL of patients.

SUMMARY

Hypersomnia in narcolepsy greatly affects the psychosocial and economic burden to the patient and society pointing to the importance of early diagnosis and biopsychosocial management. Educational programs must be directed toward professionals and the public to create greater sensitivity to the wide ranging effects of hypersomnolence on the lives of patients and their families. Research is needed on (1) innovative pharmacologic management with greater efficacy and less adverse effects and (2) the role of support groups on patients' well-being and mechanism of action. Standardized measures with high internal and external validity will make national and international comparisons more meaningful. A multidisciplinary team, with the patient as a team member, pursuing a person-centered and family-centered approach, including a monitoring strategy to identify patients' perceived barriers to accessing treatment and adhering to treatment plan, will contribute to optimal delivery of health care and improve the QOL in patients.

REFERENCES

1. Hennessy CH, Moriarty DG, Zack MM, et al. Measuring health-related quality of life for public health surveillance. Public Health Rep 1994; 109(5):665–72.
2. Kindig DA, Booske BC, Remington PL. Mobilizing Action Toward Community Health (MATCH): metrics, incentives, and partnerships for population health. Prev Chronic Dis 2010;7(4):A68.
3. Goswami M. Sleep and quality of life in narcolepsy. In: Verster JC, Pandi-Perumal SR, Streiner DL, editors. Sleep and quality of life in clinical medicine. Totowa (NJ): Humana Press; 2008. p. 93–9.
4. Parkes JD. Amphetamines and other drugs in the treatment of daytime drowsiness and cataplexy. In: Parkes JD, editor. Sleep and its disorders. London: W.B. Saunders; 1985. p. 459–82.
5. Mattson R, Calverley J. Dextroamphetamine-sulfate-induced dyskinesias. JAMA 1968;204: 400–2.
6. Segraves RT, Madsen R, Carter SC, et al. Erectile dysfunction associated with pharmacological agents. In: Segraves RT, Schoenberg HW, editors. Diagnosis and treatment of erectile disturbances: a guide for clinicians. New York: Plenum; 1985. p. 23–63.
7. Karacan I. Erectile dysfunction in narcoleptic patients. Sleep 1986;9:227–31.
8. Duquette RL, Dupuis G, Perrault J. A new approach for quality of life assessment in cardiac patients: rationale and validation of the Quality of Life Systemic Inventory. Can J Cardiol 1994;10: 106–12.
9. Browne JP, O'Boyle CA, McGee HM, et al. Individual quality of life in the healthy elderly. Qual Life Res 1994;3:235–44.
10. Calman K. Quality of life in cancer patients— a hypothesis. J Med Ethics 1984;10:124–7.
11. Levine S, Croog S. What constitutes quality of life? A conceptualization of the dimensions of life quality in health populations and patients with cardiovascular disease. In: Wegner NK, Mattson ME, Furberg CD, et al, editors. Assessment of quality of life in clinical trials of cardiovascular therapies. New York: Le Jacq Publishing Inc; 1984. p. 46–58.
12. Schipper H. Guidelines and caveats for quality of life measurement in clinical practice and research. Oncology 1990;4:51–7.
13. Williams G, Testa M. Quality of life: an important consideration in antihypertensive therapy. In: Hollenberg NK, editor. Management of hypertension: a multifactorial approach. Stoneham (MA): Butterworth; 1987. p. 79–100.
14. Dimenas E, Dahlof C, Jern S, et al. Defining quality of life in medicine. Scand J Prim Health Care 1990; 1:7–10.
15. Camfield L, Skevington SM. On subjective well-being and quality of life. J Health Psychol 2008; 13:764–75.
16. Siegrist J, Junge A. Measuring the social dimension of subjective health in chronic illness. Psychother Psychosom 1990;54(2–3):90–8.
17. Dijkers MP. Individualization in quality of life measurement: instruments and approaches. Arch Phys Med Rehabil 2003;84(Suppl 2):S3–14.
18. World Health Organization Quality of Life Group. Development of the WHOQOL: rationale and current status. Int J Ment Health 1994;23:24–56.
19. Goswami M. Quality of life and psychosocial issues in narcolepsy. In: Goswami M, Pandi-Perumal SR, Thorpy MJ, editors. Narcoelpsy: a clinical guide. New York: Springer; 2010. p. 189–204.
20. Koenig HG. Religion and medicine IV: religion, physical health, and clinical implications. Int J Psychiatry Med 2001;31(3):321–36.

21. McBride JL, Brooks AG, Pilkington L. The relationship between a patient's spirituality and health experiences. Fam Med 1998;30(2):122–6.

22. Hays JC, Meador KG, Branch PS, et al. The Spiritual History Scale in four dimensions (SHS-4): validity and reliability. Gerontologist 2001; 41(2):239.

23. O'Connell KA, Skevington SM. Spiritual, religious, and personal beliefs are important and distinctive to assessing quality of life in health: a comparison of theoretical models. Br J Health Psychol 2010; 15:729–48.

24. Bergner MB, Bobbitt R, Carter W, et al. The SIP: development and final revision of a health status measure. Med Care 1981;19(8):787–805.

25. McEwen J. Nottingham Health Profile: application in clinical care. J Drug Ther Res 1988;13:164–6.

26. Chambers LW. The McMaster Health Index Questionnaire: an update. In: Walker SR, Rosser RM, editors. Quality of life: assessment and application. Lancaster (England): MTP Press; 1988. p. 113.

27. Guyatt G, Walter S, Norman G. Measuring change over-time: assessing the usefulness of evaluative instruments. J Chronic Dis 1987;2:171.

28. Ware JE, Snow KK, Kosinsky M. SF-36 Health Survey: manual and interpretation guide. Lincoln (RI): QualityMetric Inc; 2000.

29. Kellner R. Symptom questionnaire. J Clin Psychiatry 1987;48:268–74.

30. Meenan RF, Gertman PM, Mason JM, et al. The arthritis impact measurement scales: further investigations of a health status measure. Arthritis Rheum 1982;25:1048.

31. Mor V, Laliberte L, Morris J, et al. The Karnofsky Performance Status Scale: an examination of its reliability and validity in a research setting. Cancer 1984;53(9):2002–7.

32. DCCT Research Group. Diabetes Control and Complications Trial (DCCT): results of feasibility study. Diabetes Care 1987;10:1.

33. Weaver TE, Laizner AM, Evans LK, et al. An instrument to measure functional status outcomes for disorders of excessive sleepiness. Sleep 1997;20: 835–43.

34. Carmines E, Zeller R. Reliability and validity assessment. Beverly Hills (CA): Sage Publications; 1979.

35. MacKeigan L, Pathak D. Overview of health-related quality-of-life measures. Am J Hosp Pharm 1992; 49(9):2236–45.

36. Waters E, Davis E, Ronen GM, et al. Quality of life instruments for children and adolescents with neurodisabilities: how to choose the appropriate instrument. Dev Med Child Neurol 2009;51:660–9.

37. Stewart AL, Ware JE. Measuring functioning and well-being. Durham (NC): Duke University Press; 1992.

38. Ware JE, Kosinsky M, Keller SD. A 12-item short-form survey: construction of scales and preliminary tests of reliability and validity. Med Care 1996;34:220–33.

39. Reimer MA, Flemons WW. Quality of life in sleep disorders. Sleep Med Rev 2003;7(4):335–49.

40. Jenkinson C, Stewart-Brown S, Peterson S, et al. Assessment of the SF-36 version 2 in the United Kingdom. J Epidemiol Community Health 1999; 53:46–50.

41. Ware JE, Gandek B. Overview of the SF-36 health survey and the International Quality of Life Assessment (IQOLA) project. J Clin Epidemiol 1998;51: 903–12.

42. Gilson BS, Gilson JS, Bergner M, et al. The Sickness Impact Profile: development of an outcome measure of health care. Am J Public Health 1975; 65(12):1304–10.

43. The WHOQOL Group. The World Health Organization Quality of Life Assessment (WHOQOL): position paper from the World Health Organization. Soc Sci Med 1995;41(10):1403–9.

44. Skevington SM. Measuring quality of life in Britain: introducing the WHOQOL-100. J Psychosom Res 1999;47:449–59.

45. Skevington SM, Carse MS, Williams AC. Validation of the WHOQOL-100: pain management improves quality of life for chronic pain patients. Clin J Pain 2001;17(3):264–75.

46. Development of the World Health Organization WHOQOL-BREF quality of life assessment. The WHOQOL Group. Psychol Med 1998;28:551–8.

47. Skevington SM, McCrate FM. Expecting a good quality of life in health: assessing people with diverse diseases and conditions using the WHOQOL-BREF. Health Expect 2012;15(1):49–62.

48. Awasthi S, Agnihotri K, Singh U, et al. Determinants of health related quality of life in school-going adolescents in Northern India. Indian J Pediatr 2011;78:555–61.

49. Baumann C, Erpelding ML, Regat S, et al. The WHOQOL-BREF questionnaire: French adult population norms for the physical health, psychological health and social relationship dimensions. Rev Epidemiol Sante Publique 2010;58:33–9.

50. Chiu WT, Huang SJ, Hwang HF, et al. Use of the WHOQOL-BREF for evaluating persons with traumatic brain injury. J Neurotrauma 2006;23: 1609–20.

51. Najafi M, Sheikhvatan M, Montazeri A, et al. Reliability of World Health Organization's Quality of Life-BREF versus Short Form 36 Health Survey questionnaires for assessment of quality of life in patients with coronary artery disease. J Cardiovasc Med (Hagerstown) 2009;10:316–21.

52. Skevington SM, Lotfy M, O'Connell KA. The World Health Organization's WHOQOL-BREF quality of life assessment: psychometric properties and results of

the international field trial. A report from the WHOQOL group. Qual Life Res 2004;13:299–310.

53. Roth B. Narcolepsy and hypersomnia. Basel (Switzerland): Karger; 1980.

54. Broughton WA, Broughton RJ. Psychosocial impact of narcolepsy. Sleep 1994;17:S45–9.

55. Goswami M, Pollak CP, Cohen FL, et al, editors. Psychosocial aspects of narcolepsy. New York: Haworth Press Inc; 1992. p. 1–203.

56. Nevsimalova S, Sonka K, Spackova N, et al. Excessive daytime somnolence and its psychosocial sequelae. Sb Lek 2002;103(1):51–7 [in Czech].

57. Bayon V, Leger D, Philip P. Socio-professional handicap and accidental risk in patients with hypersomnias of central origin. Sleep Med Rev 2009;13(6):421–6.

58. Peacock J, Benca RM. Narcolepsy: clinical features, co-morbidities & treatment. Indian J Med Res 2010;131:338–49.

59. Lindsley G. Narcolepsy, intimacy, and sexuality. In: Goswami M, Pandi-Perumal SR, Thorpy MJ, editors. Narcolepsy: a clinical guide. New York: Springer; 2010. p. 205–15.

60. Goswami M. The influence of clinical symptoms on quality of life in patients with narcolepsy. Neurology 1998;50(2 Suppl 1):S31–6.

61. Powell NB, Schechtman KB, Riley TW, et al. Sleepy driving: accidents and injury. Otolaryngol Head Neck Surg 2002;126(3):217–27.

62. Donjacour CEHM, Mets MAJ, Verster JC. Narcolepsy, driving, and traffic safety. In: Goswami M, Pandi-Perumal SR, Thorpy MJ, editors. Narcolepsy: a clinical guide. New York: Springer; 2010. p. 217–21.

63. Broughton R, Guberman A, Roberts J. Comparison of the psychosocial effects of epilepsy and narcolepsy/cataplexy: a controlled study. Epilepsia 1984;25:423–33.

64. Aldrich MS. Automobile accidents in patients with sleep disorders. Sleep 1989;12(6):487–94.

65. Kingshott RN, Jones DR, Smith AD, et al. The role of sleep-disordered breathing, daytime sleepiness, and impaired performance in motor vehicle crashes—a case control study. Sleep Breath 2004;8:61–72.

66. Ozaki A, Inoue Y, Nakajima T, et al. Health-related quality of life among drug-naïve patients with narcolepsy with cataplexy, narcolepsy without cataplexy, and idiopathic hypersomnia without long sleep time. J Clin Sleep Med 2008;4:572–8.

67. Goswami M, Glovinsky P, Thorpy MJ. Needs assessment and socio-demographic characteristics in narcolepsy [abstract]. Presented at the 5th International Congress of Sleep Research. Copenhagen (Denmark), June 28–July 3, 1987. p. 805.

68. Bayard S, Abril B, Yu H, et al. Decision making in narcolepsy with cataplexy. Sleep 2011;34:99–104.

69. Sturzenegger C, Bassetti C. The clinical spectrum of narcolepsy with cataplexy: a reappraisal. J Sleep Res 2004;13:395–406.

70. Krishnan RR, Volow MR, Miller PP, et al. Narcolepsy: preliminary retrospective study of psychiatric and psychosocial aspects. Am J Psychiatry 1984;141:428–31.

71. Teixeira VG, Faccenda JF, Douglas NJ. Functional status in patients with narcolepsy. Sleep Med 2004;5(5):477–83.

72. Vignatelli L, Plazzi G, Peschechera F, et al. A 5-year prospective cohort study on health-related quality of life in patients with narcolepsy. Sleep Med 2011;12:19–23.

73. Dauvilliers Y, Paquereau J, Bastuji H, et al. Psychological health in central hypersomnias: the French Harmony study. J Neurol Neurosurg Psychiatry 2009;80:636–41.

74. Daniels E, King MA, Smith IE, et al. Health related quality of life in narcolepsy. J Sleep Res 2001;10: 75–81.

75. Merritt SL, Cohen FL, Smith KM. Depressive symptomatology in narcolepsy. In: Goswami M, Pollak CP, Cohen FL, et al, editors. Psychosocial aspects of narcolepsy. New York: Haworth Press Inc; 1992. p. 53–9.

76. Vourdas A, Shneerson JM, Gregory CA, et al. Narcolepsy and psychopathology: is there an association? Sleep Med 2002;3(4):353–60.

77. Jara OC, Popp R, Zulley J, et al. Determinants of depressive symptoms in narcoleptic patients with and without cataplexy. J Nerv Ment Dis 2011;199:329–34.

78. Shneerson J. Narcolepsy and mental health. In: Goswami M, Pandi-Perumal SR, Thorpy MJ, editors. Narcolepsy: a clinical guide. New York: Springer; 2010. p. 239–47.

79. Bellebaum C, Daum I. Memory and cognition in narcolepsy. In: Goswami M, Pandi-Perumal SR, Thorpy MJ, editors. Narcolepsy: a clinical guide. New York: Springer; 2010. p. 223–9.

80. Ha KS, Yoo HK, Lyoo IK, et al. Computerized assessment of cognitive impairment in narcoleptic patients. Acta Neurol Scand 2007;116:312–6.

81. Rieger M, Mayer G, Gauggel S. Attention deficits in patients with narcolepsy. Sleep 2003;26(1):36–43.

82. Beusterien KM, Rogers AE, Walsleben JA, et al. Health-related quality of life effects of modafinil for treatment of narcolepsy. Sleep 1999;22(6): 757–65.

83. Stoddard RB, Goswami M, Ingalls KK. The development and validation of an instrument to evaluate quality of life in narcolepsy patients. Drug Information Journal. Amber (PA): Drug Information Association; 1996. p. 850.

84. Vignatelli L, D'Alessandro R, Mosconi P, et al. Health related quality of life with narcolepsy: the SF-36 health survey. Sleep Med 2004;5(5):467–75.

85. Vignatelli L, D'Alessandro R, Candelise L. Antidepressant drugs for narcolepsy. Cochrane Database Syst Rev 2008;1:CD003724.

86. Bruck D. The impact of narcolepsy on psychosocial health and role behaviors: negative effects and comparisons with other illness groups. Sleep Med 2001;2:437–46.

87. Ervik S, Abdelnoor M, Heier MS, et al. Health-related quality of life in narcolepsy. Acta Neurol Scand 2006;114:198–204.

88. Dodel R, Peter H, Walbert T, et al. The socioeconomic impact of narcolepsy. Sleep 2004;27:1123–8.

89. Dodel R, Peter H, Spottke A, et al. Health-related quality of life in patients with narcolepsy. Sleep Med 2007;8:733–41.

90. Droogleever Fortuyn HA, Fronczek R, Smitshoek M, et al. Prevalence and impact of severe fatigue—separate from sleepiness—in patients with narcolepsy. Sleep 2008;31:A214.

91. Ton TG, Watson NF, Longstreth WT. Narcolepsy and the sickness impact profile: a general health status measure. Sleep 2008;31:A218.

92. Weaver TE, Cuellar N. A randomized trial evaluating the effectiveness of sodium oxybate therapy on quality of life in narcolepsy. Sleep 2006;29(9):1189–94.

93. Dean B, Aguilar D, Shapiro C, et al. Impaired health status, daily functioning, and work productivity in adults with excessive sleepiness. J Occup Environ Med 2010;52:144–9.

94. Rovere H, Rossini S, Reimao R. Quality of life in patients with narcolepsy: a WHOQOL-BREF study. Arq Neuropsiquiatr 2008;66:163–7.

95. Jennum P, Knudsen S, Kjellberg J. The economic consequences of narcolepsy. J Clin Sleep Med 2009;5:240–5.

96. Jennum P, Kjellberg J. The socio-economical burden of hypersomnia. Acta Neurol Scand 2010; 121:265–70.

97. Ingravallo F, Vignatelli L, Brini M, et al. Medico-legal assessment of disability in narcolepsy: an interobserver reliability study. J Sleep Res 2008; 17:111–9.

98. Goswami M. Quality of life in narcolepsy: the importance of social support. In: Kumar VM, Mallick HN, editors. Second Interim Congress of the World Federation of Sleep Research and Sleep Medicine Societies 2005, New Delhi (India), Medimond: International Proceedings; September 22–26, 2005.

99. Wilson SJ, Frazer DW, Lawrence JA, et al. Psychosocial adjustment following relief of chronic narcolepsy. Sleep Med 2007;8:252–9.

100. Goswami M, Thorpy MJ. Occupational status of patients with narcolepsy. Sleep Research Abstracts 1988 [abstract: 184].

101. Czeisler CA. Impact of sleepiness and sleep deficiency on public health—utility of biomarkers. J Clin Sleep Med 2011;7(Suppl 5):S6–8.

Inappropriate Situational Sleepiness and the Law

Peter R. Buchanan, MD, FRACP[a,b,c], Arlie Loughnan, BA, LLB, LLM, PhD[d],
Ronald R. Grunstein, MD, PhD, FRACP[c,e,*]

KEYWORDS

- Inappropriate situational sleepiness • Medicolegal • Criminal liability • Civil liability

KEY POINTS

- Sleepiness may occur in circumstances related to personal behaviors, medical conditions and in consequence of workplace behaviors: consequent impaired performance may have legal ramifications.
- Specific legislations to take account of sleepiness-impaired performance are scarce but societies attempt due account through a range of administrative and legal instruments.
- Legal and other sanctions against impaired performance causing harm and due to sleepiness are often selectively applied on the basis of perceived moral culpability.

INTRODUCTION

Sleepiness causes adverse personal consequences and inconvenience to individuals but may also impact on performance with sequelae that have potential to cause harm to others. Such harm has individual and societal consequences and therefore the community has reasonable grounds from which to use legal and other frameworks to mitigate such adverse events and sanction against their occurrence.

Elsewhere in this issue the epidemiologic, pathophysiologic, clinical, therapeutic, and other aspects of excessive sleepiness of the clinical entity of hypersomnia are presented. Where sleepiness, mediated by impaired performance, is the promoter of potential and actual harmful outcomes, communities have reacted by amending the law and using existing legal measures to protect society in general. These protective legal constructs may be found in various fields, including criminal law, and under the omnibus category of civil law, in labor law, and health law. This article presents an overview of some aspects of the interaction between sleepiness and various facets of the law.

INAPPROPRIATE SITUATIONAL SLEEPINESS AND THE LAW: BROAD CONCEPTS

The use of the terms "hypersomnia" and "excessive daytime sleepiness" is in some ways an incomplete representation of the nature of the problem that challenges the sleepiness-law nexus. Sleepiness is an entirely appropriate physiologic response to a combination of homeostatic,

[a] Sleep and Circadian Research Group, NHMRC Centre for Integrated Research and Understanding of Sleep, Woolcock Institute of Medical Research, University of Sydney, PO Box M77, Missenden Road, New South Wales 2050, Australia; [b] Department of Respiratory Medicine, Liverpool Hospital, Elizabeth Street, Liverpool, New South Wales 2170, Australia; [c] Sleep Disorders Service, St Vincent's Clinic, 438 Victoria Street, Suite 806, Darlinghurst, Sydney, New South Wales 2010, Australia; [d] Faculty of Law F10, University of Sydney, Sydney, New South Wales 2006, Australia; [e] Sleep and Circadian Research Group, NHMRC Centre for Integrated Research and Understanding of Sleep, Woolcock Institute of Medical Research, University of Sydney and Royal Prince Alfred Hospital, PO Box M77, Missenden Road, New South Wales 2050, Australia
* Corresponding author. Sleep and Circadian Research Group, NHMRC Centre for Integrated Research and Understanding of Sleep, Woolcock Institute of Medical Research, University of Sydney and Royal Prince Alfred Hospital, PO Box M77, Missenden Road, New South Wales 2050, Australia.
E-mail address: ron.grunstein@gmail.com

Sleep Med Clin 7 (2012) 353–363
doi:10.1016/j.jsmc.2012.03.014
1556-407X/12/$ – see front matter © 2012 Elsevier Inc. All rights reserved.

circadian, and other (eg, drugs) factors. It is a normal part of life for humans to manifest sleepiness with a periodicity that approximates a 24-hour cycle: this is appropriate situational sleepiness. Excessive sleepiness mostly occurs in a daytime context but may also occur at night in individuals who are expected to be alert in occupational and other circumstances. Various subjective descriptions or definitions of excessive sleepiness have been applied in epidemiologic studies of this symptom when describing its community prevalence.[1] When "hyper" is prefixed, it refers to an exaggerated modifier of a quality or entity (in this instance "somnia," for sleep) but in an adjectival or slang sense "hyper" also passes in common parlance for an individual who is overexcited, overstimulated, or keyed up. To overcome the narrowness and confusion of some of the terms commonly in use in this area, and to go some way toward capturing what is relevant in law about sleepiness, in this article a useful umbrella term, "inappropriate situational sleepiness" (ISS), is used.

The rubric ISS suggests a degree of sleepiness that takes into account prior patterns of sleep–wake cycling over days or even weeks; the time-of-day factor (potentially related to sleep homeostasis and circadian physiology); the quality of prior sleep periods (going to the issue of presence of sleep disorders); and appropriateness of the overall contextualized wake environment (eg, consideration of the consequence of falling asleep to the individual and others).

In effect ISS does not necessarily imply some underlying disorder of sleep. In a general sense the concept of sleepiness is well understood; all humans experience it, on a daily basis. The sleep medicine scientific and clinical community has developed adequate, reliable, and accurate tests of sleepiness that have application particularly in sleep laboratories and clinical and research situations. However, there is a clear need for useful sleepiness tests with wider community application, such as at the roadside or in work situations. In a practical sense, such a test is currently lacking. The most widely accepted laboratory and clinical standard tests of measuring sleepiness, such as the multiple sleep latency test and maintenance of wakefulness test, can only be applied in controlled circumstances and indeed usually in a retrospective manner when considering most medicolegal issues.

Perhaps the most readily recognized manifestation of ISS in the medicolegal domain is impaired vehicle driving performance. There is wide recognition that a problem of impaired driving of motor vehicles and sleepiness exists, and presents potentially major individual and societal consequences.[2–4] This applies to private motor vehicles (eg, cars); to commercial (eg, truck or bus) driving; to the piloting of marine and aeronautic vehicles; and to the operation of heavy motorized nonvehicular machinery or complex amalgams (eg, cranes, nuclear and other power plant stations, and industrial complexes).

Impaired performance caused by sleepiness can also manifest without direct reference to the operation of motor vehicles or physical machinery. Judicial decision-making may be impaired in the case of sleepiness-impaired judicial officers[5]; fiscal recommendations might be scrambled by sleep-deprived financial advisers; gamblers and others may indulge in more risky behaviors[6,7]; military judgments may be awry in the case of sleepiness-impaired commanders[8]; and critical management decisions made by executives, government, and related operatives running space exploration, maritime, and other complex programs may be suboptimal.[9–12] Health workers are particularly vulnerable.[13–15] To a lesser extent (at least, to date, when compared with motor vehicle operation) the wider community also recognizes examples of impaired cognitive performance caused by ISS.

Individuals may bear direct or indirect civil or criminal liability for adverse outcomes seen to be related to ISS, and face prosecution and sanction in relevant courts or tribunals. For instance, falling asleep at the wheel of a car may result in criminal liability for dangerous driving, and a driver may incur civil liability for any harm to persons or property. Employers may also face liability when adverse outcomes accrue because of the actions of employees when those events occurred within what may be reasonably regarded as the parameters of their employees' work practices. For employers, it also may not be just a civil law issue but may also attract criminal law sanction as a form of corporate or industrial manslaughter.[16–18]

Physician liability is a particularly relevant category for healthcare providers. This has a patient-centered and a physician-centered aspect in terms of whom in the physician–patient relationship is impaired by excessive sleepiness. Liability for adverse outcomes may fall on those (nonsleepy) physicians whose medical advice or treatment and its consequences causes an adverse outcome for patients who are impaired by excessive sleepiness, and this outcome is considered reasonably foreseeable. Examples include a patient's poor performance because of his or her sleepiness resulting in injury or death, as a result of inadequate physician diagnosis or treatment of a sleep disorder, or prescription of a sleepiness-associated medication without adequate warning.

However, a physician's liability has a somewhat different focus if the physician has ISS and makes impaired medical decisions resulting in harm. These types of medical errors may give rise to criminal liability in negligence, where the medical professional's level of care has fallen far below the standard of a medical professional with his or her level of experience. The precise way in which these and other liabilities arise in respect of ISS varies across legal jurisdictions.

MEDICAL CONDITIONS NOTABLE FOR SLEEPINESS AND LEGAL CONSEQUENCES

There is a range of possible causes of ISS, with varying but generally limited recognition of specific medical conditions in law. The *International Classification of Sleep Disorders, 2nd Edition* lists three main types of disorders associated with excessive sleepiness as a major symptom: (1) narcolepsy; (2) an omnibus category of hypersomnias; and (3) behaviorally induced insufficient sleep syndrome (voluntary sleep restriction).[19] In addition, obstructive sleep apnea (OSA) is also commonly although not invariably associated with ISS.[20,21] Given the significant community prevalence of OSA[22] and its relatively low level of community diagnosis and effective treatment, OSA presents as a potentially major contributor to instances of ISS. Sleepiness may occur in other sleep medicine diagnostic categories, such as insomnia, phase-shift disorders, and parasomnias, but these and other sleepiness-associated entities usually have other more prominent symptom features.

ISS and Insufficient Sleep

Insufficient sleep is so common in many communities (estimated prevalence of 20%–40% in the adult United States population[23]) that it might almost be regarded as a character trait of such societies. With increasing industrialization and globalization of work practices, insufficient sleep may also be increasing in developing economies. Although a small proportion of such insufficient sleep may be attributable to medical sleep disorders, a substantial proportion of societal insufficient sleep is attributable to voluntary (or in some cases corporate mandated) choices about work, and domestic and social patterns of behavior (ie, behaviorally induced insufficient sleep or voluntary sleep restriction). This seems an almost inevitable aspect of the driven "24/7" lifestyle engendered by the conditions of contemporary industrialized society and its demands for maximization of production, profit, security, and so forth. It is well established that lack of sleep and concepts related to workplace sleepiness increase risk of workplace accidents. An underlying proclivity for accidents in the workplace related to fatigue and need for recovery (surrogate markers of excessive workplace sleepiness) has been documented.[24,25]

The ubiquity of behaviorally induced insufficient sleep has ensured it has largely escaped specific criminal legal response. For instance, although most jurisdictions provide for the prosecution of instances of vehicular homicide or injury on the basis of reckless behavior causing harm, and may include voluntary sleep restriction as a progenitor or the actual cause of reckless behavior, the only notable and specific legislative interdiction of such behaviorally induced insufficient sleep in relation to vehicular homicide is embodied by so-called "Maggie's Law," enacted in New Jersey in 2003 (discussed later).[26]

Healthcare Workers and ISS

Excessive sleepiness is commonplace in healthcare workers and clearly associated with increased risk of medical errors.[13,27] Such sleepiness in healthcare workers is typically a consequence of voluntary (or employer expected) sleep restriction. The international legal ramifications of this have been recently reviewed[28] and exemplified by cases where doctors have been investigated for malpractice related in part to long working hours in hospitals.[29] Efforts to mitigate the deleterious effects on work performance from prolonged work hour practices in the United States have largely devolved to professional recommendations and regulations regarding doctors-in-training.[30] Other aspects of patient care other than the work hours of junior doctors also impact on the level of medical errors, such as inadequate supervision of junior doctors and deficiency in patient hand-offs (handover). There is no national regulation in the United States pertaining to attending (consultant) physician work hours or nurses. Recognition of the adverse impact of onerous healthcare worker work hours has also led to modifications of such work practices in other countries. There is still no consensus on the overall impact of the recent introduction of less onerous hours of duty (eg, for junior doctors).[31–34]

OSA

OSA is a condition characterized by repetitive partial or complete upper airway obstructions during sleep and may be causative of a diverse range of adverse health outcomes for the affected

---

Case Report

A 32-year-old male driver returns home in the late afternoon, on his own on a 1-hour trip from his work-place at the end of the week, driving his car along a rural highway. He is seen over a 10-minute period by occupants of a following vehicle to veer repeatedly across the center line briefly and return to the correct side of the highway. This recurs until on the last such crossing his vehicle collides head-on with an oncoming vehicle traveling on its correct side of the road and whose four occupants sustain a series of injuries, including a serious permanent brain injury to one child. The 32-year-old solo driver is obese, had been earlier made aware of his snoring and restless sleep by others, and has had somewhat disturbed and restricted sleep patterns over prior weeks. During his usual work day, breakfast includes coffee as a beverage and a caffeine-containing "energy drink," and work breaks are sometimes filled by naps. Subsequent investigations rule out alcohol and other drugs and mechanical malfunctions as relevant factors, and confirm severe OSA.

Based on these facts, the driver is charged with dangerous driving and negligent driving causing grievous bodily harm. Legal issues raised in this case are likely to include the attribution of the fall-asleep accident to the (subsequently diagnosed) OSA, the question as to whether it was reasonable for an ordinary member of the public to have sought medical or other attention for the preaccident status of snoring-disrupted sleep–daytime sleepiness, the issue of whether the repeated erratic driving behavior immediately preceding the accident should have led to the driver's appropriate action of ceasing driving forthwith, and others. Some of these issues are discussed next.

---

individual. These include the complaint of excessive daytime or ISS for a substantial proportion of patients with OSA. Included also among those diverse outcomes are impaired daytime behavioral features that directly impact on performance across several domains and importantly including impaired neurocognitive function, attention deficits, and wake–sleep instability states that may allow brief or complete intrusions of sleep into daytime and waketime tasks. This resultant impaired performance in wake tasks potentially has a direct impact on the efficiency and safety of operational activities, such as driving vehicles, but also has implications for other important nondriving tasks, such as management, financial, judicial, and medical decisions. It is clear that impaired individual performance in this context has potential extrapolations for harm to self and others, with flow-through legal ramifications where a relevant legal framework is in place.[35,36]

One problematic medicolegal aspect of OSA is the issue of whether a driver can be reasonably expected to be aware of the risks associated with significant but undiagnosed and untreated OSA, an issue going to general community knowledge about the very existence of OSA. Moreover, can a patient with OSA be aware of impending OSA-related sudden sleep episodes immediately leading up to an accident? Against a background of possible long-standing neurocognitive impairment caused by the underlying condition, legal evaluation of liability in any given instance may include consideration (either as a matter of law, or a matter of jury evaluation) of whether that awareness of impending sleep gave rise to an

obligation on the driver to stop driving in the immediate circumstances.

Medical experts have questioned whether inconsistency in the outcomes of cases of this type results from the difficulty in apportioning causation to OSA in fall-asleep incidents among those with OSA.[37] However, from a legal perspective, the factor distinguishing the diverse outcomes seen in such cases is frequently the degree of moral culpability involved (eg, ignoring warnings of drowsiness, having been aware of preexisting diagnosis but not acting appropriately on that information, failure to follow medical instructions, and so forth). This means that better public awareness, diagnosis, intervention, and treatment is crucial; not only will this ensure fewer accidents, but it should also mean that where an accident occurs and prosecution follows, there is more chance of conviction and appropriate penalty. However courts may emphasize different aspects of fall-asleep accidents (see later).

Narcolepsy

There are jurisdictions that specifically recognize narcolepsy as a disorder notable for potentially unsafe levels of excessive sleepiness and increased risk for accidents, and some jurisdictions preclude individuals with narcolepsy from holding commercial motor vehicle or aviation licenses, whereas others may grant a conditional license qualified by a requirement for rigorous medical management and supervision.[38] However, the approach to narcolepsy in some European countries is not so proscriptive.[39] The situation for narcoleptic patients with respect to a private motor vehicle license is generally such that individuals may hold a private license, provided that the condition has been demonstrated to have been adequately treated and subject to ongoing appropriate medical monitoring (usually by a neurologist or sleep specialist).[35] Beyond narcolepsy there is no specific recognition of other "hypersomnia disorders."

Drugs

Use of illicit intoxicants or narcotics or inappropriate use of prescription medications, often combined with alcohol, can form the background to impaired work performance and to impaired driving. "Sleep driving" is a term used to describe individuals who, while asleep or not fully conscious, arouse, leave their beds, enter cars, and drive, often in an impaired and unsafe manner.[40] A small proportion of such cases represent instances of a variant of the non–rapid eye movement parasomnia sleepwalking. However, others are related to driving under the influence of such prescribed medications (and illicit drugs and alcohol) with a significant risk to drivers and others.[40–42]

For legal purposes, intoxication by a drug or substance is not in itself a defense to a criminal charge but it may be evidence that the defendant did not form the requisite mental state required for the offense. Traditionally, the legal approach to drug-related offending groups all intoxicants including alcohol together, and adopts a conservative approach to the way in which claims of intoxication may permit an individual to deny criminal liability. However, in recent years, some courts have carved out what is an exception to the traditional approach in the case of consumption of so-called "nondangerous" drugs. For instance, in a thin line of case law, the courts in England and Wales have concluded that intoxication by nondangerous drugs is not subject to the usual rules regarding intoxicants unless, in taking the drug, the defendant was reckless, being aware of the risk of uncontrollable conduct but going ahead anyway to take the drug.

The main United Kingdom authority for the special case of nondangerous drugs is *Hardie* (and the earlier decision it purported to follow, *Bailey*).[43,44] Hardie had taken some diazepam tablets and started a fire inside a flat. He was charged and convicted of two different criminal damage offenses. The Court of Appeal quashed Hardie's convictions, holding that, even if he had taken excessive quantities of this type of drug, this could not "in the ordinary way" raise a conclusive presumption against the admission of

intoxication for the purposes of disproving the mental state required by the offense. The Court reasoned that diazepam was "wholly different in kind from drugs which are liable to cause unpredictability or aggressiveness," stating that, if the jury found that the defendant had been unable to appreciate the risks of his actions, they should consider whether taking the (diazepam) itself was reckless.[43]

The way in which this particular vein of case law relating to intoxication by nondangerous drugs has evolved exposes courts' reliance on lay knowledge about intoxication.[45] As one commentator has argued, the category of nondangerous drugs depends on what most people are supposed to believe about the drug, rather than any actual objective, scientific-pharmacologic properties of the drug itself.[46]

LEGAL FRAMEWORKS

It is not within the scope of this manuscript to describe each of the various legal frameworks that relate to ISS and consequent sleepiness-impaired performance and that apply across multiple regional, national, and international jurisdictions. Instead the focus is principles that have some generalizability across legal systems. Many of the legal principles and practices discussed here have widespread application across common law jurisdictions.

Criminal Liability for ISS

In criminal law, ISS raises the issue of an individual's criminal responsibility (the issue of whether an individual can be held accountable for his or her actions or omissions at law). Offenses of omission and commission coinciding with or as a result of ISS are a subset of a broader set of behaviors classed as "automatistic" conduct under criminal law. At its broadest, this category of behaviors includes accidental movement and reflex actions, although offenses arising from this kind of conduct rarely if ever come to the attention of the courts because they are usually dealt with by police or prosecutorial bodies. Offending coinciding with, or resulting from, ISS including driving offenses is more common than other kinds of automatistic behavior, but it must be noted that it is still relatively unusual for such matters to come to the attention of the courts.

Automatism is the legal label given to the argument made by an individual to deny criminal liability for an offense in this sort of circumstance. In criminal law, automatism applies to conduct performed in an impaired state of consciousness or impaired control. In criminal law, an individual is presumed to be capacitous (the presumption of mental capacity).[47] This means that it is assumed that a defendant was conscious and acted or omitted to act in a volitional way at the time of the offense (for an act to count as the conduct element of an offense, it must be a freely chosen or willed act). Thus, automatism is a difficult defense to make out; a defendant has to raise some evidence of automatism before the defense is able to be left to the jury or fact-finder for evaluation. Of automatism, it has been said that "only those in desperate need of some kind of a defense" enter the "quagmire of law" that is automatism.[48]

The Australian High Court (equivalent in Australia to the United States Supreme Court) decision of *Jiminez v The Queen*[49] addressed some of the issues related to sleepiness and fall-asleep motor vehicle accidents. In this decision, the court granted an appeal against conviction of a driver involved in a fatal accident. In that case, the driver was charged and convicted of dangerous driving occasioning death after he was driving a car that crashed, killing the passenger in the front seat. Evidence indicated that the defendant driver fell asleep just before the crash. Although the precise issue on appeal was the trial judge's directions to the jury (and the technical issue of whether being asleep at the wheel constituted "driving"), the substantive issue in the case concerned the foreseeability of a sleep attack on the part of the driver (in legal parlance, whether the sleep attack was an unexpected event).

The *Jiminez* decision provides a useful illustration of the difficulties of principle in which the criminal law finds itself in relation to offenses occurring during ISS. These difficulties arise because of the requirement that a criminal defendant have performed the relevant action element (in the case of dangerous driving, the driving) at the same time as he or she had the requisite mental state (eg, recklessness or negligence). This is known as the principle of "coincidence" (requiring that the action element and mental element of the offense occur at the same point in time). The *Jiminez* court concluded that when a driver falls asleep at the wheel, the relevant period of driving is that which immediately precedes his or her falling asleep. Because the defendant could not be said to be driving at the precise time of the crash (ie, his or her actions while asleep were not conscious or voluntary as required for action element of a criminal offense), the court had to engage in a kind of subterfuge and stretch out the relevant action element to encompass the time before the crash when the defendant driver was driving dangerously (posing a risk to the public over and

above that ordinarily associated with driving) and the time at which he was asleep at the wheel.

The *Jiminez* court stressed that the issue was not whether there was warning of the onset of sleep (a subjective basis for liability) but whether in the circumstances the driving was a danger to the public (an objective basis for liability). Thus, a driver can be liable for dangerous driving even in cases where there is no warning about the onset of sleep; falling asleep while driving could be the beginning and thus the end (so to speak) of the offense of dangerous driving.

Another example of the devastating consequences of ISS is the Selby train disaster, an example of severe voluntary sleep deprivation contributing to a road vehicle accident involving two trains colliding and resulting in 12 deaths, multiple injuries, and temporary closure of a major rail line. The Leeds, United Kingdom, court held that the motor vehicle driver was at fault for his sleepiness and should have foreseen the potential consequences of his sleepiness. The driver was convicted and served a prison sentence.[50] In addition, his vehicle insurer had to assume civil liability.

Legal matrix governing sleepiness-impaired driving performance in New South Wales and other Australian states

The previously mentioned extreme cases also raise the more general issue of the obligations on an individual to report a relevant sleep condition when applying for or renewing his or her driving license. The following excerpt summarizes the current approach in Australia to the driver or applicant's duty-to-report, clearly laying out the primary responsibility to the driver or applicant: "In all States and Territories, except for Western Australia (at the time of reprint 2006), legislation requires a driver to advise the relevant Driver Licensing Authority of any permanent or long-term injury or illness that may affect his or her safe driving ability. These laws can impose penalties for failure to report. (Refer Appendix 3 [of the report] for further details).

As well as the legal obligations described above, a driver may be liable if he or she continues to drive knowing that he or she has a condition that is likely to adversely affect safe driving. Drivers should be aware that there may be long-term financial and legal consequences where there is failure to report an impairment to the Driver Licensing Authority. In the case of medical examinations requested by the Driver Licensing Authority, drivers also have a duty to declare truthfully their health status to the examining health professional."[38]

The previously mentioned Appendix 3 tabulates the relevant legislations across the various

Australian state and territory jurisdictions pertinent to the reporting of perceived driving safety impairment from the perspective of the driver, and separately from the perspective of the relevant health professional required to perform any medical examination required. By way of example, in the state of New South Wales the relevant law was the *Road Transport (Driver Licensing) Regulation 1999 c. 30 (5)* for the driver's perspective (subsequently amended 2005),[51] and its gist is summarized as follows: "The holder of a driver license must, as soon as practicable, notify the Authority of any permanent or long-term injury or illness that may impair his or her ability to drive safely." This clearly leaves the primary responsibility to the driver or applicant to recognize and declare any such impairment. Such an approach has obvious limitations.

From the examining health professional's perspective in New South Wales there are several laws (Road Transport [General] Act 2005, s. 243 [3] and [4]; Road Transport [Driver Licensing] Act 1998, s. 20; and Road Transport [Driver Licensing] Regulation 1999 c. 31) that pertain to the medical examination process. There is no mandatory reporting element to these legislative schemes in Australia but they do allow discretionary reporting and in concert provide protection to the medical examiner against civil or criminal liability for examining or reporting individuals in these circumstances. Reporting is mandatory in some jurisdictions elsewhere (eg, some Canadian provinces) but also accompanied in many such instances by legal protections that cover the reporter against legal claims from individuals so reported.

Civil Liability for ISS

Within the broad category of civil law, ISS raises issues in labor law (with liability falling to individual employees, and employers in some cases, for negligent work practices) and health law (in relation to issues of professional liability). In labor law, additional issues arise from the legal implications of shiftwork on employee health, and in the area of discrimination law (ie, relating to work and sleep hours, gender and age), and from the implications of new technologies in the workplace (alertness-promoting lighting, pharmacologic wakefulness promoters [such as the stimulant drug modafinil, which might be prescribed for management of excessive sleepiness in workers suffering from shift-work disorder]).

In civil law, liability for ISS arises under the common law (in negligence, which is part of the law of torts) and under specific statutory regimes mandating safe workplaces. In both contexts, an employee may be liable for causing injury to a coworker or another person or property, if he or she experiences ISS. In addition, an employer may be held liable if that employer knew of the employee's medical condition (if present) that gave rise to the ISS, or if he or she failed to maintain appropriate risk and safety procedures. Note here that the employers' duties extend to positive requirements that they establish and maintain safe workplaces, which in turn foster preventative actions to avoid or minimize the likelihood of harm resulting from ISS.

In general, the nature of the liability facing employees and employers is such that they will have breached their legal obligations whenever ISS leads to an injury to the employee, a coworker, or another, or whenever a particular workplace falls below the safety standard required by the law. However, the nature of the enforcement of the civil law is such that only a small proportion of breaches are investigated and a small selection of employees and employers prosecuted. This is largely a question of resources (although reporting and other issues feed into it). It means that enforcement and

---

Case Report

Mr X arrives at a busy metropolitan airport after a long, overnight international flight. He seeks to rent a car from a hire company for the purposes of a connecting drive to his destination. In the process of waiting to secure his car hire, Mr X is visibly sleepy to the hire company staff. The staff members process the hire arrangement nonetheless and Mr X successfully hires a car. Subsequently on the road, Mr X falls asleep at the wheel, has a serious accident and kills Ms Y, the driver of another car. Does the car hire company bear liability here?

The precise response to this hypothetical case scenario is likely to vary from jurisdiction to jurisdiction but it is possible to make some broad points. In general terms, if the car hire company could be thought to owe a duty of care to Ms Y as a victim, and the harm that Mr X causes because he falls asleep at the wheel is foreseeable, it is possible to hold the care hire company liable in negligence. Here, liability is analogous to that borne by a bar that continues to serve a patron who is seriously intoxicated, and which patron then commits an assault on the street on his way home. Although there may be issues of evidence and proof to resolve, it is possible to see how liability might arise in this instance.

prosecution is necessarily selective. Recent research indicates that, although these types of offenses are regarded as regulatory or quasiregulatory (ie, they do not connote the moral fault traditionally associated with liability), in making decisions about prosecution regulators are selecting those offenders whose actions (perhaps because they consist of repeated failings, or gross failure to reach the standard set by the law) seem to encode moral blameworthiness.[52] Often highly variable moral considerations also seem to have a role in these legal frameworks. Thus, from a legal perspective, although ISS raises issues under the umbrella of criminal and civil law, and although different policy considerations are driving the development of the law across the civil–criminal divide, individual differences in moral culpability help explain variation in specific instances of responsibility-attribution, and in the practices of investigation and prosecution of regulatory offenses.

Legal Context: United States

Specific legislation relating to drowsy driving is limited in the United States. Nevertheless, most states have the option to pursue prosecution for drowsy driving vehicular offenses under more general statutes, such as reckless driving, and in a preventive way many states have regulations applying curfews to young drivers. A notable exception to this generalist approach was provided in 2003 by the modification of an existing statute (the modification became known as "Maggie's law") in New Jersey.[26] This related to vehicular homicide while driving a motor vehicle or (maritime) vessel in providing that, when the driver is knowingly fatigued, with "fatigued" defined as "having been without sleep for a period in excess of 24 consecutive hours," he or she will be deemed to be reckless for the purposes of the offense of homicide. In reality this imposes a low (although nevertheless useful) level of interdiction when its basis is 24 hours of continuous total sleep deprivation and thus likely only includes the most egregious instances of voluntary sleep insufficiency.

Given that impairment of various functional capacities may occur at lower levels of total sleep deprivation and also in the context of chronic partial sleep deprivation,[53,54] Maggie's law may not prove to be as robust a restraint on individuals' impaired driving behavior as its legislators hoped. It is not known to the authors whether or not Maggie's Law has been successfully applied in a prosecution since its legislative enactment or whether other methods of assessing its success have been used.[55]

A further drowsy driving–related statute has been enacted in Massachusetts and approved in early 2007.[56] This statute is chiefly concerned with regulating (limiting) young ("junior") drivers and their permissible hours of driving, providing a legal framework for driver education programs, and in its penultimate section refers to drowsy driving: "SECTION 26. There shall be a special commission to study the impact of drowsy driving on highway safety and the effects of sleep deprivation on drivers while operating on the highways, adjacent parking areas and other areas."

A summary of the current and recent legal situations with respect to drowsy driving across the United States was documented in the National Sleep Foundation's *State of the States Report on Drowsy Driving 2007 (updated 2008)*, which surveyed the states' approach to drowsy driving issues and wherein it was noted that "Currently there are 12 bills introduced in 8 states addressing drowsy driving in various ways."[57]

Commercial motor vehicle drivers

In relation to commercial motor vehicle drivers, United States federal statute requires such drivers to undergo at least biennial medical examinations to determine the presence or otherwise of any "...established medical history or clinical diagnosis of respiratory dysfunction likely to interfere with the ability to control and drive a commercial motor vehicle safely."[58] However, the conference recommendations from which the relevant federal statute was drafted took place in 1991, and with subsequent advances in sleep medicine and other areas of science relevant to safer driving practices, there is a perceived need for a more contemporaneous framework of legislation, regulations, and guidelines for drivers, medical examiners, the transportation industry, and the public. To that end a Joint Task Force of interested parties (American College of Chest Physicians, American College of Occupational and Environmental Medicine, and National Sleep Foundation) recently developed and released a statement on *Sleep Apnea and Commercial Motor Vehicle Operators*[36] whose recommendations were endorsed by each of the individual organizations previously mentioned but to date have not been formally adopted by the Federal Motor Carrier Safety Administration.

There were to 1995 no OSA-specific regulations at the US federal level, nor regulations specific to other sleep disorders, but in respect of commercial motor carrier safety for interstate commerce (delineated under FMCSR [49 CFR 390–399]) there were clauses that contained descriptors that could have, arguably, included OSA and narcolepsy.[35] For example, there was reference to "a respiratory dysfunction likely to interfere with...ability to control and drive a motor vehicle safely, a prescription against the presence of epilepsy or any other condition which is likely to cause loss of consciousness or any loss of ability to control a motor vehicle, and that individuals have no mental, nervous, organic or functional disease or psychiatric disorder likely to interfere with...ability to drive a motor vehicle safely." In the United States, only one state before 1995 had a prohibition to drive while sleepy (but with no indication of how that condition was to be defined and evaluated). Seven states had in the mid-1990s regulations or guidelines that mentioned OSA or narcolepsy, but only two mentioned both. Details of the proffered guidelines with respect to requirement of duration of control of the condition, timing of any review process, or distinguishing between personal and commercial driving prohibitions varied considerably.

In addition to licensing statutes and regulations, occupation, health, and safety provisions within various (and mainly transportation) industries regulate hours of duty to minimize risk from ISS caused by voluntary sleep restriction to some degree, and these provisions are in many instances underpinned by an enforceable legal or regulatory framework. These hours-of-service regulations have been promulgated for commercial motor vehicle operators by the US Department of Transportation's Federal Motor Carrier Safety Administration and among several rules limit the hours of service (driving) to 10 or 11 hours after 8 or 10 hours off duty for passenger-carrying and property-carrying driving, respectively.[59]

Legal Context: Europe

It has been recognized that many medical disorders contribute to the risk for impaired driving. The weighted average of several listed medical conditions (but not including sleep disorders) considered in a recent Norwegian report[60] was 1.33; that is, any driver with a medical condition considered in the study had a 33% higher risk of accident involvement than a driver without such a medical condition. The report also then considered other conditions, such as sleep apnea or narcolepsy; depression; and consumption of cannabis, benzodiazepines, opiates, or cocaine. The highest relative risk was for sleep apnea or narcolepsy, with a figure as high as 3.71; that was the highest risk among all medical conditions considered and second only to age and gender as a general risk factor (young male drivers have a relative risk of ~7).

In a recent review of pan-European approaches to drowsy driving and associated medical conditions,[61] excessive daytime sleepiness was specifically identified in nine countries, whereas sleep apnea was specifically identified in 10 countries. In all cases, a patient with untreated OSA was considered unfit to drive. Some countries include a general "mental or physical state of incapacity to drive" rule where excessive daytime somnolence, either caused by sleep apnea or not, could be included. However, even when excessive daytime sleepiness or sleep apnea was mentioned, no criteria for severity were given nor guidelines on how to assess severity, what technical means could be used, or who should confirm the diagnosis. In some countries, after a diagnosis of sleep apnea syndrome was made, it became the physician's duty to inform the administrative authorities issuing driving licenses (mandatory reporting), whereas in other European countries the physician was expected to inform the patient (but not the authorities) that he or she was unfit to drive.

To determine the driving capacity in patients with sleep apnea, eight European countries rely on a medical certificate from a general practitioner or specialist (pneumologist or neurologist) based on symptom control and compliance with therapy. Only one country (France) requires a normalized electroencephalography-based maintenance of wakefulness test for group 2 (professional) drivers. There was thus reported in this study a wide "heterogeneity (that) concerns almost every aspect of the medical specifications, as well as many administrative aspects."[61] As far as sleep apnea is concerned, the situation had not much evolved since 2002, the date of the publication of an earlier survey.

SUMMARY

This article considers some of the medicolegal aspects of ISS. Where sleepiness mediated by impaired performance is the promoter of potential and actual harmful outcomes, communities have reacted by amending the law and using existing legal measures to curb those proclivities, and thereby protect its members.

From a legal perspective, ISS raises issues under the umbrella of criminal and civil law. The issue of the varying moral culpability of individuals involved in offending causing or coinciding with ISS is one of the key if somewhat nebulous issues in the attribution of criminal responsibility. It is also an important issue in the enforcement of legal obligations on employees and employers, which arise in the field of labor law. Here, employees and employers bear duties to avoid accidents associated with ISS as part of the wider regulatory framework governing safe workplaces. ISS is also an issue in the health law context, with treatment by sleep-deprived healthcare professionals a matter of some public concern. Although different policy considerations are driving the development of the law across the civil-criminal divide, individual differences in moral culpability seem to help explain variation in specific instances of responsibility attribution, and in the investigation and prosecution of regulatory offenses.

In terms of regulatory arrangements affecting ISS there is a diversity of laws, regulations, and guidelines across jurisdictions. A common theme may be discerned around the difficulty of determining the correct balance between the privileges of individuals to pursue their lives as private drivers or operators of workplace vehicles and machinery, and the perceived need for communities to provide a measure of protection for their members against adverse consequences of risky or dangerous behaviors. This difficulty is likely informed by a further diversity of factors including cultural values, level of recognition of the issues, and financial and political imperatives.

REFERENCES

1. Ohayon MM. Epidemiology of excessive sleepiness. In: Thorpy MJ, Billiard M, editors. Sleepiness: causes, consequences and treatment. Cambridge (United Kingdom): Cambridge University Press; 2011. p. 3–13.
2. Horne JA, Reyner LA. Sleep related vehicle accidents. BMJ 1995;310(6979):565–7.
3. Connor J, Norton R, Ameratunga S, et al. Driver sleepiness and risk of serious injury to car occupants: population based case control study. BMJ 2002;324(7346):1125.
4. Akerstedt T. Consensus statement: fatigue and accidents in transport operations. J Sleep Res 2000; 9(4):395.
5. Grunstein RR, Banerjee D. The case of "Judge Nodd" and other sleeping judges: media, society, and judicial sleepiness. Sleep 2007;30(5):625–32.
6. Venkatraman V, Chuah YM, Huettel SA, et al. Sleep deprivation elevates expectation of gains and attenuates response to losses following risky decisions. Sleep 2007;30(5):603–9.
7. Roehrs T, Greenwald M, Roth T. Risk-taking behavior: effects of ethanol, caffeine, and basal sleepiness. Sleep 2004;27(5):887–93.
8. Aoyama N, Goto E. A good night's sleep: the state of sleep in the U.S. Sleep well. Lack of sleep leads to death and loss. Tokyo (Japan): The Asahi Shimbun GLOBE; 2011.
9. Presidential Commission. Report of the Presidential Commission on the Space Shuttle Challenger accident, vol. 2, appendix G. Washington, DC: U.S. Government Printing Office; 1986.
10. Marine accident report: grounding of the U.S. tankship Exxon Valdez on Bligh Reef, Prince William Sound, near Valdez, Alaska, 1989. Washington, DC: National Transportation Safety Board; 1990.
11. U.S. Nuclear Regulatory Commission. Report on the accident at the Chernobyl Nuclear Power Station. Washington, DC: U.S. Government Printing Office; 1987.
12. Mitler MM, Carskadon MA, Czeisler CA, et al. Catastrophes, sleep, and public policy: consensus report. Sleep 1988;11(1):100–9.
13. Arnedt JT, Owens J, Crouch M, et al. Neurobehavioral performance of residents after heavy night call vs after alcohol ingestion. JAMA 2005;294(9): 1025–33.
14. Barger LK, Cade BE, Ayas NT, et al. Extended work shifts and the risk of motor vehicle crashes among interns. N Engl J Med 2005;352(2):125–34.
15. Philibert I. Sleep loss and performance in residents and nonphysicians: a meta-analytic examination. Sleep 2005;28(11):1392–402.
16. Hoey v Martin's Stock Haulage (Scone) Pty Ltd, 41 A, ed (2003).
17. Workers Compensation Act of 1987 (NSW), s 151G1987.
18. Motor Traffic Amendment (Driving Hours) Regulation of 1998 (NSW), regs 39, 771998.
19. American Academy of Sleep Medicine. The international classification of sleep disorders: diagnostic and coding manual. 2nd edition. Westchester (IL): American Academy of Sleep Medicine; 2005.
20. Kapur VK, Baldwin CM, Resnick HE, et al. Sleepiness in patients with moderate to severe sleep-disordered breathing. Sleep 2005;28(4):472–7.
21. Oksenberg A, Arons E, Nasser K, et al. Severe obstructive sleep apnea: sleepy versus nonsleepy patients. Laryngoscope 2010;120(3):643–8.
22. Young T, Palta M, Dempsey J, et al. The occurrence of sleep-disordered breathing among middle-aged adults. N Engl J Med 1993;328(17):1230–5.
23. Banks S, Dinges DF. Behavioral and physiological consequences of sleep restriction. J Clin Sleep Med 2007;3(5):519–28.
24. Swaen GM, Van Amelsvoort LG, Bultmann U, et al. Fatigue as a risk factor for being injured in an occupational accident: results from the Maastricht Cohort Study. Occup Environ Med 2003;60(Suppl 1): i88–92.
25. Akerstedt T, Philip P, Capelli A, et al. Sleep loss and accidents: work hours, life style, and sleep pathology. Prog Brain Res 2011;190:169–88.
26. An Act concerning vehicular homicide and amending N.J.S.2C:11–5, N.J.S.2C:11-5 (2003).

27. To err is human: building a safer health system. Institute of Medicine; 1999. Available at: http://www.iom.edu/Reports/1999/To-Err-is-Human-Building-A-Safer-Health-System.aspx. Accessed November 12, 2011.

28. McDonald F. Working to death: the regulation of working hours in health care. Law Policy 2008;30(1):108–40.

29. Medical Board of Queensland v Doneman, QHPT 0102004 (2004).

30. Accreditation Council for Graduate Medical Education. Common program requirements, resident duty hours. 2011. Available at: http://www.acgme.org/acWebsite/dutyHours/dh_index.asp. Accessed November 22, 2011.

31. Volpp KG, Rosen AK, Rosenbaum PR, et al. Mortality among hospitalized Medicare beneficiaries in the first 2 years following ACGME resident duty hour reform. JAMA 2007;298(9):975–83.

32. Volpp KG, Rosen AK, Rosenbaum PR, et al. Mortality among patients in VA hospitals in the first 2 years following ACGME resident duty hour reform. JAMA 2007;298(9):984–92.

33. Shetty KD, Bhattacharya J. Changes in hospital mortality associated with residency work-hour regulations. Ann Intern Med 2007;147(2):73–80.

34. Abaluck B, Landrigan CP. Sleepiness in healthcare workers. In: Thorpy MJ, Billiard M, editors. Sleepiness: causes, consequences and treatment. Cambridge (UK): Cambridge University Press; 2011. p. 204–14.

35. Pakola SJ, Dinges DF, Pack AI. Review of regulations and guidelines for commercial and noncommercial drivers with sleep apnea and narcolepsy. Sleep 1995;18(9):787–96.

36. Hartenbaum N, Collop N, Rosen IM, et al. Sleep apnea and commercial motor vehicle operators: statement from the joint Task Force of the American College of Chest Physicians, American College of Occupational and Environmental Medicine, and the National Sleep Foundation. J Occup Environ Med 2006;48(Suppl 9):S4–37.

37. Desai AV, Ellis E, Wheatley JR, et al. Fatal distraction: a case series of fatal fall-asleep road accidents and their medicolegal outcomes. Med J Aust 2003; 178(8):396–9.

38. Assessing fitness to drive. Sydney, NSW (Australia): Austroads Incorporated; 2003.

39. Philip P, Sagaspe P, Taillard J. Drowsy driving In: Principles and practice of sleep medicine. 5th edition. Philadelphia: Elsevier Saunders; 2010.

40. Southworth MR, Kortepeter C, Hughes A. Nonbenzodiazepine hypnotic use and cases of "sleep driving". Ann Intern Med 2008;148(6):486–7.

41. Pressman MR. Sleep driving: sleepwalking variant or misuse of z-drugs? Sleep Med Rev 2011;15(5):285–92.

42. Marshall NS, Buchanan PR. Z drug zombies: parasomnia, drug effect or both? Sleep Med Rev 2011; 15(5):283–4.

43. R v Hardie, 1 WLR 64 (1984).

44. R v Bailey, 1 WLR 760 (1983).

45. Loughnan A. Manifest madness: mental incapacity in criminal law. Oxford (United Kingdom): Oxford University Press; 2012.

46. Mitchell C. Intoxication, criminality and responsibility. Int J Law Psychiatry 1990;13(1–2):1–7.

47. Bratty v Attorney-General for Northern Ireland, AC 386 (1963).

48. R v Quick, Q.B. 910, 922 (1973).

49. Jiminez v The Queen, 173 CLR 572 (1992).

50. R v Hart Leeds Crown Court, (2002).

51. Road Transport (Driver Licensing) Amendment (Miscellaneous) Regulation, 2005, No 6102005.

52. Wells C, Quick O. Lacey, wells and quick reconstructing criminal law. Text and materials. 4th edition. Cambridge (UK): Cambridge University Press; 2010.

53. Van Dongen HP, Maislin G, Mullington JM, et al. The cumulative cost of additional wakefulness: dose-response effects on neurobehavioral functions and sleep physiology from chronic sleep restriction and total sleep deprivation. Sleep 2003;26(2):117–26.

54. Belenky G, Wesensten NJ, Thorne DR, et al. Patterns of performance degradation and restoration during sleep restriction and subsequent recovery: a sleep dose-response study. J Sleep Res 2003;12(1):1–12.

55. JimSix/SouthJerseyNewspapers. 2007; nj.com. Available at: http://blog.nj.com/gloucester/2007/07/maggies_law_used_to_charge_dri.html. Accessed November 27, 2011.

56. An Act Further Regulating Driver Education and Junior Operator's Licenses. 2006. Available at: http://www.malegislature.gov/Laws/SessionLaws/Acts/2006/Chapter428. Accessed January 8, 2012.

57. National Sleep Foundation. State of the States Report on Drowsy Driving: Summary of Findings November 2008

58. US Department of Transportation Federal Highway Administration, Office of Motor Carriers. Conference on Pulmonary/Respiratory Disorders and Commercial Drivers. Publication No. FHWA-MC-91-004. 1991. Available at: http://www.fmcsa.dot.gov/documents/pulmonary1.pdf. Accessed November 13, 2011.

59. Federal Motor Carrier Safety Administration. CFR Parts 385 and 395. Hours of Service of Drivers, vol. 49. Washington, DC: U.S. Department of Transportation; 2008.

60. Vaa T. Impairments, diseases, age and their relative risks of accident involvement: results from meta-analysis. Oslo (Norway): Institute of Transport Economics; 2003.

61. Alonderis A, Barbe F, Bonsignore M, et al. Medico-legal implications of sleep apnoea syndrome: driving license regulations in Europe. Sleep Med 2008;9(4):362–75.

Hypersomnia in Older Patients

Marcia E. Braun, PhD[a], Pamela Cines, MD[b],
Nalaka S. Gooneratne, MD, MSc[b,c],*

KEYWORDS

- Hypersomnia • Sleepiness • Fatigue • Older adult • Obstructive sleep apnea • Central sleep apnea
- Cognitive impairment • Institutionalized

KEY POINTS

- Hypersomnia is a common clinical complaint in older patients; distinction needs to made between napping and hypersomnia, as they are not necessarily correlated in older adults.
- As hypersomnia is known to be independently related to, or even predictive of, a broad array of disorders and diseases, and an increased risk of mortality, the assessment of excessive daytime sleepiness in older adults should be considered as part of a diagnostic plan.

Although the definition of hypersomnia in older patients is similar to that of younger populations, namely, the presence of excessive daytime sleepiness (EDS), its manifestations, etiology, consequences, and treatment differ from those of younger patients in several subtle and not so subtle ways. Several factors underlie these differences, including the impact of comorbid medical conditions and polypharmacy; age-related changes in the sleep-wake homeostatic system; lifestyle changes due to retirement; and altered expectations of acceptable health. When discussing hypersomnia in older adults, these factors form an additional layer of considerations that can help guide an appropriate evaluation and treatment plan, which minimizes the risk of unnecessary testing or treatment so as to avoid iatrogenic complications while maximizing quality of life.

This article emphasizes areas in which the evaluation and management of hypersomnia in older adults differ from those for younger adults. A general review of hypersomnia is provided. In addition, several neurologic, medical, and psychiatric comorbidities related to hypersomnia in older adults are discussed.

While there exist research and clinical definitions of hypersomnia that distinguish hypersomnia from fatigue or weakness, it is important to emphasize that older adult patients, especially those with cognitive impairment, may not necessarily be able to make this distinction. Thus an older adult patient or their caregiver may present with complaints of fatigue that may in fact represent hypersomnia, or vice versa. This distinction becomes even more important because there are no simple, inexpensive measures to objectively distinguish hypersomnia and fatigue that can readily be implemented in a clinical setting. For this reason, when evaluating hypersomnia complaints in older adults, it is also worthwhile to also consider differential diagnoses more commonly associated with fatigue. As such, while this review mainly addresses hypersomnia, it also includes at times discussion of disorders that are primarily associated with fatigue.

The authors have no conflicts of interest.

[a] Division of Sleep and Chronobiology, Unit for Experimental Psychiatry, Perelman School of Medicine, University of Pennsylvania, 1013 Blockley Hall, 423 Guardian Drive, Philadelphia, PA 19104–6021, USA; [b] Division of Geriatric Medicine, Department of Medicine, University of Pennsylvania School of Medicine, 3615 Chestnut Street, Philadelphia, PA 19104, USA; [c] Center for Sleep and Circadian Neurobiology, University of Pennsylvania School of Medicine, 3624 Market Street, Philadelphia, PA 19104, USA

* Corresponding author. Division of Geriatric Medicine, Department of Medicine, University of Pennsylvania School of Medicine, 3615 Chestnut Street, Philadelphia, PA 19104.

E-mail address: ngoonera@mail.med.upenn.edu

Sleep Med Clin 7 (2012) 365–378
doi:10.1016/j.jsmc.2012.03.011
1556-407X/12/$ – see front matter © 2012 Published by Elsevier Inc.

PREVALENCE

Data from the Sleep Heart Health Study sample of 4578 older study participants (age 65 years and older) suggests that approximately 20% of older adults complain of feeling "usually sleepy in the daytime."[1] Although it is generally anticipated that older adults have higher levels of daytime sleepiness in comparison with younger populations, this is not necessarily the case. Several studies have noted that sleepiness complaints may decrease when comparing young with old populations.[2–5] Pallesen and colleagues,[6] for example, noted that young adulthood was associated with higher rates of sleepiness. Similarly, data from the Behavioral Risk Factors Surveillance Study found that sleepiness decreased with age, and that older adults had the lowest likelihood of endorsing daytime sleepiness.[7] One factor that may underlie the reduction in daytime sleepiness with age is that healthy older adults generally have a lower 24-hour maximal total sleep capacity than do healthy younger subjects. In a 7-day study performed at an inpatient research unit that removed social, external constraints and allowed subjects to sleep for up to 16 hours per day, the total daily sleep duration was 8.9 hours in younger subjects and only 7.4 hours in older subjects, even after allowing subjects several nights to recover from baseline sleep debt.[8]

It is worth noting, however, that within the age category of older than 65 years, there can be heterogeneity as regards the prevalence of hypersomnia. Among the very old (age >75 years) or those with more severe comorbidities, the prevalence of hypersomnia tends to increase.[9] The conventional wisdom that considers daytime sleepiness as a normal aspect of aging therefore may be inaccurate in the contemporary era, where there is a growing cohort of "healthy elderly" attributable to progressive increases in life span. The hypersomnia that was common in adults older than 65 in the past may indeed have been relevant when many of these adults suffered from comorbidities, whereas in the modern era these hypersomnia symptoms are appearing in later years, such as age 75 years and older.

Paradoxically, although the complaint of daytime sleepiness may decrease, older adults are more likely to take naps,[10,11] with 64% of older subjects taking a nap compared with 45% of younger subjects.[12] Most older adults who take regular naps do not complain of EDS: analysis of the 2003 Sleep in America poll noted that 37% of regular nappers aged 65 to 74 years and 21% of regular nappers aged 75 to 84 years reported experiencing EDS (defined as "having daytime sleepiness so severe that it interferes with…daily activities").[10]

One explanation for this discrepancy is that with advancing age, there can be an altered perception of an acceptable health status.[13] In middle age, fewer than 5% of subjects consider it acceptable to have a severe impairment in their ability to perform usual activities, whereas in subjects older than 70 years, 10% to 30% consider this level of impairment acceptable.[13] This finding reflects a shift toward greater tolerance of poor health with advancing age. A similar trend may occur with hypersomnia, thus leading to a tendency to underreport the prevalence of hypersomnia despite increased evidence of hypersomnia (ie, naps).

A second explanation for the discrepancy between the rising prevalence of naps and the declining prevalence of hypersomnia complaints with age may be that an older adult has more opportunities than a younger adult to nap, which can occur in large part as a consequence of retirement. Thus, although a younger adult may feel sleepy and wish to nap, he or she is unable to do so because of work requirements. An alternative explanation, however, is that the increased prevalence of napping in older adults may help to treat their daytime hypersomnia, thus leading to reduced rates of hypersomnia, whereas in younger adults, work requirements prevent them from using a nap to relieve their sleepiness. Few studies have examined this relationship, however, and whereas anecdotal reports suggest napping increases after retirement, others have not observed this trend in cross-sectional research.[14]

A third consideration arises from the observation that a nap may be voluntary or involuntary.[15] It is possible that involuntary naps may be more strongly linked to excessive sleepiness than voluntary naps. The increased prevalence of voluntary naps could occur in cases where naps are an important element of the cultural background of the patient, such as Mediterranean cultures in which an afternoon nap or siesta may be more common and may occur in a patient who otherwise does not have symptoms of hypersomnia. There is little research on the distinction between voluntary and involuntary naps, although there is a growing appreciation that multiple physiologic, pathophysiologic, and cultural factors influence napping behavior.[15]

ASSESSMENT

One of the major challenges in identifying hypersomnia in older adults is related to assessment. Several different methods have been proposed for measuring hypersomnia, ranging from self-report measures to objective assessments. However, most these tools have not been validated in older adults.

The Epworth Sleepiness Scale (ESS), one of the most widely used tools to assess hypersomnia, was first developed in middle-aged patients and has primarily been used in the outpatient or at-home setting. Research in older adults suggests that they may have higher scores on the ESS.[16] Specific subpopulations, such as patients with Parkinson disease, may also have gaps in their assessment of sleepiness when relying solely on the ESS.[17] Use of the ESS among older adults with more significant levels of comorbidity can also be problematic. For example, 28% of inpatient older adults omitted ESS items, and 38% were unable to complete the ESS at all.[18] Despite these limitations, recent work examining the ESS in older men has demonstrated that the ESS was correlated with another commonly used measure of sleep, the Pittsburgh Sleep Quality Index.[19] Furthermore, it has been suggested that validated questionnaires assessing sleepiness during specific activities may be more useful than general questions about sleepiness because of the tendency to underreport sleepiness and sleep complaints.[20,21]

The Multiple Sleep Latency Test (MSLT) is a commonly used measure of daytime sleep propensity. Research in older adults suggests that the MSLT is fairly stable, with correlations of 0.7 to 0.87 across multiple days of testing.[22] However, although MSLT sleep-onset latency is decreased in older adults with sleepiness compared with those without sleepiness,[23] the difference is fairly small (9.3 ± 4.8 minutes and 11.9 ± 4.9 minutes, respectively [$P<.0001$]). The correlation between the MSLT and subjective measures of sleepiness, such as the ESS, is poor across all ages.[5] Furthermore, in older adults the MSLT does not correlate with performance on 13 neuropsychological measures, such as the Stroop Color-Word Naming test or the Trailmaking A/B tests.[22] One explanation for this is that daytime sleep latency in general may increase with age, going from 8.7 minutes in 20- to 30-year-old subjects up to 14.2 minutes in 66- to 83-year-old subjects,[24] a finding that has been noted in other studies.[5] These data also have ramifications when using the MSLT as a diagnostic test. One study in patients with narcolepsy noted that the number of sleep-onset rapid-eye movement (REM) episodes was decreased in older adults relative to younger subjects, and that older adults tended to have longer sleep latencies, leading the investigators to conclude that the current MSLT criteria for narcolepsy may lead to an increased percentage of false-negative MSLTs in older adults.[25]

Other tools that can assist in the diagnosis of hypersomnia include actigraphy and sleep logs, both of which allow for assessment across multiple days. Actigraphy is particularly interesting, as it provides the opportunity to gather objective information. Research in older adults with heart failure, for example, has shown significant decreases in daytime activity as measured by actigraphy in subjects who reported lack of energy.[26] This research is in its early stages, however, and clearly defined thresholds for abnormal daytime actigraphy levels in older adults are not yet available. Actigraphy can also be used to measure nap periods during the daytime, which can be particularly useful because older adults have a tendency to underreport their napping: one study identified an average of 4 naps over a 12-day period when using self-report, and 6 naps over a 12-day period when using actigraphy to provide an objective assessment.[27] However, the accuracy can vary significantly based on the actigraphy settings.[28,29]

Etiology of Hypersomnia

A broad range of factors may lead to the development of clinically significant hypersomnia. In many cases they are similar to risk factors that also occur in younger populations, but may be more common in older adults. In addition, the prevalence of various hypersomnia diagnoses in older adults differs. Whereas narcolepsy is commonly considered in the differential diagnosis for hypersomnia in a younger adult, it is rare to identify this disorder for the first time in an older adult. Instead, other hypersomnia diagnoses, such as hypersomnia due to medical condition or idiopathic hypersomnia (with or without long sleep time), may be more common in older adults. An overview is presented in **Fig. 1** for the clinical evaluation of older adults with hypersomnia, based on potential etiologic factors now discussed in more detail.

Demographic Factors

One of the major demographic changes that occur with advancing age is the opportunity to retire from full-time work. The GAZEL study, the largest study to date to examine the effects of retirement on sleep, focused primarily on the complaint of fatigue and noted significant decreases with retirement.[30] This study followed 14,104 employees of the French national gas and electricity company, starting 7 years before retirement and extending to 7 years after retirement, and observed an 81% decrease in "mental fatigue" and a 73% decrease in "physical fatigue" 1 year after retirement compared with 1 year before retirement.[30] The reduction in fatigue was most prominent in those with a chronic medical condition. Another smaller study in 40 subjects also noted a reduced

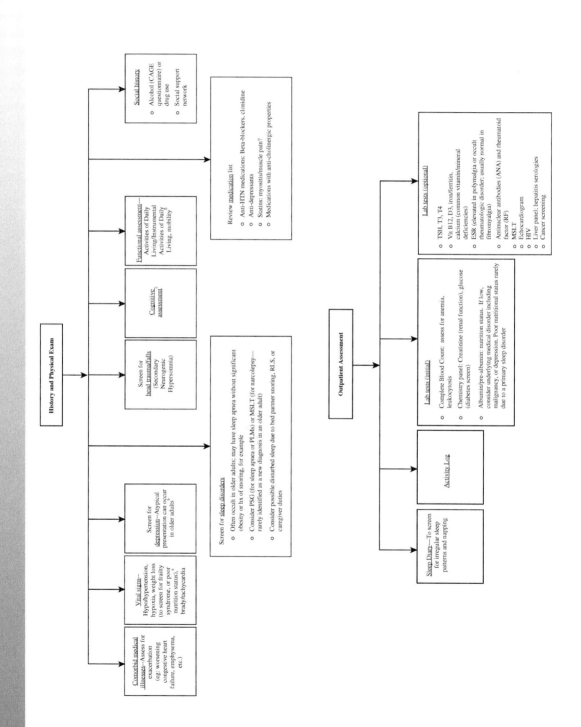

History and Physical Exam

Comorbid medical illnesses—Assess for exacerbation (eg: worsening congestive heart failure, emphysema, etc.)

Vital signs—Hypohypertension, hypoxia, weight loss (to screen for frailty syndrome, or poor nutrition status),[a] brady/tachycardia

Screen for depression—Atypical presentation can occur in older adults[a]

Screen for head trauma/falls (Secondary Neurogenic Hypersomnia)

Cognitive assessment[a]

Functional assessment—Activities of Daily Living/Instrumental Activities of Daily Living, mobility[a]

Social history
○ Alcohol (CAGE questionnaire) or drug use
○ Social support network

Screen for sleep disorders
○ Often occult in older adults; may have sleep apnea without significant obesity or hx of snoring, for example
○ Consider PSG (for sleep apnea or PLMs) or MSLT (for narcolepsy— rarely identified as a new diagnosis in an older adult)
○ Consider possible disturbed sleep due to bed partner snoring, RLS, or caregiver duties

Review medication list
○ Anti-HTN medications: Beta-blockers, clonidine
○ Anti-depressants
○ Statins: myositis/muscle pain?
○ Medications with anti-cholinergic properties

Outpatient Assessment

Sleep Diary—To screen for irregular sleep patterns and napping

Activity Log

Lab tests (initial)
○ Complete Blood Count: assess for anemia, leukocytosis
○ Chemistry panel: Creatinine (renal function), glucose (diabetes screen)
○ Albumin/pre-albumin: nutrition status. If low, consider underlying medical disorder including malignancy, or depression. Poor nutritional status rarely due to a primary sleep disorder

Lab tests (optional)
○ TSH, T3, T4
○ Vit B12, D3, iron/ferritin, calcium (common vitamin/mineral deficiencies)
○ ESR (elevated in polymyalgia or occult rheumatologic disorder; usually normal in fibromyalgia)
○ Antinuclear antibodies (ANA) and rheumatoid factor (RF)
○ MSLT
○ Echocardiogram
○ HIV
○ Liver panel; hepatitis serologies
○ Cancer screening

frequency of napping with retirement[14] although, as noted earlier, most studies show an increase in napping with advancing age.

Another change that occurs primarily in an aging population is confinement to a nursing home, a setting in which abnormal sleep patterns and hypersomnia may be common.[31] A variety of causative factors can contribute to this problem. Martin and colleagues[31] studied 492 residents of 4 nursing homes, using direct observation every 15 minutes to identify daytime sleeping and how it may relate to disturbed nighttime sleep. Those who were asleep during more than 15% of all observations over 2 days were considered to be excessively sleepy. Of the original group of nursing home residents observed in this study, 339 of 492 were noted to sleep for greater than 15% of their observations during the day. Of those residents, 194 were consented for 2 nights of wrist actigraphy, 133 of whom had disrupted nighttime sleep. Of this group, 118 went on to have 3 more days of wrist actigraphy to monitor circadian rhythms. All but 2 of this group had abnormal circadian rhythms and abnormal light exposure, receiving an average of only 10 minutes of bright light per day. In addition, residents who were asleep during a greater percentage of the daytime observations were noted to have more cognitive impairment (as measured by lower scores on the Mini-Mental State Examination), spent more time in bed and in their own rooms, engaged in fewer social and physical activities (and when engaged they required more assistance), and were involved in fewer conversations.

Medical Factors

Certain medical and psychiatric conditions that are more prevalent in the elderly are also more frequently associated with hypersomnia, thus older adults are more likely to have the International Classification of Sleep Disorders, 2nd edition (ICSD-2) diagnosis of "Hypersomnia Due to Medical Condition."[32] Asplund[33] surveyed 6143 members of the National Swedish Pensioners' Association (average age 73 years) and noted that 32% of men and 23.2% of women often experienced daytime

sleepiness. Men and women who believed themselves to be in poor health were 4.9 and 5.1 times more likely, respectively, to feel sleepy during the daytime compared with those who reported good health. Daytime sleepiness was reported more frequently in subjects who had cardiac disease, diabetes, musculoskeletal complaints, and awakenings at night due to nocturia. Similarly, those who reported taking medications to treat the aforementioned illnesses were more likely to experience daytime sleepiness. Bixler and colleagues[9] also interviewed 16,583 people about their sleep habits, daytime sleepiness, and medical comorbidities, and found that subjects with diabetes were about twice as likely as those without diabetes to experience daytime sleepiness.

Vitamin or mineral deficiencies are more common in older adults and can also contribute to hypersomnia or fatigue complaints. Vitamin deficiencies that are strongly associated with hypersomnia include deficiencies of vitamin D, B6, and B12.[34–37] Deficiencies of vitamins C and E may also lead to fatigue and supplementation of these vitamins may correspondingly reduce fatigue,[38,39] but there is less evidence to support this at present.[40] Iron or calcium mineral deficiencies that can occur in older adults may also be associated with hypersomnia or fatigue.[35,41] Screening of these deficiencies may be warranted in certain cases as part of the evaluation of hypersomnia.

Geriatric depression is a unique syndrome in comparison with depression in the general population, because it may present with atypical features[42] including symptoms such as overeating, weight gain, oversleeping, and leaden paralysis in the absence of catatonic or melancholic features.[43] As such, these patients may meet ICSD-2 criteria for "Hypersomnia Not Due to Substance or Known Physiologic Condition," especially in cases where the hypersomnia symptoms are more prominent or of more concern to the patient/caregiver than other symptoms of the underlying depression.[32] Risk factors for developing depression in older age include female sex, social isolation, widowed, divorced, or separated marital status, lower socioeconomic status, medical comorbidities, pain that is not controlled,

---

Fig. 1. Evaluation of an older adult with hypersomnolence. [a] Over 1 month, weight loss of more than 5 lb (2.3 kg) or 5% of total body weight is considered significant. Over 6 months, weight loss of more than 10% or 10 lb (4.5 kg) is significant. [b] Geriatric Depression Scale is a well-validated test. In patients with cognitive impairment, consider the Cornell Scale for Depression in Dementia. [c] Mini-Mental Status Examination, or brief assessment using the Mini-Cognitive Assessment Instrument. [d] Timed get-up-and-go test, available at http://www.hospital-medicine.org/geriresource/toolbox/pdfs/get_up_and_go_test.pdf. ESR, erythrocyte sedimentation rate; HIV, human immunodeficiency virus; HTN, hypertension; MSLT, Multiple Sleep Latency Test; PLM, periodic limb movement; PSG, polysomnography; RLS, restless legs syndrome; TSH, thyroid-stimulating hormone; Vit, vitamin.

insomnia, functional impairment, and cognitive impairment. Among subjects who reported a diagnosis of depression, regular napping was noted to be 50% higher than in subjects who did not carry this diagnosis,[10] and subjects being treated for depression are 6 times more likely than those not being treated to experience EDS.[9]

In addition to geriatric depression, vascular depression is a recently described phenomenon that is more common in the elderly.[44] This syndrome occurs in the setting of ischemic changes associated temporally with the onset of depression, and can be likened to the stepwise changes seen in vascular dementia. The diagnosis of vascular depression is different from the more researched complication of cerebral ischemia, poststroke depression. Vascular depression is more common in the elderly and, like other depression syndromes, may also be associated with hypersomnolence.

Another geriatric syndrome that may be linked to hypersomnia is the frailty syndrome. Frailty has been defined as having 3 or more of the following: (1) unintentional loss of more than 10 lb (4.5 kg) in past year or more than 5% of body weight at follow-up examination; (2) weakness as measured by grip strength in the lowest 20% of cohort adjusted for gender and body mass index; (3) poor endurance as measured by self-report of exhaustion; (4) slowness defined as the subjects in the cohort who were at the bottom 20% of time needed to walk 15 ft (4.6 m); or (5) low physical activity level as measured by subjects' self-report of activity each week.[45] In one study, the prevalence of frailty at baseline was 7%.[45] Subjects who met criteria for being frail were more likely to be African American, female, have less income and less education, and have higher rates of disability as well as cardiovascular disease, pulmonary disease, arthritis, and diabetes. Frailty was associated with higher likelihood of adverse outcomes including falls, hospitalization, institutionalization, and death.

Frailty as defined here may also be correlated with sleep disorders and hypersomnia. In a separate study, 54% of a sample of 3133 men were defined as meeting intermediate criteria for frailty (having 1 or 2 of the 5 aforementioned criteria), and 14% met the criteria for frailty (having 3 or more criteria).[46] Poor sleep quality, daytime sleepiness, shorter sleep duration, sleep fragmentation, and other objective measures were all increasingly common in the men considered frail. Others have also noted an association between daytime sleepiness and measures of frailty, with an adjusted odds ratio of 3.67.[47] Future research is needed to determine whether reversal of sleepiness will help stem the progression of frailty and related adverse consequences.

Polypharmacy is another potential contributor to poor sleep quality and hypersomnia in older populations. The ICSD-2 includes a distinct category for medication-related hypersomnia, "Hypersomnia Due to Drug or Substance (Medications)," and distinguishes this from illicit drug or alcohol-related hypersomnia ("Hypersomnia Due to Drug or Substance [Abuse]").[32] Polypharmacy can have a variety of definitions including the prescription of a certain number of medications, certain classes of medications, medications with specific properties, medications that are ineffective, and medications that are not specifically indicated. For example, about 50% of people older than 65 years take more than 5 medications. In addition, 40% of patients who receive care at home take more than 9 medications. Specific medications and classes of medications that can contribute to hypersomnia have been identified. These agents include medications with anticholinergic effects (**Table 1**; an example from each class is listed in parentheses): antihistamines (diphenhydramine), antidepressants (tricyclic antidepressants such as amitriptyline), antiemetics (promethazine), antipsychotics (olanzapine), antivertigo (meclizine), muscle relaxants (cyclobenzaprine), Parkinson therapy (benztropine), and urinary incontinence (oxybutynin).[48] β-Blockers (metoprolol) are another class of medication that can cause sleepiness. These agents are often indicated for coronary artery disease, hypertension, congestive heart failure, migraine, and tremor. Another agent used in older adults that is associated with daytime sleepiness is clonidine, for refractory hypertension. Narcotics, which can lead to daytime sleepiness, are often prescribed for pain control as contraindications to the use of other pain medications, such as nonsteroidal anti-inflammatory drugs, mount with advancing age.[49] One alternative includes using scheduled doses of acetaminophen, which may allow the clinician to avoid the use of narcotics or possibly limit narcotic use to nighttime only when the patient may need stronger pain relief to ensure sleep. Of note, there are nighttime formulations of several over-the-counter agents (in many cases including the term "PM" in the product name) that contain diphenhydramine in addition to the analgesic. Diphenhydramine can be problematic in older adults because of its side-effect profile, which includes delirium and cognitive impairment.[50] Benzodiazepines, such as lorazepam, are frequently used for symptoms of anxiety; however, to adequately treat the symptoms these medications often need to be dosed throughout the day, again leading to daytime sleepiness.

Approximately 30% to 50% of older adults will have a fall episode each year, making falls one of the most common causes of trauma and death in

Table 1
Medications associated with hypersomnia

Category or Indication	Examples
Analgesic	Diclofenac, etodolac, fentanyl, hydrocodone, ketoprofen, naproxen, oxycodone, pregabalin, tramadol
Antibiotic	Cephalosporins, norfloxacin, ofloxacin
Antidepressant	Amitriptyline, clomipramine, escitalopram, fluvoxamine, paroxetine, sertraline, trazodone, venlafaxine
Antihistamine	Dimenhydrinate, diphenhydramine, hydroxyzine, loratadine, meclizine, propoxyphene, terfenadine
Antihypertensive	Amlodipine, clonidine, prazosin
Antiparkinson	Benztropine, levodopa, pramipexole
Antipsychotic	Quetiapine, olanzapine
β-Blocker	Atenolol, carvedilol, labetolol, metoprolol, pindolol, propranolol
Cholesterol lowering	Fluvastatin, niacin
Cognitive impairment	Donepezil
Diabetes	Glipizide, metformin
Epilepsy	Gabapentin, phenytoin, topiramate, valproic acid
Gastrointestinal	Hyoscyamine, metoclopramide, promethazine
Hormone	Estrogen, progestin
Muscle relaxant	Baclofen, cyclobenzaprine, metaxalone
Sedative	Alprazolam, chlordiazepoxide, clonazepam, diazepam, eszopiclone, flurazepam, lorazepam, meprobamate, oxazepam, temazepam, triazolam, valerian, melatonin
Urinary incontinence	Oxybutynin

Based on a review of the US Pharmacopeia for medications with hypersomnia (drowsiness, somnolence, sleepiness, unusually tired, unusual tiredness, fatigue) identified as being "more common."

this population.[51] Furthermore, falls in older adults are more likely than falls in younger adults to be associated with head or neck trauma.[52] This finding increases the risk of subsequently developing "Posttraumatic Hypersomnia" (ICSD-2 diagnosis) in older adults. As such, a history of falls is an important aspect of evaluating older adults with hypersomnia.

Sleep Disorders

Hypersomnia has been associated with disruptions in nighttime sleep caused by a broad range of age-related changes, including shifts in sleep architecture (ie, phase shifts, decreases in slow-wave sleep [SWS] or REM sleep), increased prevalence rates of various sleep disorders (ie, insomnia, sleep apnea, restless legs syndrome), or sleep fragmentation.[20,53–55] These hypersomnias are generally classified in the ICSD-2 under the specific causative sleep disorder and are not included in the general category of "Hypersomnias of Central Origin."[32]

Pack and colleagues[23] examined risk factors for EDS in older adults, with diagnoses of sleep disorder confirmed using polysomnography. These investigators identified the following factors that increased the risk for daytime sleepiness (adjusted analyses): apnea-hypopnea index (odds ratio [OR] for 20-events/h increase) 1.4 (1.1–1.9); Pittsburgh Sleep Quality Index self-report of overall sleep quality (OR for 1-point increase) 2.3 (1.6–3.6); percent time in REM sleep (OR for 6.8% increase) 1.4 (1.1–1.9); pain or physical discomfort 3 times or more per week 5.9 (2.2–19.0); any wheezing or whistling from chest at night 3.2 (1.4–8.0); use of medications with sleepiness as a common side effect 1.9 (1.1–3.3); and male sex 1.9 (1.0–3.5). Periodic limb movements were not associated with hypersomnia in this study. As it is beyond the scope of this article to discuss each of these disorders, we will focus instead on specific aspects related to older adults.

Disruptions in sleep may be due to changes in sleep structure that can take place with advancing age, including circadian rhythm dysregulation[56–58] and weakening of the homeostatic sleep system.[59] Whereas clinicians generally tend to think of older adults as more likely to have advanced sleep-phase disorder, research suggests that many also have delayed sleep-phase disorder.[58] Insomnia symptoms (including unrefreshing sleep) may also lead to daytime sleepiness.[60] However, some insomnia patients may have a hyperarousal component that reduces their daytime sleep propensity, resulting in increased daytime alertness as measured by longer MSLT values compared with controls.[61] These patients may present with complaints of daytime fatigue, therefore fatigue scales are recommended as part of the research evaluation of insomnia.[32,62] In older adults, sleepiness assessment using measures such as the Functional Outcomes of Sleepiness Questionnaire suggest increased levels of sleepiness in those with insomnia; however, there is considerable overlap between those with and without insomnia, and specific cutoff points could not be identified that distinguish either group effectively.[63]

Sleep-disordered breathing and associated disorders (eg, obstructive sleep apnea [OSA], central apnea, and mixed sleep apnea become more common with advancing age: nearly 20% of older adults have sleep-disordered breathing when using a criteria of an apnea-hypopnea index of 15 events or more per hour, compared with approximately 10% of younger subjects, for example.[64] Decreases in the quality of nighttime sleep and increased daytime sleepiness[65] may be the result of oxygen desaturation related to episodes of apnea and hypopnea caused by coexisting snoring and sleep disruptions,[66] although findings have not always been consistent.[55,66] Instead, some investigators suggest that a third variable, such as obesity, may actually mediate the relationship between daytime sleepiness and sleep-disordered breathing.[9,55] Dixon and colleagues[66] found sleepiness remained even after treatment of OSA in obese individuals, and contend that this may be due to multiple comorbidities associated with obesity. Similar findings were obtained for a group of diabetic patients. Chasens and colleagues[67] found that those patients reporting greater daytime sleepiness also had a higher body mass index, rated their own health more poorly, had poorer sleep quality, and had more comorbidities. Treatment of sleep-disordered breathing can lead to reductions in daytime sleepiness, even in patients with cognitive impairment.[68]

Although sleep disorders are often thought of as isolated diagnoses, older adults may have multiple sleep disorders. These patients are particularly vulnerable to daytime sleepiness effects, with one study showing the most prominent functional impairments from daytime sleepiness occurring in subjects with both insomnia and sleep-disordered breathing relative to subjects that had either disorder alone or no sleep disorders.[69]

CONSEQUENCES OF DAYTIME SLEEPINESS

There is compelling evidence of the negative effects of daytime sleepiness on health and well-being. Across all age groups, hypersomnia has been independently linked to consequences that range from functional and cognitive impairment to being at an increased risk of mortality, and these risks become particularly important during old age.[69,70] Identifying EDS, either as a symptom of a disease or disorder or as a consequence of poor sleep, is difficult because of the competing risk from comorbidity associated with existing diseases or disorders.[71] In this context, it becomes difficult to identify any specific effect that is independently associated with daytime sleepiness.[67,71] However, within an older population, hypersomnia has been found to be related to increased incidences of health-related disorders and comorbidities, as well as being independently associated with an overall decline in functional outcomes.[69] This section provides an overview of the consequences of EDS within the elderly population.

Functional Outcomes

Older adults who experience extreme daytime sleepiness typically describe having a reduction in quality of life and a decline in day-to-day functioning. As mentioned previously, for some adults, changes in social status (ie, retirement) may result in greater amounts of unstructured free time and a reduction in the number and availability of available friends or colleagues, resulting in less daily social contact, more free time, less purpose, and increased daytime sleepiness.[72] It has been reported that individuals who do experience the greatest daytime sleepiness are more sedentary, exercise less, are less vigilant, have more relationship problems, have lower overall subjective well-being, and have more symptoms of depression.[1,69,73–75] When daytime sleepiness is combined with comorbidities (eg, type 2 diabetes), as is common with advancing age, the impact on physical daytime functioning (ie, walking up and down stairs, writing with a pen or pencil) and psychological functioning (ie, depressive symptomatology) is even more pronounced, making daytime sleepiness a threat to functional well-being in later life.[67]

Falls

The elderly typically have less strength and poorer balance, and are more likely to fall after slipping or tripping than are younger adults or children.[76] For the elderly who are already physically frail, who have reduced cognitive functioning, or who have impaired balance, the addition of being sleepy during the day decreases alertness and increases the risk of fall-related injuries.[77,78] Indeed, even after taking into account additional factors of age, comorbidities, medications, and depressive symptoms, EDS still remains significantly related to the number of falls experienced by older adults.[79] In addition, the risk of injury after falling becomes greater with age and is associated with many sleepiness-related factors, such as disrupted nighttime sleep,[80] residual sleepiness from psychotropic, benzodiazepines, and antidepressant medications,[79,81] and deconditioning due to a lack of physical activity.[76] These fall-related injuries are also a leading cause of placement into long-term health care facilities and increased risk of mortality.[76] Treatment of underlying sleep disorders, such as sleep-disordered breathing, with associated reductions in hypersomnia, may reduce the risk of falls in older adults.[82]

Napping

Hypersomnia that leads to long naps is associated with increased illness, falls, and mortality.[54,83] In a community-dwelling sample of elderly women, abnormal daytime sleepiness was associated with greater risk of falls, and nappers who had 3 or more napping hours per week reported 2 or more hip fractures over a period of 1 year when compared with nonnappers.[84] The effect of napping, however, may actually depend on the length of the nap and the stage of sleep from which one awakens. Shorter naps of between 10 and 45 minutes are less likely to consist of slow-wave sleep and may be more refreshing than longer naps, which may result in feelings of inertia on awakening and increase the risk of falling.[85] In addition, taking long daily naps increases the total amount of sleep received each day, and sleeping more than 9 hours in a 24-hour day is also associated with poorer quality of life and poorer self-rated health for the elderly.[86]

Depression

Although insomnia has a more prominent relationship with depression than does daytime sleepiness,[87] EDS has been found to independently predict some types of depression (eg, bipolar depression, seasonal affective disorder).[88] Even so, hypersomnia and decreased daytime energy levels are commonly considered symptoms of depression[56,89] and may be associated with a physiologic stress response on circadian rhythms[56,88] that may contribute to circadian dysregulation,[89] or may be a result of antidepressant treatment.[90] Although the exact mechanisms linking daytime

sleepiness to depression are not known, daytime sleepiness has been found to predict future depression independent of both insomnia and the use of antidepressant medication.[88] Such findings from this recent longitudinal study suggest that the relationship between daytime sleepiness and depression may in fact be different to the relationship between insomnia and depression.[88]

Cardiovascular Disease

EDS has also been identified as an independent risk factor for morbidity and cardiovascular mortality in older adults.[91,92] In a prospective study, Goldstein and colleagues[73] reported that even though daytime sleepiness remained stable across a 5-year period, healthy men and women between the ages of 55 and 80 years who had more sleepiness at baseline were more likely to have a diagnosis of hypertension by the 5-year follow-up. In addition, while investigating different types of sleep disturbances that included difficulty falling asleep, awakening frequently during the night, snoring, and waking too early in the morning, Newman and colleagues[92] found only daytime sleepiness to be independently associated with all incident cardiovascular morbidity and mortality, myocardial infarction, and chronic heart failure. Daytime sleepiness is also independently associated with increased risk of cardiovascular-related mortality, suggesting that a robust relationship exists between sleepiness and cardiovascular disease.[93]

Dementia

Age-related daytime sleepiness may also lead to cognitive decline,[65] future cognitive disorders, and even the development of dementia.[83,94] Foley and colleagues[95] found men between the ages of 71 and 93 years who were within a normal cognitive range at baseline and but reported EDS not only had a greater decline in cognitive functioning 3 years later, but were also more likely to be diagnosed with incident dementia, having an estimated relative risk of dementia of 2.19 (95% confidence interval 1.37–3.50) when compared with participants without daytime sleepiness. Having the most severe daytime sleepiness, however, has come to be strongly predictive of future dementia.[83,96] One group of aging men reporting frequent daytime sleepiness at baseline was 3 times more likely to develop vascular dementia at the 10-year follow-up than the men who did not have daytime sleepiness at baseline.[96] Other current research suggests that frequent daytime sleepiness may actually be a prodromal symptom of vascular dementia,[96] Alzheimer disease,[94] or Parkinson disease,[97] suggesting EDS may also become a predictor of future cognitive disease.

Mortality

The gravest consequence of hypersomnia is its relationship to increases in risk of mortality. As previously discussed, the risk of mortality from daytime sleepiness may depend on the underlying cause of sleepiness and any comorbidities. There are many possible mediating factors in this relationship, including gender differences, depression, and risk of cardiovascular disease.[60,93,98]

Although EDS has repeatedly been identified as an independent risk factor for increased mortality,[60,92,93,99] when sleep-disordered breathing and daytime sleepiness are both present the mortality rate is further increased.[100] One study of older adults noted that those with sleep-disordered breathing and EDS were at 2.3 times greater risk of mortality than individuals having only one or neither of these conditions, even after controlling for other known risk factors such as age, ethnicity, and comorbidities.[100]

Treatment

Light therapy is often used by itself or alongside pharmacotherapy to synchronize circadian rhythms, and may also have daytime alerting effects.[56] Whereas light therapy in the evening is an effective treatment for phase-advanced circadian-related insomnia in older adults, light treatment given earlier in the day can help reduce daytime sleepiness.[101] This factor may be particularly important for the elderly in long-term care facilities where daytime lighting is often not optimal.[102,103]

Napping was previously mentioned as an adverse consequence of hypersomnia. However, for healthy adults (ie, without insomnia) a daytime nap may be beneficial and mitigate the neurocognitive effects of daytime sleepiness. In these individuals, there can be improved alertness and cognitive performance immediately following the nap that continues into the next day.[104,105] Napping has also been shown to improve mood and to reduce both subjective and objective sleepiness.[106] In addition, for healthy adults, long daily sleep time may not necessarily dictate poor daytime functioning or EDS,[107] but may be a way of compensating for a disrupted or short nighttime sleep.[108]

Conversely, exercise and increased physical activity can also reduce daytime sleepiness. For example, a lack of physical activity has been correlated with increased daytime sleepiness in both a community sample and in long-term care facilities, such as nursing homes, where residents'

sleep and circadian rhythms are frequently disrupted.[74,109] In fact, using an intervention design, Martin and colleagues[109] found increasing daytime activities, maintaining a routine bedtime, and reducing nighttime noise and light were effective in decreasing daytime sleepiness for nursing home residents. Similar results of decreased sleepiness following the implementation of an exercise program were also found in a group of community-dwelling women with a history of heart failure.[110]

Several medications can be used to reduce daytime sleepiness. Some agents, such as stimulants (ie, amphetamines, methylphenidates, dextroamphetamines), enhance wakefulness during the daytime, but these medications may also have a disruptive effect on nighttime sleep, with common side effects that include irritability, tremor, headaches, and heart palpitations.[111] Other alerting drugs (ie, modafinil) act in a manner different to that of stimulants, and do not affect nighttime sleep.[112] However, these agents have not been extensively studied in older adults.

SUMMARY

Hypersomnia is a common clinical complaint in older patients. A distinction needs to made between napping and hypersomnia, as they are not necessarily correlated in older adults. Although frequently thought to have a compensatory relationship with insomnia or other sleep disorders, hypersomnia is now known to be independently related to, or even predictive of, a broad array of disorders and diseases, as well as to an increased risk of mortality. In this respect, the assessment of EDS in older adults should be considered as part of a diagnostic plan rather than dismissed as inconsequential. However, the challenge of assessing and managing daytime sleepiness still remains, because of the multiple potential etiologic factors in older adults.

ACKNOWLEDGMENTS

The authors would like to thank Frances Pack and Yasmina Ahmed for their assistance in preparing **Table 1**.

REFERENCES

1. Whitney CW, Enright PL, Newman AB, et al. Correlates of daytime sleepiness in 4578 elderly persons: the Cardiovascular Health Study. Sleep 1998;21(1):27–36.
2. Young TB. Epidemiology of daytime sleepiness: definitions, symptomatology, and prevalence. J Clin Psychiatry 2004;65(Suppl 16):12–6.

3. Ford DE, Kamerow DB. Epidemiologic study of sleep disturbances and psychiatric disorders. An opportunity for prevention? JAMA 1989;262(11): 1479–84.

4. Kim H, Young T. Subjective daytime sleepiness: dimensions and correlates in the general population. Sleep 2005;28(5):625–34.

5. Geisler P, Tracik F, Cronlein T, et al. The influence of age and sex on sleep latency in the MSLT-30—a normative study. Sleep 2006;29(5):687–92.

6. Pallesen S, Nordhus IH, Omvik S, et al. Prevalence and risk factors of subjective sleepiness in the general adult population. Sleep 2007;30(5): 619–24.

7. Grandner MA, Martin JL, Patel NP, et al. Age and sleep disturbances among American men and women: data from the U.S. behavioral risk factor surveillance system. Sleep 2012;35(3):395–406.

8. Klerman EB, Dijk DJ. Age-related reduction in the maximal capacity for sleep—implications for insomnia. Curr Biol 2008;18(15):1118–23.

9. Bixler EO, Vgontzas AN, Lin HM, et al. Excessive daytime sleepiness in a general population sample: the role of sleep apnea, age, obesity, diabetes, and depression. J Clin Endocrinol Metab 2005;90(8):4510–5.

10. Foley DJ, Vitiello MV, Bliwise DL, et al. Frequent napping is associated with excessive daytime sleepiness, depression, pain, and nocturia in older adults: findings from the National Sleep Foundation '2003 Sleep in America' Poll. Am J Geriatr Psychiatry 2007;15(4):344–50.

11. Ancoli-Israel S, Martin JL. Insomnia and daytime napping in older adults. J Clin Sleep Med 2006; 2(3):333–42.

12. Buysse DJ, Browman KE, Monk TH, et al. Napping and 24-hour sleep/wake patterns in healthy elderly and young adults. J Am Geriatr Soc 1992;40(8): 779–86.

13. Brouwer WB, van Exel NJ, Stolk EA. Acceptability of less than perfect health states. Soc Sci Med 2005;60(2):237–46.

14. Webb WB, Aber WR. Relationships between sleep and retirement-nonretirement status. Int J Aging Hum Dev 1984;20(1):13–9.

15. Vitiello MV. We have much more to learn about the relationships between napping and health in older adults. J Am Geriatr Soc 2008;56(9):1753–5.

16. Gander PH, Marshall NS, Harris R, et al. The Epworth Sleepiness Scale: influence of age, ethnicity, and socioeconomic deprivation. Epworth sleepiness scores of adults in New Zealand. Sleep 2005;28(2):249–53.

17. Hagell P, Broman JE. Measurement properties and hierarchical item structure of the Epworth Sleepiness Scale in Parkinson's disease. J Sleep Res 2007;16(1):102–9.

18. Frohnhofen H, Popp R, Willmann V, et al. Feasibility of the Epworth Sleepiness Scale in a sample of geriatric in-hospital patients. J Physiol Pharmacol 2009;60(Suppl 5):45–9.

19. Spira AP, Beaudreau SA, Stone KL, et al. Reliability and validity of the Pittsburgh Sleep Quality Index and the Epworth Sleepiness Scale in older men. J Gerontol A Biol Sci Med Sci 2012;67A(4): 433–9.

20. Punjabi NM, Haponik E. Ask about daytime sleepiness! J Am Geriatr Soc 2000;48(2):228–9.

21. Gooneratne NS, Dean GE, Rogers AE, et al. Sleep and quality of life in long-term lung cancer survivors. Lung Cancer 2007;58:403–10.

22. Bliwise DL, Carskadon MA, Seidel WF, et al. MSLT-defined sleepiness and neuropsychological test performance do not correlate in the elderly. Neurobiol Aging 1991;12(5):463–8.

23. Pack AI, Dinges DF, Gehrman PR, et al. Risk factors for excessive sleepiness in older adults. Ann Neurol 2006;59(6):893–904.

24. Dijk DJ, Groeger JA, Stanley N, et al. Age-related reduction in daytime sleep propensity and nocturnal slow wave sleep. Sleep 2010;33(2):211–23.

25. Dauvilliers Y, Gosselin A, Paquet J, et al. Effect of age on MSLT results in patients with narcolepsy-cataplexy. Neurology 2004;62(1):46–50.

26. Maurer MS, Cuddihy P, Weisenberg J, et al. The prevalence and impact of anergia (lack of energy) in subjects with heart failure and its associations with actigraphy. J Card Fail 2009;15(2):145–51.

27. Dautovich ND, McCrae CS, Rowe M. Subjective and objective napping and sleep in older adults: are evening naps "bad" for nighttime sleep? J Am Geriatr Soc 2008;56(9):1681–6.

28. Kanady JC, Drummond SP, Mednick SC. Actigraphic assessment of a polysomnographic-recorded nap: a validation study. J Sleep Res 2011;20(1 Pt 2):214–22.

29. Kawada T, Suzuki H, Shimizu T, et al. Agreement in regard to total sleep time during a nap obtained via a sleep polygraph and accelerometer: a comparison of different sensitivity thresholds of the accelerometer. Int J Behav Med 2011. [Epub ahead of print].

30. Westerlund H, Vahtera J, Ferrie JE, et al. Effect of retirement on major chronic conditions and fatigue: French GAZEL occupational cohort study. BMJ 2010;341:c6149.

31. Martin JL, Webber AP, Alam T, et al. Daytime sleeping, sleep disturbance, and circadian rhythms in the nursing home. Am J Geriatr Psychiatry 2006;14(2):121–9.

32. American Academy of Sleep Medicine. International classification of sleep disorders: diagnostic and coding manual. 2nd edition. Westchester (IL): American Academy of Sleep Medicine; 2005.

33. Asplund R. Daytime sleepiness and napping amongst the elderly in relation to somatic health and medical treatment. J Intern Med 1996;239(3):261–7.

34. Heap LC, Peters TJ, Wessely S. Vitamin B status in patients with chronic fatigue syndrome. J R Soc Med 1999;92(4):183–5.

35. Hoeck AD, Pall ML. Will vitamin D supplementation ameliorate diseases characterized by chronic inflammation and fatigue? Med Hypotheses 2011; 76(2):208–13.

36. Yamada N. Treatment of recurrent hypersomnia with methylcobalamin (vitamin B12): a case report. Psychiatry Clin Neurosci 1995;49(5–6):305–7.

37. McCarty DE. Resolution of hypersomnia following identification and treatment of vitamin D deficiency. J Clin Sleep Med 2010;6(6):605–8.

38. Asha Devi S, Prathima S, Subramanyam MV. Dietary vitamin E and physical exercise: I. Altered endurance capacity and plasma lipid profile in ageing rats. Exp Gerontol 2003;38(3):285–90.

39. Cheraskin E, Ringsdorf WM Jr, Medford FH. Daily vitamin C consumption and fatigability. J Am Geriatr Soc 1976;24(3):136–7.

40. Hale WE, Perkins LL, May FE, et al. Vitamin E effect on symptoms and laboratory values in the elderly. J Am Diet Assoc 1986;86(5):625–9.

41. Verdon F, Burnand B, Stubi CL, et al. Iron supplementation for unexplained fatigue in non-anaemic women: double blind randomised placebo controlled trial. BMJ 2003;326(7399):1124.

42. McCullough PK. Geriatric depression: atypical presentations, hidden meanings. Geriatrics 1991; 46(10):72–6.

43. American Psychiatric Association. Diagnostic and statistical manual of mental disorders: DSM-IV-TR. 4th edition. Washington, DC: American Psychiatric Association; 2000.

44. Santos M, Kovari E, Hof PR, et al. The impact of vascular burden on late-life depression. Brain Res Rev 2009;62(1):19–32.

45. Fried LP, Tangen CM, Walston J, et al. Frailty in older adults: evidence for a phenotype. J Gerontol A Biol Sci Med Sci 2001;56(3):M146–56.

46. Ensrud KE, Blackwell TL, Redline S, et al. Sleep disturbances and frailty status in older community-dwelling men. J Am Geriatr Soc 2009; 57(11):2085–93.

47. Vaz Fragoso CA, Gahbauer EA, Van Ness PH, et al. Sleep-wake disturbances and frailty in community-living older persons. J Am Geriatr Soc 2009;57(11): 2094–100.

48. Chew ML, Mulsant BH, Pollock BG, et al. Anticholinergic activity of 107 medications commonly used by older adults. J Am Geriatr Soc 2008;56(7):1333–41.

49. Gloth FM 3rd. Pharmacological management of persistent pain in older persons: focus on opioids and nonopioids. J Pain 2011;12(3 Suppl 1):S14–20.

50. Agostini JV, Leo-Summers LS, Inouye SK. Cognitive and other adverse effects of diphenhydramine use in hospitalized older patients. Arch Intern Med 2001;161(17):2091–7.

51. Soriano TA, DeCherrie LV, Thomas DC. Falls in the community-dwelling older adult: a review for primary-care providers. Clin Interv Aging 2007; 2(4):545–54.

52. Sterling DA, O'Connor JA, Bonadies J. Geriatric falls: injury severity is high and disproportionate to mechanism. J Trauma 2001;50(1):116–9.

53. Carskadon MA, Brown ED, Dement WC. Sleep fragmentation in the elderly: relationship to daytime sleep tendency. Neurobiol Aging 1982;3(4):321–7.

54. Mesas AE, Lopez-Garcia E, Leon-Munoz LM, et al. Sleep duration and mortality according to health status in older adults. J Am Geriatr Soc 2010; 58(10):1870–7.

55. Johansson P, Alehagen U, Svanborg E, et al. Sleep disordered breathing in an elderly community-living population: relationship to cardiac function, insomnia symptoms and daytime sleepiness. Sleep Med 2009;10(9):1005–11.

56. Chellappa SL, Schroder C, Cajochen C. Chronobiology, excessive daytime sleepiness and depression: is there a link? Sleep Med 2009;10(5):505–14.

57. Black J, Duntley SP, Bogan RK, et al. Recent advances in the treatment and management of excessive daytime sleepiness. CNS Spectr 2007; 12(2 Suppl 2):1–14 [quiz: 15].

58. Youngstedt SD, Kripke DF, Elliott JA, et al. Circadian abnormalities in older adults. J Pineal Res 2001;31(3):264–72.

59. Buysse DJ, Monk TH, Carrier J, et al. Circadian patterns of sleep, sleepiness, and performance in older and younger adults. Sleep 2005;28(11):1365–76.

60. Hays JC, Blazer DG, Foley DJ. Risk of napping: excessive daytime sleepiness and mortality in an older community population. J Am Geriatr Soc 1996;44(6):693–8.

61. Stepanski E, Zorick F, Roehrs T, et al. Daytime alertness in patients with chronic insomnia compared with asymptomatic control subjects. Sleep 1988; 11(1):54–60.

62. Buysse DJ, Ancoli-Israel S, Edinger JD, et al. Recommendations for a standard research assessment of insomnia. Sleep 2006;29(9):1155–73.

63. Gooneratne NS, Bellamy SL, Pack F, et al. Case-control study of subjective and objective differences in sleep patterns in older adults with insomnia symptoms. J Sleep Res 2011;20(3):434–44.

64. Young T, Shahar E, Nieto FJ, et al. Predictors of sleep-disordered breathing in community-dwelling adults: the Sleep Heart Health Study. Arch Intern Med 2002;162(8):893–900.

65. Crowley K. Sleep and sleep disorders in older adults. Neuropsychol Rev 2011;21(1):41–53.

66. Dixon JB, Dixon ME, Anderson ML, et al. Daytime sleepiness in the obese: not as simple as obstructive sleep apnea. Obesity (Silver Spring) 2007; 15(10):2504–11.

67. Chasens ER, Sereika SM, Burke LE. Daytime sleepiness and functional outcomes in older adults with diabetes. Diabetes Educ 2009;35(3): 455–64.

68. Chong MS, Ayalon L, Marler M, et al. Continuous positive airway pressure reduces subjective daytime sleepiness in patients with mild to moderate Alzheimer's disease with sleep disordered breathing. J Am Geriatr Soc 2006;54(5): 777–81.

69. Gooneratne NS, Weaver TE, Cater JR, et al. Functional outcomes of excessive daytime sleepiness in older adults. J Am Geriatr Soc 2003;51(5):642–9.

70. Bloom HG, Ahmed I, Alessi CA, et al. Evidence-based recommendations for the assessment and management of sleep disorders in older persons. J Am Geriatr Soc 2009;57(5):761–89.

71. Welch HG, Albertsen PC, Nease RF, et al. Estimating treatment benefits for the elderly: the effect of competing risks. Ann Intern Med 1996;124(6): 577–84.

72. Kutner NG, Bliwise DL, Zhang R. Linking race and well-being within a biopsychosocial framework: variation in subjective sleep quality in two racially diverse older adult samples. J Health Soc Behav 2004;45(1):99–113.

73. Goldstein IB, Ancoli-Israel S, Shapiro D. Relationship between daytime sleepiness and blood pressure in healthy older adults. Am J Hypertens 2004;17(9):787–92.

74. Chasens ER, Sereika SM, Weaver TE, et al. Daytime sleepiness, exercise, and physical function in older adults. J Sleep Res 2007;16(1):60–5.

75. Yokoyama E, Saito Y, Kaneita Y, et al. Association between subjective well-being and sleep among the elderly in Japan. Sleep Med 2008;9(2):157–64.

76. Rubenstein LZ. Falls in older people: epidemiology, risk factors and strategies for prevention. Age Ageing 2006;35(Suppl 2):ii37–41.

77. Chen YY, Wu KC. Sleep habits and excessive daytime sleepiness correlate with injury risks in the general population in Taiwan. Inj Prev 2010; 16(3):172–7.

78. Dauvilliers Y. Differential diagnosis in hypersomnia. Curr Neurol Neurosci Rep 2006;6(2):156–62.

79. Brassington GS, King AC, Bliwise DL. Sleep problems as a risk factor for falls in a sample of community-dwelling adults aged 64-99 years. J Am Geriatr Soc 2000;48(10):1234–40.

80. Stone KL, Ancoli-Israel S, Blackwell T, et al. Actigraphy-measured sleep characteristics and risk of falls in older women. Arch Intern Med 2008; 168(16):1768–75.

81. Stone KL, Ensrud KE, Ancoli-Israel S. Sleep, insomnia and falls in elderly patients. Sleep Med 2008;9(Suppl 1):S18–22.

82. Onen F, Higgins S, Onen SH. Falling-asleep-related injured falls in the elderly. J Am Med Dir Assoc 2009;10(3):207–10.

83. Ohayon MM, Vecchierini MF. Daytime sleepiness and cognitive impairment in the elderly population. Arch Intern Med 2002;162(2):201–8.

84. Stone KL, Ewing SK, Lui LY, et al. Self-reported sleep and nap habits and risk of falls and fractures in older women: the study of osteoporotic fractures. J Am Geriatr Soc 2006;54(8):1177–83.

85. Tassi P, Muzet A. Sleep inertia. Sleep Med Rev 2000;4(4):341–53.

86. Magee CA, Caputi P, Iverson DC. Relationships between self-rated health, quality of life and sleep duration in middle aged and elderly Australians. Sleep Med 2011;12(4):346–50.

87. Buysse DJ, Germain A, Nofzinger EA, et al. Mood disorders and sleep. In: Stein DJ, Kupfer DJ, Schatzberg AF, editors. The American psychiatric publishing textbook of mood disorders. Washington, DC: American Psychiatric Publishing; 2006. p. 717–37.

88. Jaussent I, Bouyer J, Ancelin ML, et al. Insomnia and daytime sleepiness are risk factors for depressive symptoms in the elderly. Sleep 2011;34(8): 1103–10.

89. van den Berg JF, Luijendijk HJ, Tulen JH, et al. Sleep in depression and anxiety disorders: a population-based study of elderly persons. J Clin Psychiatry 2009;70(8):1105–13.

90. Fava M. Daytime sleepiness and insomnia as correlates of depression. J Clin Psychiatry 2004; 65(Suppl 16):27–32.

91. Goldstein MR. Should elderly individuals who frequently nap take beta-blockers and/or aspirin? Arch Intern Med 2000;160(5):710 [author reply: 711–2].

92. Newman AB, Spiekerman CF, Enright P, et al. Daytime sleepiness predicts mortality and cardiovascular disease in older adults. The Cardiovascular Health Study Research Group. J Am Geriatr Soc 2000;48(2):115–23.

93. Empana JP, Dauvilliers Y, Dartigues JF, et al. Excessive daytime sleepiness is an independent risk indicator for cardiovascular mortality in community-dwelling elderly: the three city study. Stroke 2009;40(4):1219–24.

94. Bonanni E, Maestri M, Tognoni G, et al. Daytime sleepiness in mild and moderate Alzheimer's disease and its relationship with cognitive impairment. J Sleep Res 2005;14(3):311–7.

95. Foley D, Monjan A, Masaki K, et al. Daytime sleepiness is associated with 3-year incident dementia and cognitive decline in older Japanese-American men. J Am Geriatr Soc 2001;49(12): 1628–32.

96. Elwood PC, Bayer AJ, Fish M, et al. Sleep disturbance and daytime sleepiness predict vascular dementia. J Epidemiol Community Health 2011; 65(9):820–4.

97. Eaton WW, Badawi M, Melton B. Prodromes and precursors: epidemiologic data for primary prevention of disorders with slow onset. Am J Psychiatry 1995;152(7):967–72.

98. Kolettis TM, Papathanasiou A, Tziallas D, et al. Afternoon nap, meal ingestion and circadian variation of acute myocardial infarction. Int J Cardiol 2008;123(3):338–40.

99. Bursztyn M, Stessman J. The siesta and mortality: twelve years of prospective observations in 70-year-olds. Sleep 2005;28(3):345–7.

100. Gooneratne NS, Richards KC, Joffe M, et al. Sleep disordered breathing with excessive daytime sleepiness is a risk factor for mortality in older adults. Sleep 2011;34(4):435–42.

101. Wolkove N, Elkholy O, Baltzan M, et al. Sleep and aging: 2. Management of sleep disorders in older people. CMAJ 2007;176(10):1449–54.

102. Fukuda N, Kobayashi R, Kohsaka M, et al. Effects of bright light at lunchtime on sleep in patients in a geriatric hospital II. Psychiatry Clin Neurosci 2001;55(3):291–3.

103. Riemersma-van der Lek RF, Swaab DF, Twisk J, et al. Effect of bright light and melatonin on cognitive and noncognitive function in elderly residents of group care facilities: a randomized controlled trial. JAMA 2008;299(22):2642–55.

104. Campbell SS, Murphy PJ, Stauble TN. Effects of a nap on nighttime sleep and waking function in older subjects. J Am Geriatr Soc 2005;53(1): 48–53.

105. Dhand R, Sohal H. Good sleep, bad sleep! The role of daytime naps in healthy adults. Curr Opin Pulm Med 2006;12(6):379–82.

106. Milner CE, Cote KA. Benefits of napping in healthy adults: impact of nap length, time of day, age, and experience with napping. J Sleep Res 2009;18(2): 272–81.

107. Kline CE, Zielinski MR, Devlin TM, et al. Self-reported long sleep in older adults is closely related to objective time in bed. Sleep Biol Rhythm 2009;8: 42–51.

108. Horne J. Sleepiness as a need for sleep: when is enough, enough? Neurosci Biobehav Rev 2010; 34(1):108–18.

109. Martin JL, Marler MR, Harker JO, et al. A multicomponent nonpharmacological intervention improves activity rhythms among nursing home residents with disrupted sleep/wake patterns. J Gerontol A Biol Sci Med Sci 2007;62(1):67–72.

110. Gary RA, Cress ME, Higgins MK, et al. Combined aerobic and resistance exercise program improves task performance in patients with heart failure. Arch Phys Med Rehabil 2011;92(9):1371–81.

111. Guilleminault C, Brooks SN. Excessive daytime sleepiness: a challenge for the practising neurologist. Brain 2001;124(Pt 8):1482–91.

112. Dinges DF, Weaver TE. Effects of modafinil on sustained attention performance and quality of life in OSA patients with residual sleepiness while being treated with nCPAP. Sleep Med 2003;4(5): 393–402.

Hypersomnia in Children

Suresh Kotagal, MD[a,b,c],*

KEYWORDS

• Hypersomnia • Children • Adolescents • Narcolepsy • Kleine-Levin syndrome • Hypocretin

KEY POINTS

- Further refinements are needed in the diagnostic testing of childhood daytime sleepiness.
- It is not known whether the multiple sleep latency test in childhood should use 4 or 5 naps.
- Longitudinal studies are needed to determine if treating sleepiness by medications corresponds with improved neuropsychological function. Given the small number of patients with childhood narcolepsy at each sleep center, a consortium-based approach is needed for gathering prospective high-quality evidence regarding optimum treatment measures, be they pharmacologic or nonpharmacologic in nature.

Daytime sleepiness is an important symptom of impaired health during childhood and adolescence. It is consequent to a set of diverse pathophysiologic circumstances. The initial manifestations are often underrecognized by parents, school authorities, and health professionals alike. The consequences of daytime sleepiness are significant, especially from the standpoint of its impact on mood, learning, behavior, and dexterity.[1,2] The purpose of this article is to provide an overview of childhood daytime sleepiness, with an emphasis on clinical assessment and management. In areas where there is insufficient evidence in childhood, the author has extrapolated information from adult sleep literature.

HOW PREVALENT IS CHILDHOOD DAYTIME SLEEPINESS

Nevéus and colleagues[3] conducted a questionnaire survey in 1413 Swedish children aged 6 to 10 years and found a 4% prevalence rate for daytime sleepiness. When Yang and colleagues[4] conducted the validated School Sleep Habits Survey in a sample of 1457 Korean school children aged 9 to 19 years, they found that 6.6% of the respondents admitted to daytime sleepiness being a "very big problem." As seniority in school increased from the 5th to the 12th grade, so also did the prevalence of daytime sleepiness. The increase in prevalence of daytime sleepiness with advancing grade levels in children and adolescents is also supported by Ohayon and colleagues.[5] Using a telephone survey, the investigators sampled 1125 French, British, German, and Italian adolescents aged 15 to 18 years.[5] A prevalence rate of 19.9% was found for daytime sleepiness, with 11.9% of the sample complaining also of difficulty waking up in the morning. Although Yang and colleagues[4] believe that sleepiness was slightly more prevalent in girls than in boys, gender differences in prevalence of childhood daytime sleepiness have not been definitively established. The key point established by survey instruments is that daytime sleepiness is a significant pediatric health problem, with prevalence ranging from 4% in preadolescents to almost 20% in high school seniors.[3–5]

WHAT FACTORS PREDISPOSE TO CHILDHOOD DAYTIME SLEEPINESS

A convergence of multiple factors increases the vulnerability of teenagers to daytime sleepiness.

[a] Department of Neurology, Mayo Clinic, 200 First Street Southwest, Rochester, MN 55905, USA; [b] Department of Pediatrics, Mayo Clinic, 200 First Street Southwest, Rochester, MN 55905, USA; [c] Center for Sleep Medicine, Mayo Clinic, 200 First Street Southwest, Rochester, MN 55905, USA
* Division of Child Neurology, Mayo Clinic, 200 First Street Southwest, Rochester, MN 55905.
E-mail address: Kotagal.suresh@mayo.edu

Sleep Med Clin 7 (2012) 379–389
doi:10.1016/j.jsmc.2012.03.010
1556-407X/12/$ – see front matter © 2012 Elsevier Inc. All rights reserved.

Concurrent with maturation, children and adolescents show a tendency to sleep fewer hours at night. In a longitudinal study of 493 healthy children and adolescents, Iglowstein and colleagues[6] found that the mean sleep duration in 10-year-old children was 9.9 hours (standard deviation [SD], 0.6), whereas the mean sleep duration in 16-year-old adolescents had decreased to around 8.1 hours (SD, 0.7). When this reduced total sleep time is juxtaposed with the need for teenagers to wake up between 5:30 AM and 6:30 AM to arrive at school by around 7:30 AM, the end result can be daytime sleepiness.

Dim-light melatonin onset (DLMO) is a physiologic marker for the time of sleep onset. DLMO shifts to a later time in the evening in older adolescents in comparison with preadolescents. In a study by Taylor and colleagues,[7] the mean DLMO time was found to be 2033 hours (SD, 49 minutes) in 9 prepubertal children who were of Tanner stage I sexual development (mean age, 11.1 years), whereas the mean DLMO time had shifted to 2129 hours in 11 pubertally mature adolescents who were of Tanner stage V (mean age, 13.9 years). The resulting physiologic delay in sleep onset to a later time of the night predisposes to sleep deprivation, especially on school nights. Wolfson and Carskadon[8] surveyed about 3000 high school students in New England using the School Sleep Habits Survey and found that students who self-reported higher grades reported more total sleep time and earlier bedtimes on school nights than children with lower grades (P<.001). Furthermore, early school start times are associated with decreased total sleep time, increased daytime sleepiness, and poorer school performance.[9]

The intrusion of technological devices, such as televisions, computers, cell phones, video games, and the Internet, into the bedroom tends to further postpone the sleep-onset time on school nights and leads to insufficient night sleep, with consequent daytime sleepiness. Sadeh and colleagues[10] have evaluated the effect of relative sleep restriction by an average of 41 minutes on school children. The investigators found that even a very moderate but accumulated sleep deficit (eg, watching one more television show) can have adverse neurobehavioral effects, especially when it comes to executive functioning.

A disruption of key central wake-promoting mechanisms, as seen in narcolepsy-cataplexy, can also lead to excessive daytime sleepiness (EDS). Patients with narcolepsy-cataplexy lose hypocretin (orexin)-secreting neurons from the dorsolateral region of the hypothalamus. These hypocretin neurons have widespread projections to the forebrain and brainstem. Hypocretin promotes alertness and locomotor activity.[11,12] Immune-mediated or anatomic lesions of the hypothalamus and rostral midbrain (such as neoplasms, inflammation, or trauma) can be associated with hypersomnia by virtue of alterations in the balance between the sleep-enhancing and wakefulness-promoting influences. Saper and colleagues[13] have proposed the concept of autonomic regulation via a sleep-wake switch. The investigators postulate that the tuberomammillary nucleus (histaminergic in nature), the locus coeruleus (noradrenergic in nature), and the raphe system (serotonergic in nature) work together to enhance alertness. They have a reciprocal relationship with the sleep-promoting neurons of the ventrolateral preoptic (VLPO) nucleus, which are γ-aminergic in nature. Some cells in the VLPO (termed VLPO cluster) promote non–rapid eye movement sleep, whereas other cells (VLPO extended) facilitate rapid eye movement (REM) sleep. Hypocretin (orexin) serves to stabilize the relationship between these 2 sets of physiologically opposing influences.

WHAT ARE THE CONSEQUENCES OF DAYTIME SLEEPINESS

Similar to adults, adolescents with daytime sleepiness manifest changes in behavior and a decline in performance.[2,14] Conversely, the treatment of sleep disruption by improving sleep hygiene or treating specific sleep disorders results in improvements in daytime performance.[15] Ha and colleagues[16] performed objective computerized testing on 24 patients with narcolepsy (being treated with stimulants, mean age 30.7 ± 12.8 years, mean intelligence quotient of 119, 79% male) and 24 matched controls. The patients with narcolepsy performed more frequent omission and commission errors on a vigilance test and more omission errors on a continuous performance test.

Stores and colleagues[17] studied psychosocial problems in children with narcolepsy (n = 42) and nonnarcolepsy hypersomnia (EDS, n = 18) along with 23 age-matched controls. The investigators observed that patients with both narcolepsy and EDS exhibited more behavioral difficulties than controls on the Strengths and Difficulties Questionnaire. Both groups (patients with narcolepsy and nonnarcolepsy hypersomnia) showed more depressed mood on the Child Depression Inventory and lower quality of life on the Child Health Questionnaire's mental health subscale when compared with controls. These findings suggest that deficits in mood, behavior, and quality of life were more related to hypersomnia than specifically to narcolepsy. Furthermore, patients with narcolepsy seem to show impaired quality of life, more from sleepiness and less from cataplexy.[18]

This may be a moot issue, but it is hard to sort out from studies in the literature whether the cognitive and behavioral changes in children with EDS are a consequence of hypersomnia, nocturnal sleep disruption, or both. Furthermore, are the sequelae of nocturnal sleep disruption occurring in association with hypoxemia (as in obstructive sleep apnea) similar to those related to sleep fragmentation without gas exchange abnormalities as seen in periodic limb movement disorder or anxiety? These questions remain unanswered and are methodologically difficult to study.

CLINICAL ASSESSMENT

To make an accurate sleep diagnosis, it is essential to combine a carefully elicited history with appropriate screening questionnaires and sleep laboratory studies. The history should determine whether the hypersomnolence is constant or episodic; the latter is observed in Kleine-Levin syndrome (KLS). Circumstances under which the child becomes sleepy should be elicited in a child with narcolepsy; for example, there may be a history of falling asleep in the classroom or during conversations. The impact of sleepiness on daily function, such as decline in grades, negative moods, accidents, and social withdrawal, should also be studied. Ancillary symptoms, such as cataplexy, hypnagogic hallucinations, and sleep paralysis, indicate narcolepsy. Habitual snoring, mouth breathing, and weight gain may suggest obstructive sleep apnea–hypopnea syndrome. A habitual inability to fall asleep until the early morning hours and not being able to awaken until the late morning hours is common in delayed sleep phase syndrome. Feelings of sadness may point to underlying depression, although sometimes depressed moods may be consequent to the sleepiness itself. The medication history helps understand potential iatrogenic influences on sleepiness and decides what medications could be used for future treatment.

There are about 27 pediatric sleep-wake questionnaires that have had their psychometric properties validated.[19] These questionnaires can be also incorporated into the clinical assessment. These scales evaluate circadian rhythms, sleep apnea, periodic limb movements, restless legs, dreams, and daytime sleepiness to variable degrees. They usually contain questions that can be answered on a 4- to 5-point Likert scale. The commonly used questionnaires that address sleepiness include the Child Sleep Habits Questionnaire,[20]

the Sleep Disorders Inventory for Students,[21] the Sleep Disturbance Scale for Children,[22] the Pediatric Sleep Questionnaire,[23] the Cleveland Adolescent Sleepiness Scale,[24] and the Pediatric Daytime Sleepiness Scale (PDSS)[25] (**Table 1**). The author prefers the PDSS because of its simplicity. This is an 8-item questionnaire, with each question to be answered on a scale of 0 to 4. The higher the score, the greater the degree of sleepiness, with the highest score being 32. A percentile score can be assigned for the degree of sleepiness. Pediatric sleep questionnaires are useful in clinical practice. Nevertheless, they possess the same limitations that are common to all survey instruments, such as recall bias. Furthermore, patients who are sleepy are not able to accurately estimate their degree of sleepiness. A certain bias may also influence survey instruments such as the Child Sleep Habits Questionnaire,[20] which are completed primarily by the parent. How well does questionnaire-determined hypersomnia correlate with objective tests for sleepiness? In a level I study of children with obstructive sleep apnea–hypopnea syndrome, Chervin and colleagues[26] found a significant but weak correlation of sleepiness between the Pediatric Sleep Questionnaire sleep latency and the multiple sleep latency test (MSLT; $r = -0.23$, $P = .006$).

Wrist actigraphy and sleep logs maintained for 2 to 3 weeks are used to assess suspected delayed sleep phase syndrome or inadequate sleep hygiene. Nocturnal polysomnography (PSG) indicates suspected obstructive sleep apnea–hypopnea syndrome and sleep-related epilepsy. Whenever there is a concern about possible narcolepsy or idiopathic hypersomnia, the MSLT is performed the day after PSG. This test consists of a series of 4 to 5 nap opportunities that are provided at 2-hourly intervals. The electroencephalogram (EEG), eye movements, and submental electromyogram are monitored during each 20-minute nap opportunity. The test measures the speed at which the patient falls asleep (sleep latency). A mean sleep latency (MSL) is derived by averaging the values from all the 4 or 5 nap opportunities.[27] In preadolescent children, the normal MSL is often in the 16- to 18-minute range, decreasing to about 14 minutes during adolescence. Reference values for MSL as measured on the MSLT are provided in **Table 2**. In narcolepsy, the MSL is usually less than 8 minutes.[28,29] When the MSL is less than 8 minutes, a urine drug screen should be obtained to exclude hypersomnolence from drug-seeking behavior. In patients with narcolepsy, REM at sleep onset (SOREMP) is encountered in 2 or more nap opportunities.

Table 1
Survey instruments commonly used for assessing daytime sleepiness

Name	Authors	Year Published	Age Range of Patients (y)	Who Completes the Questionnaire	Total/Sleepiness Items	Remarks
Sleep Disturbance Scale for Children	Bruni et al[22]	1996	5–15	Parent	27	Internal consistency α = 0.79 Test-retest reliability r = 0.71
Pediatric Sleep Questionnaire	Chervin et al[23]	2000	2–18	Parent	22/4	Internal consistency for sleepiness subscale α = 0.66 Test-retest reliability r = 0.66
PDSS	Drake et al[25]	2003	11–15	Patient	8/8	Internal consistency α = 0.81
Cleveland Adolescent Sleepiness Questionnaire	Spilsbury et al[24]	2007	12–15	Patient	16/16	Internal consistency α = 0.89
Children's Sleep Habits Questionnaire	Owens et al[20]	2000	4–10	Parent	35/8	Internal consistency α = 0.65 (control population) and 0.70 (clinic population) Test-retest reliability r = 0.69
School Sleep Habits Survey	Wolfson and Carskadon[8]	1998	13–17	Patient	140/15	Internal consistency α = 0.73

Table 2
Reference values for the MSLT

Tanner Stage	General Corresponding Age (y)	MSL (min)	SD
Stage I	≤10	18.8	1.8
Stage II	10–12	18.3	2.1
Stage III	11.5–13.0	16.5	2.8
Stage IV	13–14	15.5	3.3
Stage V	≥14	16.2	1.5
Older teenagers	≥14	15.8	3.5

Data from Carskadon MA. The second decade. In: Guille-minault C, editor. Sleeping and waking disorders: indications and techniques. Menlo Park (CA): Addison Wesley; 1982. p. 99–125.

INADEQUATE SLEEP HYGIENE

Inadequate sleep hygiene may be free standing or superimposed on other sleep disorders. Onset is usually around adolescence. Bed-onset and sleep-onset times are delayed. With the morning wake-up times remaining relatively unchanged between 6 AM and 7 AM because of school, the total sleep time becomes truncated, leading to insufficient sleep and secondary daytime sleepiness.[10,30]

The factors that contribute to delayed bed onset include excessive caffeine or nicotine intake, illicit substance abuse, excessive late-night physical activity, watching television in the bedroom at bedtime, working on the computer while in bed, using cell phones while in bed to chat with friends at night, text messaging while in bed, and so forth.

The management of delayed bed onset includes a discussion with the patient (and the parents when appropriate) on the importance of getting adequate sleep at night, making a clear separation between activities of wakefulness and the process of falling asleep, building an approximately 30-minute buffer of quiet time between wakefulness and sleep onset, and using relaxing activities that do not involve technology. The issues of avoiding caffeine, nicotine, and the use of illicit substances should be addressed when indicated.

PERIODIC HYPERSOMNIA

Periodic hypersomnia, also termed KLS or recurrent hypersomnia, is generally seen in adolescents. This disorder is predominant in males, with a mean age of onset of around 15 years.[31] Patients develop periods of sleepiness lasting 1 to 2 weeks, during which they may sleep 18 to 20 hours a day and also manifest cognitive and mood disturbances in association with compulsive hyperphagia and hypersexual behavior, with an intervening 2 to 4 months of normal alertness and behavior. Incomplete and atypical forms of the disorder in which anorexia or insomnia predominate have also been recognized. Hyperphagia can manifest in the form of binge eating and may actually be associated with a 2- to 5-kg increase in body weight. There is a predilection to consume chocolate and other high-calorie food items. Nocturnal PSG, when the patient is symptomatic, shows decreased sleep efficiency, shortened REM latency, and decreased percentage of time spent in stage N3 and REM sleep. The MSLT shows moderately shortened MSL, in the 5- to 10-minute range, but without the 2 or more SOREMPs observed in narcolepsy. There may be diffuse slowing on the EEG. Structural brain imaging and evaluation of the cerebrospinal fluid (CSF) for inflammatory markers show a negative result. Brain scintigraphy may disclose areas of hypoperfusion in the thalamic, hypothalamic, and frontotemporal regions.[31] Periodic hypersomnia may gradually subside over 2 to 3 years, or evolve into classic depression, bringing up the issue of whether the disorder is a variant of depression. A disturbance of hypothalamic function has been hypothesized but not established. In a 14-year-old girl with KLS, Podesta and colleagues[32] have documented a 2-fold reduction in CSF levels of hypocretin during the period in which she was symptomatic in comparison with when she was not symptomatic. The association of KLS with the histocompatibility antigen DQB1*0201 has not been replicated in large case series.[31] Familial clustering and a potential Jewish founder effect seem to support the role for potential genetic susceptibility factors.[31] There is no satisfactory treatment, although lithium,[33] sodium valproate,[34] and lamotrigine[35] have been reported to be modestly effective in case reports.

NARCOLEPSY

The characteristic clinical features of narcolepsy are chronic daytime sleepiness, fragmented night sleep, and superimposition of REM sleep phenomena onto wakefulness in the form of hypnagogic hallucinations (vivid dreams at sleep onset), sleep paralysis, and cataplexy (sudden loss of skeletal muscle tone in response to emotional triggers, such as laughter, fright, or surprise). Based on an epidemiologic survey performed in Olmsted County, Minnesota, the incidence of narcolepsy in the United States (with and without cataplexy) has been estimated at 1.37 per 100,000 persons per year (1.72 for men and 1.05 for women).[36] The incidence is highest in the second and third decades of life, followed by a gradual decline thereafter. In the same study, the prevalence of narcolepsy was approximately 56 persons per 100,000. There are no published data on the relative prevalence in childhood of narcolepsy-cataplexy compared with narcolepsy without cataplexy. It is the author's opinion, however, based on clinical experience, that the former is far more common than the latter in childhood. This is an issue that needs further study.

Although the onset of narcolepsy is generally in the latter half of the first or second decade of life, cases with onset of extreme sleepiness and cataplexy even before ages 5 or 6 years have been reported.[37] Daytime sleepiness may be overlooked by parents, schoolteachers, and physicians alike. Children who are sleepy may be mistaken for being lazy. These children frequently also exhibit mood swings and inattentiveness. Cataplexy is present in about two-thirds of patients with narcolepsy. Cataplexy attacks generally last for a few seconds to minutes and are characterized by loss of tone in the antigravity muscles and absence of muscle stretch reflexes in the face of fully preserved consciousness. Mild cataplexy may present with transient ptosis, the jaw dropping open, and a slight drooping of the neck. More severe episodes may be followed by unsteadiness and falling. The most common triggers for cataplexy are laughter, excitement, and the anticipation of a reward. Although cataplexy can be subtle, the examiner needs to ask leading questions about episodic muscle weakness in the lower extremities or neck and trunk. Children younger than 7 or 8 years may be unable to articulate a reliable history of cataplexy, hypnagogic hallucinations, or sleep paralysis. Narcolepsy may be variably associated with periodic limb movement disorder.[38] The patients exhibit less circadian drive–dependent alertness during the daytime and sleepiness at night. In rare instances, secondary narcolepsy may develop after closed head injury, primary brain tumors, lymphomas, or viral encephalitis.[39]

The presence of the histocompatibility antigen DQB1*0602 in close to 100% of persons with narcolepsy-cataplexy, as compared with a 12% to 32% prevalence in the general population, indicates a genetic susceptibility. This indication per se, however, is insufficient to precipitate the clinical syndrome; monozygotic twins can remain discordant for developing narcolepsy.[40] In genetically susceptible individuals who are DQB1*0602 positive, acquired life stresses such as minor head injury, systemic illnesses such as infectious mononucleosis, and bereavement may trigger narcolepsy. These stresses have been reported to occur in about two-thirds of patients: the two-hit hypothesis.

Hypocretin deficiency is the key pathophysiologic event in narcolepsy-cataplexy.[41] Hypocretin (orexin) is a peptide that is produced by neurons of the dorsolateral hypothalamus. Hypocretins 1 and 2 (synonymous with orexins A and B) are peptides that are synthesized from preprohypocretin. Hypocretin neurons have widespread projections to the forebrain and brainstem. This peptide promotes alertness and increases motor activity and basal metabolic rate.[42] Of significance is the autopsy finding by Thannickal and colleagues[43] in human narcolepsy. The study reported that a reduction of 85% to 95% was observed in the number of hypocretin-secreting neurons in the hypothalamus, whereas melanin-concentrating hormone neurons that are intermingled with hypocretin neurons remained unaffected, thus suggesting a targeted neurodegenerative process. It is hypothesized that degeneration of the hypocretin-producing cells of the hypothalamus (perhaps predisposed to HLA DQB1*0602 positivity) provokes a decrease in forebrain noradrenergic activation, which in turn decreases alertness. A corresponding decrease of noradrenergic activity in the brainstem leads to disinhibition of brainstem cholinergic systems, thus triggering cataplexy and other phenomena of REM sleep, such as hypnagogic hallucinations and sleep paralysis. Other manifestations of hypocretin deficiency that are seen in the early stages of childhood narcolepsy-cataplexy are increased appetite, binge eating, obesity (presumably related to hypocretin deficiency), and precocious puberty.[44]

The decrease in the secretion of hypocretin-1 that is characteristic of human narcolepsy-cataplexy is reflected in the CSF. Using a radioimmunoassay, Nishino and colleagues[41] found that the mean level of hypocretin-1 was 280.3 ± 33.0 pg/mL in healthy controls and 260.5 ± 37.1 pg/mL in neurologic controls, whereas in those with narcolepsy, hypocretin-1 was either undetectable or less than 100 pg/mL. Low to absent levels of hypocretin-1 were found in 32 of 38 patients with narcolepsy, who were also HLA DQB10*0602 positive. Patients with narcolepsy who were also HLA DQB1*0602 negative tend to have normal to high CSF hypocretin-1 levels. In another study of patients with narcolepsy with cataplexy, narcolepsy without cataplexy, and idiopathic hypersomnia, Kanbayashi and colleagues[45] found that 9 patients with narcolepsy-cataplexy who had CSF hypocretin deficiency were HLA DQB1*0602 positive, including 3 preadolescents. By contrast, patients with narcolepsy without cataplexy and idiopathic hypersomnia showed normal CSF hypocretin levels. The application of CSF hypocretin-1 assays for the diagnosis of narcolepsy-cataplexy is most useful when an HLA DQB1*0602–positive patient with suspected narcolepsy-cataplexy is already receiving central nervous system stimulants or selective serotonin reuptake inhibitors on initial presentation and when discontinuation of these medications for the purpose of obtaining a PSG and MSLT is medically unsafe or impractical.

Are narcolepsy with cataplexy and narcolepsy without cataplexy 2 presentations of the same disorder, or do they represent 2 distinct entities? This is an intriguing question, the answer to which is not known. Deficiency of CSF hypocretin-1 level is seen only in narcolepsy-cataplexy. Furthermore, HLA DQB1*0602–positive status, although seen in about 30% of the general population, occurs in narcolepsy-cataplexy but not in narcolepsy without cataplexy. These findings therefore suggest that the 2 forms of narcolepsy are pathophysiologically distinct. On the other hand, older literature suggests that narcolepsy is a unitary phenomenon, with cataplexy sometimes developing 5 to 10 years after onset of daytime sleepiness. However, the PSG features described later are common to both subtypes.

A combined battery of nocturnal PSG and MSLT is still the most widely accepted method for diagnosing narcolepsy. The nocturnal PSG shows almost immediate sleep onset, possible REM-onset sleep (occurring within 15 minutes of sleep onset), increased arousals, elevated periodic limb movement index, and absence of any other significant sleep pathology, such as obstructive sleep apnea. REM sleep behavior disorder or REM sleep without atonia may also be present.[37,46] The MSLT is performed the day after the nocturnal PSG. The MSLT consists of the provision of 4 daytime nap opportunities in a darkened quiet environment at 2-hourly intervals, for example, 0900, 1100, 1300, and 1500 hours. The patient should be drug free for at least 2 weeks. Owing to their REM sleep–suppressant effect, drugs with very long half-lives, such as fluoxetine, may have to be stopped for protracted periods (such as 3–4 weeks, provided it is safe to do so). The time between lights out and sleep onset is defined as sleep latency. In narcolepsy, the MSL that is derived from averaging the sleep latency of the 4 naps is less than 8 minutes. Furthermore, the transition from wakefulness to sleep is directly into REM sleep during at least 2 of the 4 nap opportunities. By way of reference, in unaffected children the MSL ranges from 16 to 18 minutes (see **Table 2**). The MSLT is generally invalid in children younger than 5 to 6 years because it may be difficult to differentiate physiologic daytime napping from pathologic daytime sleepiness. In these patients, as well as in situations when the psychotropic medication that the patient is already receiving cannot be stopped, testing for reduction in the CSF hypocretin-1 level of less than 110 pg/mL (diagnostic for narcolepsy-cataplexy) is indicated.[41]

The management requires a combination of lifestyle changes and pharmacotherapy. A planned daytime nap of 20 to 30 minutes at school and another nap in the afternoon on returning home may enhance alertness. The patient should observe regular sleep onset and morning wake-up times, avoid alcohol, and exercise regularly. To minimize the risk of accidents, the patient should stay away from sharp moving objects. Driving should be avoided until daytime alertness has been brought into the normal or near normal range. Drugs commonly used in the management of daytime sleepiness and cataplexy are listed in **Table 3**. Besides selective serotonin reuptake inhibitors, emotional and behavioral problems that commonly accompany childhood narcolepsy may also require supportive psychotherapy. Because of possible underlying immune dysregulation, patients with narcolepsy-cataplexy have been treated in small open-label series using intravenous immunoglobulin G, with variable results.[47] Modification of T-cell function has not yet been targeted.

IDIOPATHIC HYPERSOMNIA

Idiopathic hypersomnia is a disorder characterized by chronic nonimperative sleepiness in association with long unrefreshing naps and difficulty reaching full alertness even after napping. In severe cases, there may be sleep drunkenness. Night sleep is qualitatively and quantitatively normal, with excellent sleep efficiency. In the MSLT the patients exhibit pathologic daytime sleepiness, with the MSL being in the 5- to 10-minute range. However, 2 or more sleep-onset REM periods that are characteristic of narcolepsy are not seen. Bassetti and Aldrich[48] reviewed 42 cases of idiopathic hypersomnia. Hypersomnia began at a mean age of 19 ± 8 years (range, 6–43 years). As is evident from this series, the onset of the condition may sometimes be in childhood. The onset of hypersomnia was associated with symptoms such as insomnia, weight gain, viral illness, or head injury. The naps lasted 30 minutes or more and were generally not refreshing. The management of sleepiness calls for treatment measures similar to those for narcolepsy.

Table 3
Drugs commonly used for treating narcolepsy

Symptom/Drug	Dosage
Daytime Sleepiness	
Modafinil[a]	100–400 mg/d in 2 divided doses
Armodafinil[b]	150–300 mg/d in 2 divided doses
Methylphenidate hydrochloride	5–10 mg, 1–2 times/d, to a maximum of 60 mg/d
Dextroamphetamine	5–10 mg, 1–2 times/d, to a maximum of 40 mg/d
Methamphetamine	5–25 mg/d in 2 divided doses
Amphetamine/dextroamphetamine mixture	10–40 mg once a day
Lisdexamfetamine	30 mg once daily to a maximum of 70 mg/d
Cataplexy	
Sodium oxybate[b]	3–9 g in 2 divided doses at night
Venlafaxine[b]	35–75 mg/d in divided doses
Fluoxetine	10–30 mg once every morning
Sertraline	25–200 mg once every morning
Clomipramine	25–100 mg/d in divided doses
Imipramine	25–75 mg/d in divided doses
Protriptyline	5–15 mg/d in divided doses
Periodic Limb Movements	
Elemental iron	1–2 mg/kg in 1–2 divided doses
Gabapentin	100–300 mg at bedtime
Clonazepam	0.5–1.0 mg at bedtime
Levodopa-carbidopa[b]	1–2 tablets of 25/100 or 50/200 mg at bedtime
Pramipexole[b]	0.125–0.250 mg at bedtime
Ropinirole[b]	0.25–0.50 mg at bedtime

[a] Usage is off-label for individuals younger than 16 years.
[b] Usage is off-label.

DELAYED SLEEP PHASE DISORDER

Delayed sleep phase disorder (DSPD) is a circadian rhythm disturbance related to dysfunction of the suprachiasmatic nucleus, which serves as the circadian timekeeper. The disorder typically has onset in adolescence, with predominance in men. Patients have a constitutional difficulty in advancing (phase advancing) sleep and can only fall asleep at progressively later times at night.[49] Patients are frequently misdiagnosed as having severe insomnia. Sleep-onset time may be delayed past midnight into the early morning hours. Once asleep, and if allowed to sleep uninterrupted, patients show normal sleep quantity and quality. Most patients are obligated to wake up by 6:30 AM or 7:00 AM to attend school, which results in chronic sleep deprivation, sleep drunkenness on awakening, daytime sleepiness along with variable degrees of depression, and personality changes.

In an unsuccessful attempt to regulate their sleep-wake function, patients with DSPD may abuse stimulants during the daytime and hypnotics at night.

Polymorphisms in the *hPer* gene, arylalkylamine-N-acetyltransferase gene, HLA-DR1 gene, and *hClock* gene have been associated with increased predisposition to DSPD. There is increased clustering of DSPD within some families.

DSPD must be differentiated from school avoidance seen in adolescents with delinquent and antisocial behavior because these individuals may be able to fall asleep at an earlier hour at night in the controlled sleep laboratory setting. Sleep logs combined with wrist actigraphy for 2 to 3 weeks are helpful in establishing the diagnosis.

Bright light therapy is helpful in advancing the sleep-onset time. The therapy involves the provision of 8000 to 10,000 lux of bright light via a light box for 20 to 30 minutes immediately on awakening in the morning. The light box is kept at a distance of 18 to 24 in from the face, leading to a gradual advancement (shifting back) of the sleep-onset time at night. Bright light therapy may be combined with melatonin that is administered about 5 to 5.5 hours before the required bedtime, in a dose of 0.5 mg. Diminished exposure to light in the evening, such as by using sunglasses, may also facilitate earlier sleep onset at night. The other therapeutic option is one of gradually delaying bedtime by 3 to 4 hours per day until it becomes synchronized with socially acceptable sleep-wake times and then adhering to this schedule (phase advancing, chronotherapy). Over time, however, all patients with DSPD remain at a risk for drifting forward to progressively later and later bedtimes. Daytime stimulants, such as modafinil (100–400 mg/d in 2 divided doses), may also improve daytime alertness. The physician may also need to write a letter to the school requesting a late midmorning school start time on medical grounds. General and specific measures used to treat common childhood disorders associated with hypersomnia are shown in **Table 4**.

CHALLENGES AND OPPORTUNITIES

Further refinements are needed in the diagnostic testing for childhood daytime sleepiness. It is not known whether the MSLT in childhood should use 4 or 5 naps. Is there any significance in the sequence of appearance of SOREMPs on the MSLT, that is, is there a greater likelihood of narcolepsy if REM-onset sleep is seen in naps 3 and 4 rather than in naps 1 and 2? Does the shortening of initial REM latency on the nocturnal PSG have a predictive value for childhood narcolepsy? There is limited availability of testing for CSF hypocretin level in aiding narcolepsy-cataplexy diagnosis in preschool-aged children, an age group in which the MSLT is invalid. Evidence of the utility of PSG and the MSLT in the diagnosis of daytime sleepiness is sparse, and comprises mainly of level 3 or 4 studies. For example, 10 studies have been published to date with regard to the MSLT in childhood hypersomnia, 9 pertaining to narcolepsy and 1 to KLS. One study can be categorized as having level 1 evidence, 2 as having level 3 evidence, and 7 as having level 4 evidence. There is thus a need to generate studies of better evidentiary quality. Longitudinal studies are needed to determine whether treating sleepiness with medication corresponds with improved neuropsychological function. Given the small number of patients with childhood narcolepsy at each sleep center, a consortium-based approach is needed for gathering prospective high-quality evidence regarding optimum treatment measures, be they pharmacologic or nonpharmacologic in nature.

Table 4
Management approach for common disorders associated with hypersomnia

Condition	Nonpharmacologic	Pharmacologic
Narcolepsy	Regular exercise Regular sleeping-waking schedules Avoiding alcohol Psychological counseling for emotional support	Excessive sleepiness: modafinil/armodafinil, salts of methylphenidate, dextroamphetamine Cataplexy: sodium oxybate, protriptyline, venlafaxine, or clomipramine Depression: a selective serotonin reuptake inhibitor
Idiopathic hypersomnia	Regular exercise Regular sleeping-waking schedules Avoiding alcohol Psychological counseling for emotional support	Modafinil/armodafinil, salts of methylphenidate, dextroamphetamine
Recurrent hypersomnia (KLS)	—	Lithium or lamotrigine (off-label usage)
Delayed sleep phase syndrome	Bright light therapy, with 8000–10,000 lux during the first 20–30 min on awakening in the morning Daytime exercise	Melatonin, 0.5 mg, about 5.5–6 h before the desired bedtime Modafinil, 100–200 mg, on awakening to counter residual sleepiness

REFERENCES

1. Paruthi S, Chervin RD. Approaches to the assessment of arousals and sleep disturbance in children. Sleep Med 2010;11:622–7.
2. Beebe DW. Cognitive, behavioral, and functional consequences of inadequate sleep in children and adolescents. Pediatr Clin North Am 2011;58:649–65.
3. Nevéus T, Cnattinqius S, Olsson U, et al. Sleep habits and sleep problems among a community sample of school children. Acta Paediatr 2001;90:1450–5.
4. Yang CK, Kim JK, Patel SR, et al. Age-related changes in sleep/wake patterns among Korean teenagers. Pediatrics 2005;115(Suppl):250–6.
5. Ohayon MM, Roberts E, Zulley J, et al. Prevalence and patterns of problematic sleep among older adolescents. J Am Acad Child Adolesc Psychiatry 2000;39:1549–56.
6. Iglowstein I, Jenni OG, Molinari L, et al. Sleep duration from infancy to adolescence: reference values and generational trends. Pediatrics 2003;111:302–7.
7. Taylor DJ, Jenni OG, Acebo C, et al. Sleep tendency during extended wakefulness: insights into adolescent sleep regulation and behavior. J Sleep Res 2005;14:239–44.
8. Wolfson AR, Carskadon MA. Sleep schedules and daytime functioning in adolescents. Child Dev 1998;69:879–87.
9. Wolfson AR, Carskadon MA. Understanding adolescents' sleep patterns and school performance: a critical appraisal. Sleep Med Rev 2003;7:491–506.
10. Sadeh A, Gruber R, Raviv A. The effects of sleep restriction and extension on school-age children: what a difference an hour makes. Child Dev 2003; 74:444–55.
11. Samson WK, Bagley SL, Ferguson AV, et al. Orexin receptor subtype activation and locomotor behavior in the rat. Acta Physiol (Oxf) 2010;198:313–24.
12. España RA, Scammell TE. Sleep neurobiology from a clinical perspective. Sleep 2011;34:845–58.
13. Saper CB, Scammell TE, Lu J. Hypothalamic regulation of sleep and circadian rhythms. Nature 2005; 437:1257–63.
14. Beebe DW, Rose D, Amin R. Attention, learning, and arousal of experimentally sleep-restricted adolescents in a simulated classroom. J Adolesc Health 2010;47:523–5.
15. O'Brien LM. The neurocognitive effects of sleep disruption in children and adolescents. Child Adolesc Psychiatr Clin N Am 2009;18:813–23.
16. Ha KS, Yoo HK, Lyoo IK, et al. Computerized assessment of cognitive impairment in narcoleptic patients. Acta Neurol Scand 2007;116:312–6.
17. Stores G, Montgomery P, Wiggs L. The psychosocial problems of children with narcolepsy and those with excessive daytime sleepiness of uncertain origin. Pediatrics 2006;118:e1116–23.
18. Bayon V, Leger D, Phillip P. Socio-professional handicap and accidental risk in patients with hypersomnias of central origin. Sleep Med Rev 2009;13:421–6.
19. Spruyt K, Gozal D. Pediatric sleep questionnaires as diagnostic and epidemiological tools: a review of currently available tools. Sleep Med Rev 2011;15: 19–32.
20. Owens JA, Spirito A, McGuinn M. The Children's Sleep Habits Questionnaire (CSHQ): psychometric properties of a survey instrument for school-aged children. Sleep 2000;23:1043–51.
21. Luginbuehl M, Bradley-Klug KL, Ferron J, et al. Pediatric sleep disorders: validation of the sleep disorders inventory for students. Sch Psychol Rev 2008; 37:409–31.
22. Bruni O, Ottaviano S, Guidetti V, et al. The Sleep Disturbance Scale for Children (SDSC). Construction and validation of an instrument to evaluate sleep disturbances in childhood and adolescence. J Sleep Res 1996;5:251–61.
23. Chervin RD, Hedger K, Dillon JE, et al. Pediatric sleep questionnaire (PSQ): validity and reliability of scales for sleep-disordered breathing, snoring, sleepiness, and behavioral problems. Sleep Med 2000;1:21–32.
24. Spilsbury JC, Drotar D, Rosen CL, et al. The Cleveland adolescent sleepiness questionnaire: a new measure to assess excessive daytime sleepiness in adolescents. J Clin Sleep Med 2007;3:603–12.
25. Drake C, Nickel C, Burduvali E, et al. The pediatric daytime sleepiness scale (PDSS): sleep habits and school outcomes in middle-school children. Sleep 2003;26:455–8.
26. Chervin RD, Ruzicka DL, Giordani BJ, et al. Sleep-disordered breathing, behavior, and cognition in children before and after adenotonsillectomy. Pediatrics 2006;117:769–78.
27. Littner MR, Kushida C, Wise M, et al. Practice parameters for clinical use of the multiple sleep latency test and the maintenance of wakefulness test. Sleep 2005;28:113–21.
28. Dauvilliers Y, Gosselin A, Paquet J, et al. Effect of age on MSLT results in patients with narcolepsy-cataplexy. Neurology 2004;62:46–50.
29. Guilleminault C, Pelayo R. Narcolepsy in prepubertal children. Ann Neurol 1998;43:135–42.
30. Malone SK. Early to bed, early to rise? An exploration of adolescent sleep hygiene practices. J Sch Nurs 2011;27:348–54.
31. Arnulf I, Lecendreux M, Franco P, et al. Kleine-Levin syndrome: state of the art. Rev Neurol (Paris) 2008; 164:658–68 [in French].
32. Podesta C, Ferreras M, Mozzi M, et al. Kleine-Levin syndrome in a 14-year-old girl: CSF hypocretin-1 measurements. Sleep Med 2006;7:649–51.
33. Poppe M, Friebel D, Reuner U, et al. The Kleine-Levin syndrome—effects of treatment with lithium. Neuropediatrics 2003;34(3):113–9.

34. Adhlakha A, Chokroverty S. An adult onset patient with Kleine-Levin syndrome responding to valproate. Sleep Med 2009;10:391–3.

35. Surges R, Walker MC. A case of late-onset Kleine-Levin syndrome responding to lamotrigine. Sleep Med 2009;10:394.

36. Silber MH, Krahn LE, Olson EJ, et al. The epidemiology of narcolepsy in Olmsted County, Minnesota: a population-based study. Sleep 2002;25:197–202.

37. Kotagal S, Paruthi S. Narcolepsy in childhood. In: Goswami M, Pandi-Perumal SR, Thorpy MJ, editors. Narcolepsy: a clinical guide. New York: Humana Press; 2010. p. 55–67.

38. Bahamam A. Periodic leg movements in narcolepsy patients: impact on sleep architecture. Acta Neurol Scand 2007;115:351–5.

39. Autret A, Lucas F, Henry-Lebras F, et al. Symptomatic narcolepsies. Sleep 1994;17(Suppl 1):21–4.

40. Mignot E, Lin L, Rogers W, et al. Complex HLA-DR and -DQ interactions confer risk of narcolepsy-cataplexy in three ethnic groups. Am J Hum Genet 2001;68:686–99.

41. Nishino S, Ripley B, Overeem S, et al. Hypocretin (orexin) deficiency in human narcolepsy. Lancet 2000;355:39–40.

42. Nishino S, Ripley B, Overeem S, et al. Low cerebrospinal fluid hypocretin (orexin) and altered energy homeostasis in human narcolepsy. Ann Neurol 2001;50:381–8.

43. Thannickal TC, Moore RY, Neinhuis R, et al. Reduced number of hypocretin neurons in human narcolepsy. Neuron 2000;27:469–74.

44. Kotagal S, Krahn LE, Slocumb N. A putative link between childhood narcolepsy and obesity. Sleep Med 2004;5:147–50.

45. Kanbayashi T, Inoue Y, Chiba S, et al. CSF hypocretin-1 (orexin-A) concentrations in narcolepsy with and without cataplexy and idiopathic hypersomnia. J Sleep Res 2002;11:91–3.

46. Nevsimalova S, Prihodova I, Kemlink D, et al. REM behavior disorder (RBD) can be one of the fist symptoms of childhood narcolepsy. Sleep Med 2007;8:784–6.

47. Dauviliers Y, Carlander B, Rivier F, et al. Successful management of cataplexy with intravenous immunoglobulins at narcolepsy onset. Ann Neurol 2004;56:905–8.

48. Bassetti C, Aldrich MS. Idiopathic hypersomnia: a series of 42 patients. Brain 1997;120:1423–35.

49. Sack RL, Auckley D, Auger RR, et al. Circadian rhythm sleep disorders: part II, advanced sleep phase disorder, delayed sleep phase disorder, free-running disorder, and irregular sleep-wake rhythm. An American Academy of Sleep Medicine review. Sleep 2007;30:1484–501.

Index

Note: Page numbers of article titles are in **boldface** type.

A

Accidents, risk of, with insufficient sleep, 318

Acquired immunodeficiency syndrome (AIDS), comorbid with narcolepsy, 298–299

Actigraphy, in narcolepsy diagnosis, 275

Alcohol, hypersomnias caused by, 200

Amphetamines, in hypersomnia treatment, 337

Animal models, of pathophysiology of narcolepsy, 264–265

Antidepressants, hypersomnias caused by, 199

Antiepileptic drugs, hypersomnias caused by, 200

Antihistamines, hypersomnias caused by, 199–200

Antihypertensive drugs, hypersomnias caused by, 200

Antipsychotics, hypersomnias caused by, 199

Anxiety, in narcolepsy, 272

Anxiolytics, hypersomnias caused by, 199

Apnea. See Obstructive sleep apnea.

Appetite, comorbid dysregulation in narcolepsy, 292–294
  compulsive eating in Kleine-Levin syndrome, 303–306

Armodafinil, in hypersomnia treatment, 337

Arousal, dopamine neurotransmission and, 184
  regulatory mechanisms of sleep and, 180–182

Autoimmune disorders, of nervous system, hypersomnia and, 258–259

Autoimmunity, in pathophysiology of narcolepsy, 266–267

Automatic behavior, in narcolepsy, 271

B

Behavioral management, of hypersomnia, **323–331**
  age considerations in, 326–327
    older adults, 326–327
    young adults, 326
  cognitive-behavioral intervention for, 329
  in context of parent disorder, 327–329
    circadian rhythm sleep disorders, 327–328
    idiopathic hypersomnia, 288, 327
    narcolepsy, 327, 346–348
    sleep apnea, 327
    unipolar and bipolar depression, 328–329
  options for, 325–326
    distracting technologies, 326
    exercise, 325–326
    napping, 326

sleep diaries, 325
sleep hygiene, 326

Behaviorally induced insufficient sleep syndrome, 251–252, **313–323**
  consequences of sleep deprivation, 316–319
    neurobehavioral effects, 316–317
    physiologic effects, 317–319
    risk of accidents, 317
    sleep architecture and physiologic sleepiness, 316
  epidemiology of, 315–316
  factors affecting risk of and adaptation to insufficient sleep, 319–320
  in differential diagnosis of hypersomnias, 191–193
  management, 320

Biomarkers, of narcolepsy and other hypersomnias, **233–248**
  basic sleep physiology and symptoms of, 235–236
  changes in other neurotransmitter systems in, 243–244
  discovery of hypocretin deficiency in, 236–238
  histamine and, 244–246
  hyprocretin involvement in symptomatic, 241–243
  hyprocretin ligand and narcolepsy phenotype, 239–241
  neurobiology of wakefulness, 234–235
  pathophysiology with normal hyprocretin levels, 238

Bipolar depression, behavioral management of, 328–329

Brain injury, secondary neurogenic hypersomnia after traumatic, 257

Brainstem lesions, hypersomnia as a consequence of, 182–183

Breathing disorders, sleep-related, in differential diagnosis of hypersomnias, 193–194

C

Caffeine, in hypersomnia treatment, 337

Cardiovascular disease, as consequence of hypersomnia in older adults, 373

Cataplexy, in narcolepsy, 268–269
  in children, 269

Central nervous system (CNS) hypersomnia
  Kleine-Levin syndrome. See Kleine-Levin syndrome.
  narcolepsy. See Narcolepsy.